A Photoguide of Common Skin Disorders
Diagnosis and Management

A Photoguide of Common Skin Disorders
Diagnosis and Management

Herbert P. Goodheart, MD

Assistant Clinical Professor
Department of Medicine
Division of Dermatology
Albert Einstein College of Medicine
Bronx, New York

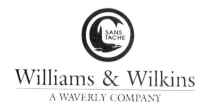

Williams & Wilkins
A WAVERLY COMPANY

BALTIMORE • PHILADELPHIA • LONDON • PARIS • BANGKOK
BUENOS AIRES • HONG KONG • MUNICH • SYDNEY • TOKYO • WROCLAW

Editor: Timothy Y. Hiscock
Development Editor: Jane Velker
Managing Editor: Danielle Hagan
Marketing Manager: Daniell T. Griffin
Project Editor: Ulita Lushnycky

351 West Camden Street
Baltimore, Maryland 21201-2436 USA

Rose Tree Corporate Center
1400 North Providence Road
Building II, Suite 5025
Media, Pennsylvania 19063-2043 USA

Printed in the United States of America

First Edition, 1999

Library of Congress Cataloging-in-Publication Data

Goodheart, Herbert P.
    A photoguide of common skin disorders: diagnosis and management /
Herbert P. Goodheart. — 1st ed.
        p.   cm.
    Index.
    ISBN 0-683-30257-4
    1. Skin--Diseases--Handbooks, manuals, etc.   2. Primary care
(Medicine)--Handbooks, manuals, etc.   3. Skin--Diseases--Atlases.
I. Title.
    [DNLM: 1. Skin Diseases--diagnosis atlases.   2. Skin Diseases-
-therapy atlases.   WR 17G652p   1999]
RL74.G66   1999
616.5'0022'2--dc21
DNLM/DLC
for Library of Congress   98-26292
                                                                                             CIP

0-683-30257-4

The publishers have made every effort to trace the copyright holders for borrowed material. If they have inadvertently overlooked any, they will be pleased to make the necessary arrangements at the first opportunity.

To purchase additional copies of this book, call our customer service department at **(800) 638-0672** or fax orders to **(800) 447-8438.** For other book services, including chapter reprints and large quantity sales, ask for the Special Sales department.

Canadian customers should call **(800) 665-1148,** or fax **(800) 665-0103.** For all other calls originating outside of the United States, please call **(410) 528-4223** or fax us at **(410) 528-8550.**

Visit Williams & Wilkins on the Internet: *http://www.wwilkins.com* or contact our customer service department at **custserv@wwilkins.com.** Williams & Wilkins customer service representatives are available from 8:30 am to 6:00 pm, EST, Monday through Friday, for telephone access.

99 00 01 02 03
1 2 3 4 5 6 7 8 9 10

To Karen, David, and Bernie and to my mother, Rose Goodheart.

To the health care providers who care for the whole patient—those who have an ongoing love for the art, as well as the science, of medicine. To David H. Henry, MD, hematologist–oncologist at Allegheny–Graduate Hospital, Philadelphia, Pennsylvania, who continually exemplifies this tradition in this time of information overload, and to Mike Fisher, MD, at the Albert Einstein College of Medicine, whose wise and patient instruction ignited my love for dermatology.

As a second-year medical student, I recall studying cardiology one evening when my brother Andrew asked me to look at a rash that developed on his trunk. I did not have a clue as to how to make *any* dermatologic diagnosis. So, after Andrew accused my father of wasting tuition money on my evidently inadequate education, I thought it proper to register for a dermatology elective in my fourth year. I reasoned that, regardless of whatever field I would ultimately choose, I would inevitably be confronted with some cutaneous dilemmas. It was with tremendous fortune that I subsequently trained at the Albert Einstein College of Medicine in the Bronx, New York, under the tutelage of Michael Fisher, MD, who still heads an illustrious division of dermatology. It was during my training that I befriended the attending physician, Dr. Herb Goodheart. Herb always provided special insights, wisdom, and compassion in the evaluation of even the most rudimentary dermatologic disorders. He is a stellar teacher and dermatologist, who has compiled his years of perspicacity into this guide to dermatology.

As we approach the twenty-first century, the landscape of American medicine and dermatology is changing at an accelerating pace. Even though we can now comprehend many skin disorders at a molecular level and have advanced our therapeutic realm to include laser technology and immunobiology, the cornerstone of all dermatologic endeavors will always be careful clinical observation. As venues of practice shift toward a greater proportion of primary dermatologic care being delivered by nondermatologists, resources for these providers must be accessible, comprehensible, and practical. Dr. Goodheart's guide to dermatology is divided into common disorders, the interrelationship between the skin and systemic disease, basic and advanced dermatologic procedures, and a very useful appendix providing patient handout material in both English and Spanish. Importantly, it combines features of an atlas with Herb's pithy perspectives, as though he is standing over your shoulder in the dermatology clinic. Those who utilize this guide will come to appreciate many of the finer points and opinions that Dr. Goodheart provides and even more so when becoming more facile with the discipline. Use this guide as a primer, an atlas, a consultant, and as a supplement to more in-depth dermatology texts and medical literature. Your dermatologic knowledge base will flourish, your appreciation of the field will blossom, and most importantly, your patients will benefit from your expertise.

Warren R. Heymann, MD
Head Division of Dermatology
UMDNJ—Robert Wood Johnson School of Medicine at Camden

In dermatology, the naked eye is our primary tool, and because virtually every skin disorder is visible, the photographic image is an essential teaching aide.

Despite the commonplace occurrence of skin disorders, making a correct dermatologic diagnosis is a customary stumbling block for many in the health care professions. It is rather unusual to find the nondermatologist who is comfortable diagnosing or managing most skin problems; in fact, many admit to the frequent approach of trial and error. Medical schools simply do not emphasize the teaching of dermatology. Skin diseases are generally considered less life-threatening and are of lower priority than most of the conditions seen in teaching hospitals. Frequently, this can result in mistreatment, a delay in appropriate treatment, or a referral to a dermatologist.

This book is intended to be an accessible reference for nondermatologists such as family physicians, physician assistants, nurse practitioners, and medical students. Its focus has been limited intentionally to the diagnosis and management of the most common skin problems encountered in an outpatient setting.

The purpose of this photo guide is to provide some much needed assistance to the nondermatologist who, in the future, will be on the frontline in treating skin problems.

Herbert P. Goodheart, M.D.

I would like to acknowledge the many people without whose advice and support this book would never have been possible. I am especially indebted to Warren Heymann, MD, for reviewing each chapter; he is a veritable walking encyclopedia of dermatologic knowledge. I'd also like to give a special thanks to Gay Young who recognized the potential of my original "photoguides" and brought them to the attention of Williams & Wilkins.

I am also grateful to all the wonderful people at Williams & Wilkins. Jonathan Pine and Molly Mullen gave me a warm welcome to Baltimore and continued to be supportive throughout the process of publishing this book. Paula Brown, Melissa Carton, Danielle Hagan, and Ulita Lushnycky each offered her own insight and expertise to the project. I especially wish to thank Jane Velker, my skillful and talented editor at Williams & Wilkins, with whom I've had a seamless working relationship. From the beginning, she understood the purpose of this book and has been a major proponent of some of my less traditional ideas.

My gratitude is also extended to Cassandra Venable for her ongoing advice and review of material. Eileen Rubinstein, Rick Dura, Justin Burk, Mor Erlich, Carlos Cohen, and my contributors all helped compensate for my particular deficiencies. I thank present and former colleagues at CHP, including Dee Guiliano, Sandra Mamis, Kristina Heitzman, Barbara Lozier, Susan Mirabel, Janet Clear, and Ruth Telford. They have helped make my dermatologic education enjoyable, and they have reinforced for me the notion that teaching is learning. My thanks to John Charde, whose openness to new ideas coupled with his concern for patient care, first gave me the idea for this book. And I thank my most important teachers of all—my patients.

Mary Ruth Buchness, MD

Chief
Dermatology
Saint Vincent's Hospital and Medical Center
New York, New York
Associate Professor of Dermatology and Medicine
New York Medical College
Valhalla, New York

Peter G. Burk, MD

Clinical Associate Professor of Medicine (Dermatology)
Albert Einstein College of Medicine
Bronx, New York
Director
Dermatology Service
Montefiore Medical Center
Bronx, New York

Steven R. Cohen, MD

Chairman
Department of Dermatology
Beth Israel Medical Center
New York, New York
Professor of Medicine
Division of Dermatology
Albert Einstein College of Medicine
Bronx, New York

Herbert P. Goodheart, MD

Assistant Clinical Professor
Department of Medicine
Division of Dermatology
Albert Einstein College of Medicine
Bronx, New York

Fredric Haberman, DO

Assistant Clinical Professor
Department of Medicine
Division of Dermatology
Albert Einstein College of Medicine
Attending Physician
Montefiore Medical Center
Bronx, New York
Director
Haberman Dermatology Institute
New York, New York.

Kenneth Howe, MD

Assistant Clinical Professor
Department of Medicine
Division of Dermatology
Albert Einstein College of Medicine
Bronx, New York
Department of Dermatology
Beth Israel Medical Center
New York, New York

CONTENTS

PART IV
Dermatologic Procedures

PART V
Appendices

PART I

ILLUSTRATED GLOSSARY

A description using correct dermatologic terms enables the practitioner to formulate a differential diagnosis and communicate information to others.

LESIONS

Primary Lesions

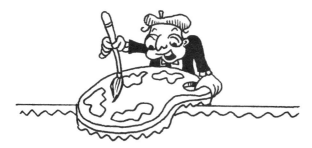

Macules are simply a change in color of the skin (you can't feel them and, if you close your eyes, they "disappear"). They come in many shapes and sizes.

Examples include freckles, postinflammatory pigmentary alteration, and vitiligo.

Patches are large macules.

Examples include melasma and vascular nevus ("salmon patch"). There is some confusion regarding patches; some dermatologists refer to a patch as a large macule, while others refer to patches as macules with overlying fine scale; for example, pityriasis rosea and mycosis fungoides.

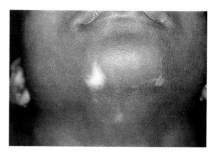

Macule. Vitiligo.

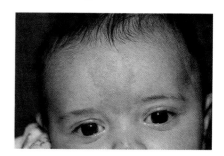

Patch. Vascular nevus ("salmon patch").

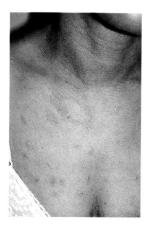

"Patch." Note herald patch of pityriasis rosea on chest.

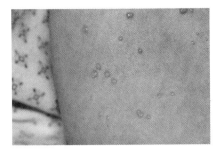

Papule. Molluscum contagiosum.

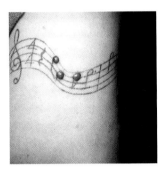

Macular and papular components. Tattoo with macular blue and yellow components and a red papular component.

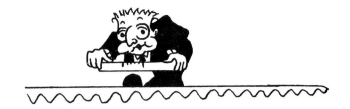

Papules are solid lumps generally 1 cm or less in diameter.

Examples include warts, nevi (moles), and molluscum contagiosum.

"Maculopapule" is a contradiction in terms and use of the term should be discouraged (an eruption may be described as being macular **and** papular, rather than "maculopapular.")

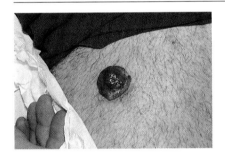

Nodule. Pyogenic granuloma.

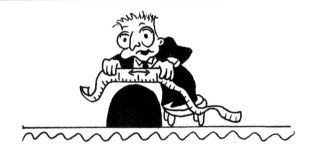

Nodules are solid lumps generally 1 cm or more in diameter. Nodules may be seen as an elevation or can be palpated within the skin.

Examples include erythema nodosum, basal cell carcinoma, and pyogenic granuloma.

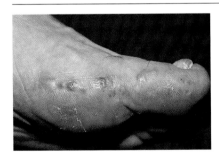

Vesicle. Acute inflammatory tinea pedis.

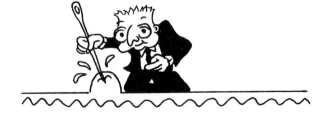

Vesicles (small blisters) are fluid-filled lesions generally 1 cm or less in diameter, such as herpes simplex, chickenpox, and acute tinea pedis.

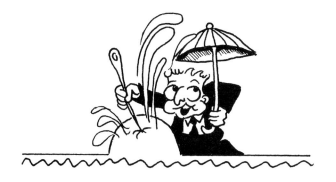

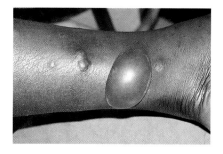

Bulla. Bullous insect bite reaction.

Bullae (large blisters) are fluid-filled lesions generally 1 cm or more in diameter, such as herpes zoster, second-degree burns, and insect bite reactions.

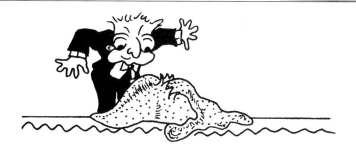

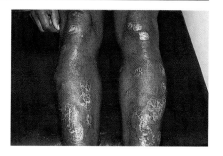

Pustule. Acneiform lesion.

Pustules are lesions that contain purulent, cloudy material (sometimes they may contain a hair and are then called follicular pustules).

Examples include acne and folliculitis.

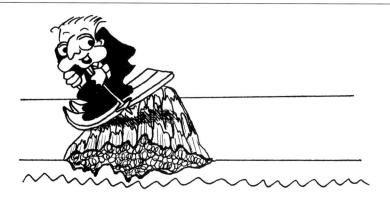

Plaque. Silvery psoriatic plaques.

Plaques are solid, elevated, flat-topped, plateaulike lesions that cover a fairly large area; they may arise from papules that join together or arise de novo.

Examples include psoriasis and chronic eczematous dermatitis.

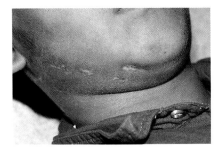

Atrophic plaque. Morphea.

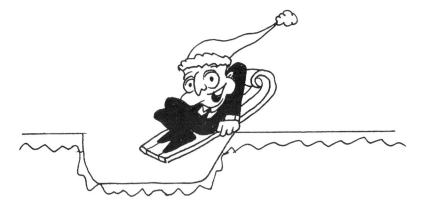

Atrophic plaques are depressed plaques. Atrophic plaques often form large erosions or even ulcers. Discoid lupus erythematosus, pyoderma gangrenosum, and morphea (localized scleroderma) often form atrophic plaques.

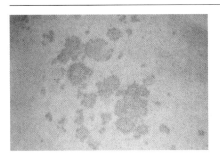

Wheal. Urticaria.

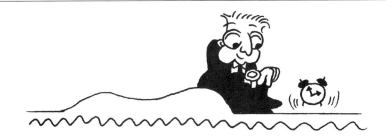

Wheals are raised flesh-colored or erythematous papules or plaques that are transient lesions. Wheals generally last less than 24 hours, during which time they may change shape and size. Wheals include urticaria (hives) and angioedema.

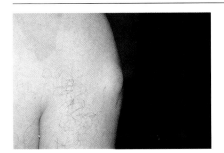

Cyst. Pilomatricoma.

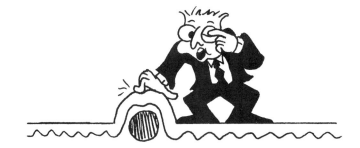

Cysts are walled-off lesions containing fluid or semisolid material. (They feel like an eyeball.)

Examples include pilar and epidermoid cysts.

Secondary (modified) Lesions

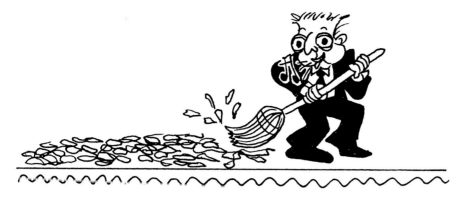

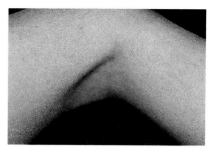

Scale. Ichthyosis vulgaris.

Scales (desquamation) derive from the outer layer of epidermis, which is imperceptibly shed daily. In many dermatologic conditions, the scale becomes obvious. *Examples include ichthyosis, seborrheic dermatitis and psoriasis.*

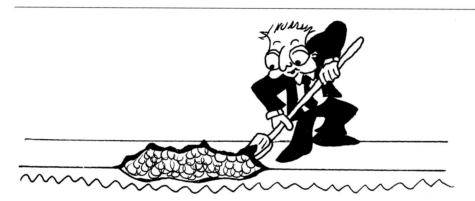

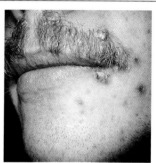

Crust. Impetigo.

Crusts (scabs) are formed from blood, serum, or other dried exudate. Honey-colored crusts (impetiginization) are a sign of superficial infection. Infected insect bites and impetigo are examples of crusts.

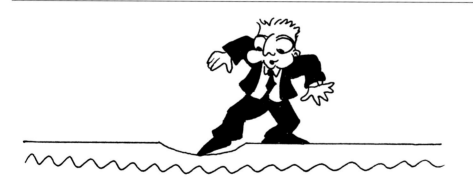

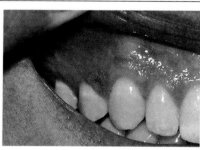

Erosion. Aphthous ulcer.

Erosions are shallow losses of tissue involving only the epidermis ("topsoil"). Erosions are nonscarring and often accompany blisters and pustules. For example, aphthous stomatitis ("canker sores") and the secondary lesions of herpes simplex and herpes zoster.

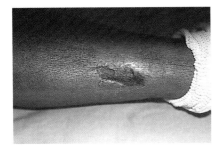

Ulcer. Coumarin necrosis (ulcer with hemorrhagic crust).

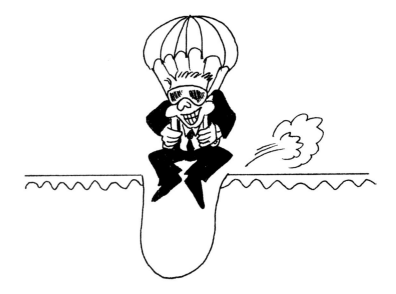

Ulcers are defects deeper than erosions. Ulcers involve the dermis or deeper layers and usually heal with scarring.

Examples include venous stasis ulcer, pyoderma gangrenosum, and the chancre of primary syphilis.

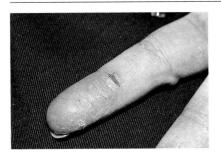

Fissure. Hand eczema.

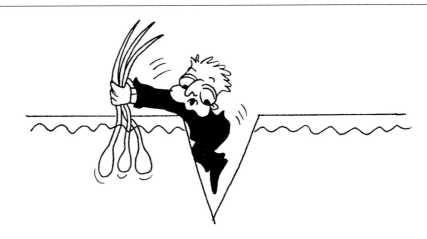

Fissures are linear ulcers or cracks in the skin, such as eczema of fingers and intertrigo.

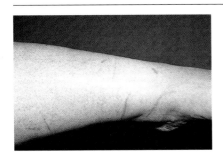

Excoriation. Cat scratches in patient with lichen planus.

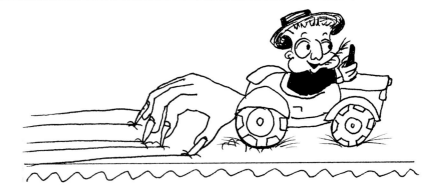

Excoriations are linear erosions induced by scratching.

Examples of excoriations are seen in insect bites and eczema.

Diseased skin has a limited number of clinical manifestations, and many dermatoses tend to occur in characteristic shapes, distributions, and arrangements and reaction patterns.

More than one reaction pattern, shape, and configuration may be present on the skin of one patient or become manifest as a dermatosis evolves. For example, a drug eruption that began in what might be characterized as a vascular reaction pattern may change into a scaly slightly erythematous eruption that would be described 2 weeks later as being papulosquamous.

Reaction Patterns

The system of using reaction patterns is often inexact, and there is a great deal of overlap; however, using reaction patterns often helps greatly in formulating a differential diagnosis.

Papulosquamous (erythemosquamous) reaction patterns refer to eruptions in which the primary lesions consist of either papules with scale or macules with scale (following strict definition, a macule with scale would be a patch or plaque).

Examples include psoriasis, tinea corporis, tinea versicolor, pityriasis rosea, lichen planus, parapsoriasis, mycosis fungoides, and candidiasis.

Eczematous reaction patterns are a little more difficult than papulosquamous patterns to describe (see Chapter 2, "Eczematous Rashes") because they may have various presentations and, at times, may be impossible to distinguish from papulosquamous patterns.
- **Acute** examples include erythematous "juicy" papules or plaques and/or weeping vesicobullous lesions.
- **Subacute** examples consist of crusts (scabs), excoriations, drying papulovesicles, or pustules, scale, and erythema.
- **Chronic.** The hallmark lesion of chronic eczematous dermatitis is lichenification, a plaque with an exaggeration of the normal skin markings that looks like the bark of a tree.

Vesicobullous reaction patterns consist of blisters; however, lesions, when noted at an early stage, may be erythematous macules or papules that later become fluid-filled. A second-degree burn is a good example.

Dermal reaction patterns. Lesions or eruptions are confined to the dermis.

Examples include granuloma annulare and cutaneous sarcoidosis.

Subcutaneous reaction patterns. Lesions or eruptions are confined to the cutis (subcutaneous tissue).

Examples include erythema nodosum and lipomas.

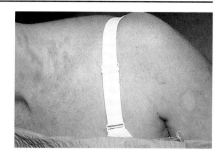

Papulosquamous reaction pattern. Pityriasis rosea.

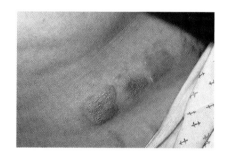

Acute eczematous reaction pattern. Contact dermatitis.

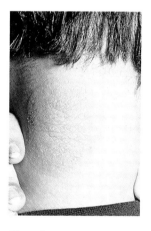

Chronic eczematous reaction pattern. Lichen simplex chronicus.

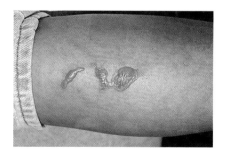

Vesicobullous reaction pattern. Second-degree burn from coffee.

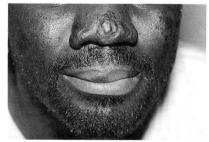

Dermal reaction pattern. Cutaneous sarcoidosis.

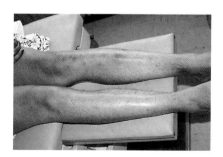

Subcutaneous reaction pattern. Erythema nodosum. (Slide courtesy of Peter G. Burk, M.D.)

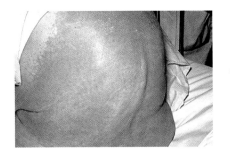

Vascular reaction pattern. Drug reaction.

Vascular reaction patterns refer to erythema and/or edema as a result of changes in the vasculature such as vasodilatation.

Examples include first-degree burns, drug rash, viral exanthem, urticaria, and erythema multiforme.

Shape of Lesions

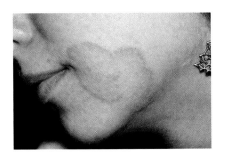

Annular lesion. Tinea faciale.

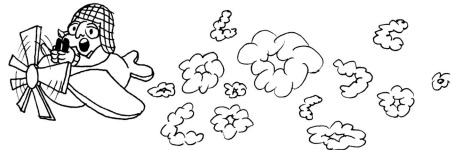

Annular and **arciform** are terms used to describe lesions that are ring-shaped or semiannular, such as granuloma annulare and tinea corporis (ringworm). Annular and arciform lesions are frequently noted in urticaria.

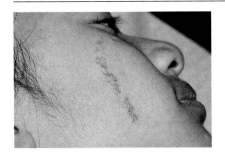

Linear lesion. Epidermal nevus.

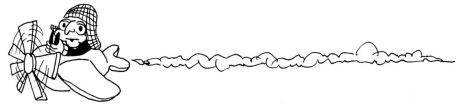

Linear shapes may be due to exogenous agents, developmental processes, or infections.

Examples include poison ivy, the Köebner (isomorphic) reaction, herpes zoster, dermographism, epidermal nevi, sporotrichosis, and lymphangitis.

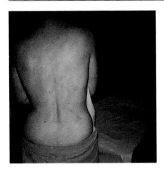

Serpiginous lesion. Jellyfish sting.

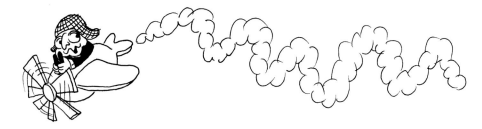

Serpiginous (snakelike) eruptions suggest an exogenous cause, such as cutaneous larvae migrans and jellyfish stings.

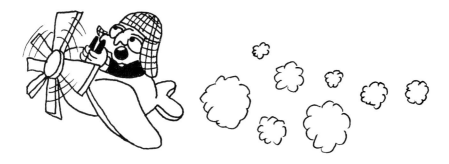

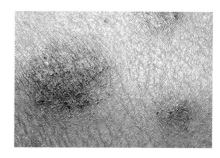

Nummular is a term that describes coin-shaped lesions, including psoriasis, eczematous dermatitis, and discoid lupus erythematosus.

Configuration

Arrangement (configuration) of lesions is the relationship of multiple lesions to one another.

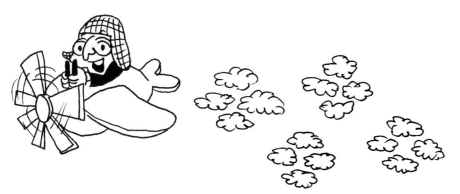

Grouped lesion. Recurrent herpes simplex.

Grouped lesions (e.g., "herpetiform," "zosteriform" vesicles) occur in herpes simplex and herpes zoster infections, insect bites, and autoinoculation of flat warts.

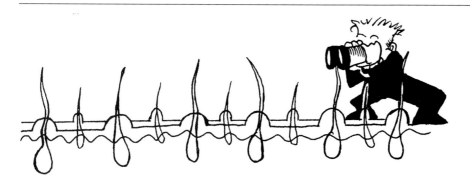

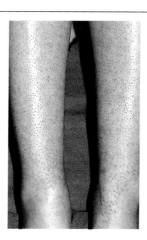

Follicular arrangement of lesions in a pattern involving hair follicles. Lesions are often papular or pustular with a central emerging hair and are spaced fairly equal distances apart.

Examples include folliculitis, furunculosis, pseudofolliculitis barbae, and acne keloidalis.

Follicular lesion. Follicular eczema.

TOPICAL THERAPY AND TOPICAL STEROIDS

General Principles Of Topical Therapy

BASICS

- Topical therapy is generally safer than systemic therapy.
- Creams are generally more popular than ointments because they are less greasy; however, they are usually less potent than ointments.
- There is no direct correlation between the quantity of a topical preparation applied and the degree of its penetration or potency; in fact, the thicker that a preparation is applied, the more of it is wasted because **only the thin layer that is in intimate contact with the skin is absorbed; the rest gets rubbed off.** More is not always better.
- With the exception of sun screens and some moisturizers, once or twice daily applications are usually sufficient for most preparations.

VEHICLES

- Vehicles, or bases in which the active drug is combined, vary in their ability to "deliver" to the target sites in the skin.
- The rate of penetration and absorption of a topical preparation into the skin depends on how occlusive its vehicle is and how readily the vehicle releases the active chemical.
- The vehicle should be cosmetically acceptable, be nonsensitizing, and must hold the drug in stable solution.

Wet dressings
- There is some validity to the old adage, "if it's dry, wet it; if it's wet, dry it."
- Wet dressings help dry wounds, aid debridement of wounds by removing debris (serum, crusts), and have a nonspecific antifungal and antibacterial effect, especially when chemicals, such as aluminum sulfate, silver nitrate, acetic acid (vinegar is a dilute acetic acid), and potassium permanganate, are added to them.
- Application of **Burow's solution** (aluminum sulfate and calcium acetate) or even **plain unsterilized tap water** help dry out weeping lesions (e.g., poison ivy, tinea pedis, herpes simplex and zoster) and oozing impetiginized lesions (e.g., impetigo, infected venous stasis ulcers).

Topical steroids
- **Topical steroids have two basic mechanisms of action: antiinflammatory and antimitotic.**
  - Antiinflammatory properties are of particular importance when they are used to treat eczematous and other primarily inflammatory conditions.
  - **Antimitotic** properties of topical steroids help reduce the buildup of scale (e.g., in the treatment of psoriasis, a condition that is both inflammatory and hyperproliferative [has rapid cell division]).

BASICS

- Topical steroids are used to treat most inflammatory dermatoses; they are a mainstay of therapy in dermatology, and, when used properly, they are safe.
- **It is only necessary to become familiar with one, or, at most, two agents from each potency group to be able to manage the vast majority of dermatoses.**

Potency.

The unwanted effects of topical steroids are directly related to their potencies.
- Fluorinated topical steroids are generally more potent than nonfluorinated. For example, triamcinolone acetonide, which contains a fluoride ion, is 100 times more potent than nonfluorinated hydrocortisone.
- Occlusion increases hydration, and hydration increases penetration, which, in turn, increases effective potency.
- If possible, **the lowest potency steroid should be used for the shortest possible time period.** Conversely, one should avoid using a preparation that is not potent enough to treat an intended condition.
  - For severe dermatoses, a very potent steroid may be used to initiate therapy, followed by a less potent preparation for maintenance ("downward titration").
  - If possible, extra measures should be taken to avoid the use of potent fluorinated compounds when treating children and the elderly.
  - Only nonfluorinated, mild topical steroids should be applied to the face, and they should be used only for short periods of time, if possible, so as to avoid atrophy and steroid rosacea. (This is a rule that can be broken; for example, in treating a severe acute contact dermatitis of the face, a superpotent topical steroid used for a brief period of time may be preferable to using a mild ineffective topical steroid or employing systemic steroids).
  - Thin eyelid skin requires the least potent preparations for the shortest periods of time. The intertriginous areas similarly respond to lower potencies because the apposition of skin surfaces acts like an occlusive dressing. The scrotum is also an area of high absorption.
- There are generic preparations in every potency group, and generic preparations are more economical than the proprietary preparation. (For example, large amounts of triamcinolone cream and ointment may be purchased in 16-oz (1- lb) jars at considerable savings.) However, there is some concern about the bioequivalence between proprietary and generic formulations.

Tachyphylaxis

- Tachyphylaxis, or tolerance, often occurs, and the medication may lose its efficacy with continued use; this is seen primarily in the treatment of psoriasis when very strong topical steroids are used.
- To help minimize tachyphylaxis, dosing may be cycled (pulse dosing) or used intermittently (intermittent dosing). Another option is to use a less potent topical steroid for maintenance.
  - In pulse dosing, the preparation is used until clearing of the dermatosis and is then resumed upon recurrence.
  - In intermittent dosing, the preparation is used at certain times (e.g., on weekends).

A CREAM, AN OINTMENT, A GEL, OR A LOTION?

- **Creams** are often preferred by patients for aesthetic reasons; however, their water content makes them more drying than ointments.
- Generally, **ointments** (oil in water) preparations and gels are more potent than creams or lotions, but their inherent greasiness often makes them cosmetically unacceptable. Ointments are more useful for dry skin conditions because of their occlusive properties; they are more lubricating and tend to be less irritating and less sensitizing.
- **Lotions, gels, aerosols,** and **solutions** are useful on hairy areas and are easier to apply to large areas.

DELIVERY (PERCUTANEOUS PENETRATION)

Topical steroids are ineffective unless they are absorbed into the skin. Percutaneous penetration varies among individual patients and can be manipulated by changing the drug used, the vehicle used, the length of exposure, and the anatomic surface area to which the drug is applied. Percutaneous penetration also depends on whether the skin is inflamed and is, therefore, less of a barrier to penetration (e.g., eczematous skin). Penetration also varies with the presence or absence of occlusive dressings.

- **The barrier to cutaneous penetration is the stratum corneum**. The thicker the stratum corneum (e.g., on the palms, soles, elbows, and knees), the harder it is for the topical steroid to penetrate the skin.
- Penetration is markedly enhanced (10- to 100-fold) by **hydrating the stratum corneum**. This can be accomplished by:
  - **Soaking or bathing an affected area in water** before the application of a topical steroid, which increases the skin's penetrability (Figure I.1)
  - **Using occlusive dressings** (Figure I.2) after the topical steroid has been applied
    - Occlusive dressings may be left on as the patient sleeps or kept on for several hours while the patient is awake. A "nonbreathing" material, such as polyethylene wrap (Saran Wrap, Handi-Wrap), which is held in place by adhesive tape, or a sock can be used.
    - Other materials and methods include:
    - A plastic shower cap may be used when treating the scalp.
    - Rubber or vinyl gloves or finger cots may be used for the hands and fingers.
    - Baggies may be used for the feet.
    - Cordran Tape is a steroid-impregnated tape that is useful for occlusive therapy when treating relatively small areas.

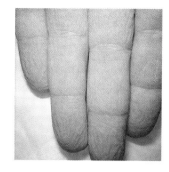

Figure I.1.
Note the after-bath "wrinkled fingers," which develop from the skin increasing its surface area to accommodate the water that has been absorbed.

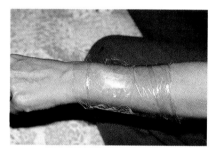

Figure I.2.
Occlusion. Topical steroid cream has been applied and covered with a "nonbreathing" polyethylene wrap.

SIDE EFFECTS

- **Epidermal atrophy** is a local reaction demonstrated by shiny, thinned skin and telangiectasia; this is rapidly reversible when topical steroids are discontinued. Striae, or linear atrophic scars, may occur after repeated use of a potent topical steroid in one area. These are permanent scars, which are seen most commonly in intertriginous areas such as the axillae and groin where the skin is generally thin, moist, and occluded (Figure I.3).
- **Acneiform eruptions** of the face (rosacealike dermatitis and perioral dermatitis; Figure I.4) may occur as a result of regular use of topical fluorinated corticosteroids on the face. This is manifested by persistent erythema, papules, pustules, and telangiectasia. This condition generally flares once the steroid is withdrawn and may not clear entirely for several months.
- **Ecchymoses** may occur on the dorsal forearms, particularly in the elderly after prolonged topical steroid use (Figure I.5).
- **Tinea incognito**. Topical steroids reduce the inflammation and itching of tinea without killing the fungus; thus, the clinical signs of fungal infections may be missed or obscured.

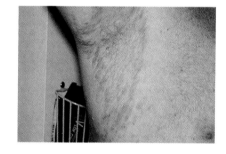

Figure I.3.
Striae. Linear atrophic scars occurring after repeated use of a potent topical steroid.

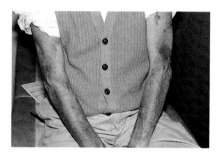

Figure I.5.
Ecchymoses. Purpura on the dorsal forearms after prolonged topical steroid use.

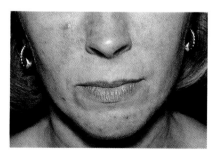

Figure I.4.
Rosacealike dermatitis.

- **Hypersensitivity reactions.** Allergic contact dermatitis to the steroid molecule may occur and may easily be overlooked; the hypersensitivity may be evoked by the steroid, the vehicle, or both and is often not suspected clinically. A clue to its presence is a lack of the expected antiinflammatory effect of the topical steroid.
- **Other**, less common, side effects include hypopigmentation, excess facial hair growth, and delayed wound healing.
- **Systemic effects.** Extensive widespread use and occlusion of potent topical steroids influence the risk of systemic adverse effects. Fortunately, these rarely occur; in fact, hypothalamic–pituitary–adrenal axis suppression is quickly reversible and unlikely to cause the same side effects as systemic steroids.

TOPICAL STEROIDS (THE "SHORT LIST")

The following agents should provide more than enough treatment options for the conditions discussed in this book.

POTENCY	GENERIC NAME	BRAND NAME
SUPERPOTENT	Clobetasol propionate Flurandrenolide Diflorasone diacetate ointment	Temovate Cordran Tape Psorcon
VERY STRONG	Fluocinonide cream, ointment Desoximetasone gel	Lidex Topicort
STRONG	Triamcinolone acetonide Betamethasone valerate	Kenalog Betatrex
MEDIUM	Hydrocortisone valerate cream	Westcort
MILD–MEDIUM	Desonide	DesOwen
MILD	Hydrocortisone	Hytone, Cortaid, Cortizone

CLASSIFICATION, STRENGTH, AND VEHICLE OF SOME COMMONLY USED TOPICAL STEROIDS (THE "LONG LIST")

There are a vast array of topical steroids available. However, all of them in the same group have roughly the same potency; they differ primarily in vehicle and price.

GENERIC NAME	BRAND NAME
Group I, Superpotent	
Betamethasone dipropionate cream/ointment 0.05%	Diprolene
Clobetasol propionate cream/ointment 0.05%	Temovate
Diflorasone diacetate ointment 0.05%	Psorcon
Halobetasol propionate ointment 0.05%	Ultravate
Flurandrenolide	Cordran Tape 4 mg/sq cm
Group II, Very High Potency	
Amcinonide ointment 0.1%	Cyclocort
Betamethasone dipropionate ointment 0.05%	Diprosone
Desoximetasone cream/ointment 0.25%, gel 0.05%	Topicort
Diflorasone diacetate ointment 0.05%	Florone, Maxiflor
Fluocinonide cream/ointment/gel 0.05%	Lidex
Halcinonide cream/ointment 0.1%	Halog
GROUP III, HIGH POTENCY	
Betamethasone dipropionate cream 0.05%	Diprosone
Betamethasone valerate ointment 0.1%	Valisone
Diflorasone diacetate cream 0.05%	Florone, Maxiflor
Triamcinolone acetate ointment 0.1%, cream 0.5%	Aristocort A
GROUP IV, MID–HIGH POTENCY	
Desoximetasone cream 0.05%	Topicort LP
Fluocinolone acetonide cream 0.2%	Synalar-HP
Fluocinolone acetonide ointment 0.025%	Synalar
Hydrocortisone valerate ointment 0.2%	Westcort
Triamcinolone acetonide ointment 0.1%	Kenalog, Aristocort
GROUP V	
Betamethasone dipropionate lotion 0.05%	Diprosone
Betamethasone valerate cream/lotion 0.1%	Valisone
Fluocinolone acetonide cream 0.025%	Synalar
Flurandrenolide cream 0.05%	Cordran SP
Hydrocortisone butyrate cream 0.1%	Locoid
Hydrocortisone valerate cream 0.2%	Westcort
Triamcinolone acetonide cream/lotion 0.1%	Kenalog
Triamcinolone acetonide cream 0.025%	Aristocort
GROUP VI	
Alclometasone dipropionate cream/ointment 0.05%	Aclovate
Betamethasone 17-valerate lotion 0.1%	Valisone
Desonide cream 0.05%	Tridesilon, DesOwen
Fluocinolone acetonide cream/solution 0.01%	Synalar
Mometasone furoate cream/ointment 0.1%	Elocon
GROUP VII	
Hydrocortisone cream/ointment/lotion 0.5%, 1.0%, 2.5%	Hytone, Cortaid, Cortizone

ACNE AND RELATED DISORDERS

Acne Vulgaris (common Acne)

BASICS

- Acne, a disorder of the pilosebaceous unit, is the most common skin problem of teenagers. It may begin before puberty in either sex or it may present initially in adulthood, primarily in women. The condition tends to be more severe in males than in females.
- Acne tends to be hereditary and is less likely to occur in Asians and dark-skinned people.
- Acne may be aggravated by a number of things, including emotional stress and certain medications. Women often experience flare-ups prior to menstruation. Despite persistent myths, acne is neither caused by, nor exacerbated by, certain types of food or a dirty face.

Pathogenesis
of acne is multifactorial and includes:
- Increased sebum production due to androgenic activity
- Abnormal follicular keratinization, resulting in comedo (blackhead and whitehead) formation
- Growth of *Propionibacterium acnes*, which flourishes in sebum and produces irritating free fatty acids, resulting in inflammation

Treatment
is aimed at several of the pathogenetic factors, and two or more therapeutic agents are often used simultaneously.

DESCRIPTION OF LESIONS

- For descriptive and therapeutic purposes, acne may be regarded as being **inflammatory** (Figure 1.1) or **noninflammartory (comedonal)** (Figure 1.2) or a combination of both (Figure 1.4).
- Designations of **mild, moderate,** and **severe** are also useful.
  - **Mild acne** consists of open **comedones**, or blackheads, and closed comedones, or whiteheads, and occasional papules (Figure 1.3).
  - **Moderate acne** is more inflammatory, with multiple papules, pustules, or both (papulopustular acne). These lesions may occur in addition to comedones (Figure 1.4).
  - **Moderate to severe** acne has a greater degree and number of inflammatory lesions: papules, pustules, and, possibly, cysts (cystic acne), with evidence of scarring (Figure 1.5).
  - **Severe cystic acne** (acne conglobata, nodular acne) consists of papules, pustules, acne cysts, abscesses, and scarring (Figures 1.6 and 1.7).

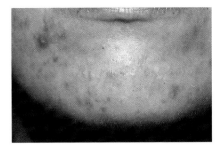

Figure 1.1
Inflammatory acne.

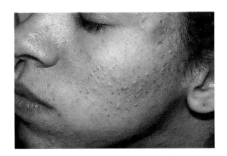

Figure 1.2
Comedonal acne.

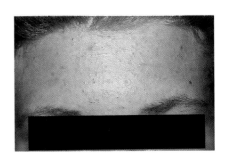

Figure 1.3
Mild acne showing open and closed comedones and ossasional papules.

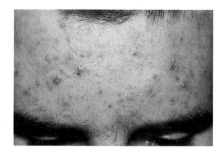

Figure 1.4.
Moderate acne with multiple papules
and pustules in addition to comedones.

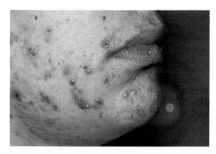

Figure 1.5.
Moderate to severe acne with papules,
pustules, nodules, cysts, and scars.

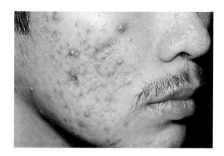

Figure 1.6.
Severe cystic acne on face.

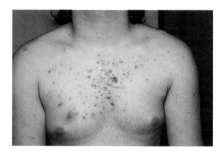

Figure 1.7.
Severe cystic acne on trunk.

DISTRIBUTION OF LESIONS

Acne is located in areas of maximal sebaceous gland activity: **face, neck, chest, shoulders, back,** and **upper arms**.

CLINICAL MANIFESTATIONS

- Paramount are the negative psychologic effects of acne (e.g., lowered self-esteem) and their impact on employment and social functioning.
- Lesions may heal with atrophic or pitted ("ice-pick") scars, hypertrophic scars, or even keloids.
- Postinflammatory hyperpigmentation may occur, particularly in dark-complexioned patients.
- Cystic lesions may be painful and tender.
- Severe, unremitting disease is more prevalent in adult males.
- Some women have acne that persists well past adolescence; others have their initial episode in their 20s or 30s.
- Some women may note improvement of acne during pregnancy or while taking birth control pills; others may note a worsening of acne under these conditions.
- Acne tends to improve in summer months.

DIAGNOSIS

- Acne is generally easy for the patient and practitioner to recognize; however, specific underlying causes for acne and look-alikes (acneiform conditions) should be considered.
- Hormonal tests are recommended for female patients whose acne is not responding to treatment and who have other signs of excess androgenic hormones, such as male characteristics (e.g., facial hair) or irregular menstrual periods.

DIFFERENTIAL DIAGNOSIS

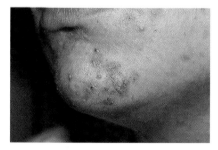

Figure 1.8.
Folliculitis. Note the papules and pustules with central hair.

Folliculitis
(Figure 1.8)
- Papules and/or pustules with central hairs
- No comedones

Keratosis pilaris (see Chapter 2, "Eczematous Rashes")
- Rough-textured, skin-colored papules, which may be acneiform (having papules and pustules)
- Most often occur on upper, outer arms, back, thighs, and lateral face
- No comedones

Rosacea and perioral dermatitis (see below)
- Seen in adults; may be seen, albeit infrequently, in children
- Most often occurs on central third of face or perioral area
- No comedones

MANAGEMENT

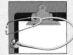

General principles

- Treatment of acne **should be individualized** and frequently involves a trial-and-error approach, beginning with those agents that are known to be most effective and least expensive and known to have the fewest side effects.
- It should be determined first if the acne is inflammatory or noninflammatory or is a combination of both features.
- Mild acne can often be managed successfully with over-the-counter remedies.
- Because topical antibiotics are most effective in preventing the formation of **new** acne lesions, a maximal therapeutic response may require at least 6 to 8 weeks.
- Every effort should be made to control acne with topical preparations alone; oral medications may be tapered or discontinued as soon as control is achieved. Topical retinoid therapy may cause a worsening of acne initially, and improvement may not be noted for 8 to 12 weeks.
- Inflammatory lesions should be approached first because they are usually the first to respond and their quick disappearance can be helpful in obtaining compliance in teenagers.
- Each topical agent should be used at different times of the day, unless two agents are combined (e.g., the erythromycin–benzoyl peroxide combination, Benzamycin Topical Gel).
- The topical agents most often used in conjuction with each other are tretinoin, benzoyl peroxide, and antibiotics. Tretinoin increases the penetration of other topical preparations, and benzoyl peroxide used together with 3% erythromycin appears to have a synergistic effect.
- A pill with a low androgenic potential, such as Ortho Tri-Cyclen or Demulen, should be considered for women who are taking oral contraceptives.
- The patient should be advised not to squeeze or pick lesions.
- There is no scientific basis for the understanding that "oil-based" cosmetics "clog pores" and cause acne; however, oil-free or water-based products are generally recommended.
- Severe cystic acne cannot be cured but often can be effectively treated and controlled with isotretinoin (Accutane). **Isotretinoin has severe teratogenic side effects and should not be used by women who are pregnant; it should only be administered by those who are familiar with its potential side effects.**

Mode of action

Topical agents

- **Retinoids** are primarily comedolytic and also have anti-inflammatory effects.
- **Benzoyl peroxide** preparations are potent antibacterial agents, which help to control inflammatory and noninflammatory lesions.
- **Clindamycin** and **erythromycin** are topical antibacterial agents, which help to control inflammatory lesions. Drug resistance to both of these agents has been reported, and the **combination of 3% erythromycin and 5% benzoyl peroxide gel (Benzamycin Topical Gel)** may be indicated to prevent resistance to erythromycin because no resistance has been reported with benzoyl peroxide.

- **Azelaic acid (Azelex)** is used for inflammatory facial acne in patients unable to tolerate benzoyl peroxide or tretinoin
- Other topical agents used to treat mild acne include **salicylic acid, sodium sulfacetamide, alpha-hydroxy acids, resorcinol, astringents, soaps,** and **cleansers.** These agents act as exfoliants or as antibiotics.

Oral antibiotics
- Use is in patients with moderate-to-severe inflammatory acne and those in whom topical therapy is insufficient.
- Gram-negative folliculitis has been seen after long-term use of oral antibiotics.

Management of comedonal acne

Topical retinoids.
Tretinoin (Retin-A) and adapalene (Differin Gel) may be used alone or in conjunction with benzoyl peroxide. The newer retinoid, adapalene, is as effective as tretinoin but appears to be better tolerated in patients with sensitive skin, causing less erythema, scaling, and burning.
- The retinoid should be:
  - Started with tretinoin 0.025% cream or adapalene 0.1% gel at bedtime
  - Increased to higher concentrations as tolerated
  - Applied as a pea-sized amount over the entire face
- There may be redness and scaling in the first few weeks.
- Patients with sensitive skin may begin using the agent every other night and then increase the frequency of application as tolerated.
- In the first few weeks, the acne may appear to be worsening; the patient must be cautioned to be diligent in continuing the medication, which may require 8 to 12 weeks for maximal effects.
- If the patient is fair-skinned or plans to be in the sun, sunscreens should be applied accordingly.
- Mild soaps should be used for routine facial washing.
- It is generally advised not to prescribe topical retinoids during pregnancy, despite the fact that no untoward reactions from them have been documented.

Benzoyl peroxide
- This agent may be used to treat mild comedonal and inflammatory acne. The patient should:
  - Begin with a low-strength 2.5% or 5% preparation alone or in conjunction with a topical retinoid
  - Apply a thin layer once or twice daily to the entire affected area
- Benzoyl peroxide may cause irritation and burning.
- It may bleach clothing, particularly if it is applied to the trunk.

Management of mild inflammatory acne
- Treatment involves application of the following agents:
  - Benzoyl peroxide alone
  - A combination of 3% erythromycin and 5% benzoyl peroxide (Benzamycin Topical Gel) twice daily
  - Topical 1% clindamycin or 2% erythromycin twice daily, which also may be used in conjunction with benzoyl peroxide
- Topical antibiotics are applied to the entire affected area.
- The agents may cause slight dryness and irritation.
- Bacterial resistance has been reported.
- A topical retinoid may be added at bedtime, if necessary.

Management of moderate to severe acne
- **Oral antibiotics are used in addition to topical antibiotics**. The dosage should be increased or decreased in 4 to 8 weeks, depending upon the patient's response. If possible, the clinician should try to taper medication to topical agents alone. Oral antibiotics include:
    - Tetracycline, starting at 500 mg to 1g per day, in divided doses
    - Erythromycin, 500 mg twice daily or 333 mg twice or three times daily
    - Minocycline, 50 mg to 100 mg twice daily
    - Doxycycline, 50 mg to 100 mg twice daily
- Tetracycline must be taken on an empty stomach (1 hour before or 2 hours after meals).
- Tetracycline, minocycline, and, particularly, doxycycline may cause photosensitivity (and sunscreens should be advised, if necessary).
- Tetracycline and minocycline should not be used before the age of 10 years to avoid permanent teeth staining. Nor should they be used during pregnancy or in lactating women.
- Minocycline may also cause pigmentary changes in the skin and vertigolike symptoms at higher doses.
- Both tetracycline and erythromycin may contribute to candidal vaginitis.
- Gastrointestinal upset may also occur occasionally with the use of tetracycline, minocycline, doxycycline, and erythromycin.
- It is unclear whether antibiotics interfere with the absorption of oral contraceptives. Women should be made aware of this so they can decide if they wish to use an alternative or additional form of birth control if they take oral antibiotics and oral contraceptives simultaneously.

Management of severe acne
- **Oral antibiotics are used in addition to topical antibiotics.**
- If there is a poor response, if oral antibiotics must be used continually for a long time period (2 or more years), or if there is evidence of progressive scarring nodular acne, the use of **isotretinoin (Accutane)** should be considered in consultation with or by referral to a dermatologist.

Other therapeutic modalities include:
- **Acne surgery**, which consists of removing comedones with an extractor
- **Intralesional injections of corticosteroids** into cystic or nodular lesions, which help to promote more rapid resolution of larger lesions
- **Abscess incision and drainage**
- **Chemical peels**
- **Dermabrasion**
- **Punch grafts**
- **Injectable fillers, such as collagen**
- **Hormonal therapy with systemic antiandrogens, such as spironolactone and oral contraceptives**

POINTS TO REMEMBER

- Compliance is often a problem in teenagers so it is important to explain clearly the treatment regimen, make it simple, and give the patient written instructions. The patient also should be advised to call the health care provider with any questions or problems.
- In darkly pigmented people, the severity of inflammation may be equivalent to, although not as apparent, as it is in those with lighter complexions. Consequently, patients with dark skin may be as concerned about the acne-related pigmentary changes as they are about the acne itself. Evidence of scarring should be treated more aggressively in these patients because even mild acne can heal with significant scarring.
- Blackheads represent oxidized melanin, not dirt.
- Patients may need reassurance that acne is not caused by dirty skin, greasy foods, or sweets.

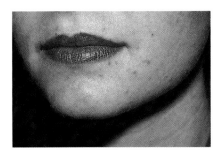

Figure 1.9.
Female adult-onset acne.

FEMALE ADULT-ONSET ACNE (Figure 1.9)

BASICS

- In all dermatologist offices, the complaint "acne, at my age!" is a daily utterance by women in whom acne suddenly appears or in whom acne has not resolved by the age of 20. Proposed explanations for the apparent increased incidence of acne in women have been attributed to the recent entry of women in the work force and its attendant stress, women having children at a later age, and the use of oral contraceptives.
- It should be kept in mind that acne may also be associated with androgen excess in female patients with menstrual problems and hirsutism (e.g., polycystic ovarian disease, androgen-secreting tumors).

DESCRIPTION OF LESIONS

- Inflammatory papules and pustules Few comedones

DISTRIBUTION OF LESIONS

is frequently perioral

CLINICAL MANIFESTATIONS

include a flare-up of acne 2 to 7 days prior to the onset of menses or at midcycle

DIAGNOSIS

is made through physical examination and by taking a careful menstrual and drug history

MANAGEMENT

General principles
- **Topical antibiotics,** such as 1% clindamycin, 2% erythromycin, or benzoyl peroxide plus erythromycin (Benzamycin Topical Gel), are applied.
- If necessary, topical retinoids or topical azelaic acid may be added.
- If necessary, systemic antibiotics are used.

Pregnancy.
Topical erythromycin is the safest choice.

Patient on oral contraceptives.
An agent with a low androgenic potential should be recommended, if it is not medically contraindicated.

Cosmetic use
is probably much less a problem to women's skin as previously thought and only rarely cause adult acne; oil-based preparations actually do not "clog the pores" of the skin.

DRUG-INDUCED ACNE

BASICS

- Drug-induced acne (or drug-exacerbated acne) has been linked to topical or systemic steroids, anabolic steroid use in weight lifters and other athletes, lithium, oral contraceptives, phenytoin, isoniazid, and iodides.
- Long-term use of potent topical steroids on the face may produce a rosacealike eruption.

DESCRIPTION OF LESIONS

- Inflammatory papules and pustules, which are usually monomorphic
- Folliculitislike lesions in systemic steroid-induced acne
- No comedones (unless patient also has coexisting acne vulgaris)

DISTRIBUTION OF LESIONS

- Primarily on the trunk, shoulders, and upper arms in systemic steroid–induced acne (Figure 1.10)
- On the face in topical steroid–induced acne

CLINICAL MANIFESTATIONS

- Gradual resolution of acne on discontinuing the offending agent
- Possible marked initial flare-up of facial acne on discontinuing topical steroid

DIAGNOSIS

is made by taking a careful patient history inquiring about drug use.

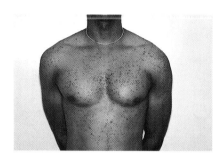

Figure 1.10.
Steroid acne. Note multiple uniform papules and scattered pustules.

 MANAGEMENT

- The offending agent should be discontinued, if possible.
- The acne should be treated with benzoyl peroxide and/or topical antibiotics.
- Systemic antibiotics should be used, if necessary.

MECHANICAL, OR CONTACT ACNE

BASICS

Mechanical, or contact, acne may erupt at sites exposed to physical trauma or occlusion (e.g., it can be caused by chin straps, (Figure 1.11) pomades, shoulder pads, bra straps, and so forth).

DESCRIPTION OF LESIONS

Lesions are comedonal and/or papulopustular

DISTRIBUTION OF LESIONS

The lesions are located under the occluded area in mechanical and pomade acne

CLINICAL MANIFESTATIONS, DIAGNOSIS, AND MANAGEMENT

are similar to those for drug-induced acne

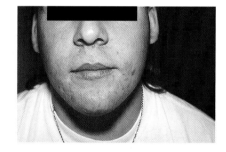

Figure 1.11.
Mechanical, or contact, acne caused by a football chin strap.

NEONATAL ACNE

(Figure 1.12) is a self-limiting form of acne, which is seen mainly in male infants. It occurs from the stimulation of maternal androgens and requires no treatment.

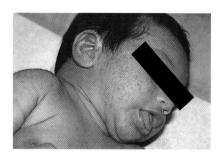

Figure 1.12.
Neonatal acne. Acneiform lesions in typical distribution on nose and cheeks.

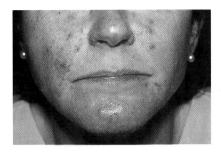

Figure 1.13.
Inflammatory papules and pustules, central one-third of face.

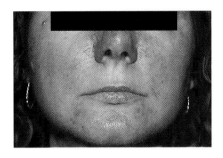

Figure 1.14.
"Pre-rosacea" erythema and telangiectasias.

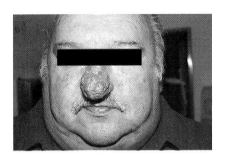

Figure 1.15.
Rhinophyma

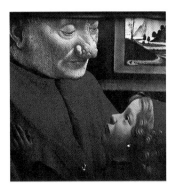

Figure 1.16.
Ghirlandaio's portrait of an old man with his grandson (showing a tender human relationship, despite the appearance of the nose).

BASICS

- **Rosacea** is a common acnelike facial eruption that consists of erythematous **papules**, **pustules**, and **telangiectasias** involving the central third of the face (Figure 1.13).
- It is most often seen in fair-skinned individuals of northern European descent. It is a chronic problem, usually presenting between 30 to 50 years of age. Women are three times more likely to be affected than men; it is unusual in dark-skinned people.
- Rosacea is considered to be an **idiopathic** vascular hyperresponsiveness to various stimuli such as heat, cold, emotional stress, sunlight, and certain foods. Several investigators believe that *Helicobacter pylori* found in the stomach may cause or exacerbate rosacea; *Demodex* mites that are often found in the hair follicle in patients with rosacea have also been implicated.

DESCRIPTION OF LESIONS

The typical progression of **lesions of rosacea** begin as facial flushing over the nose and cheeks, followed by persistent **erythema** and **telangiectasias** (Figure 1.14) that are later manifested as inflammatory **papules**, **pustules**, and possibly **nodules**.

DISTRIBUTION OF LESIONS

Rosacea has a predilection for the convex areas of the face. It is usually, but not always, **bilaterally symmetrical**.

CLINICAL MANIFESTATIONS

- Rosacea may initially manifest as a tendency to blush or flush easily, producing "rosy cheeks." Later, persistent facial erythema and fine telangiectasias develop, which may later progress to inflammatory lesions consisting of papules and pustules.
- Rosacea may be accompanied by **rhinophyma**, a sebaceous hyperplasia of the nose that is seen predominantly in men (Figures 1.15 and 1.16). Rosacea may affect the eyes, resulting in blepharoconjunctivitis, keratitis, and, less commonly, more serious ocular complications.

DIAGNOSIS

- Acnelike lesions appearing *de novo* on the face of an adult male are almost invariably rosacea.
- Rosacea may be difficult to distinguish from acne in adult females.

DIFFERENTIAL DIAGNOSIS

Adult acne
may coexist with, or be impossible to distinguish from, rosacea. The presence or absence of the following findings may be helpful in differentiating the two:
- Comedones (blackheads and whiteheads) are not seen in rosacea (Figure 1.17).
- There is a lack of facial flushing and telangiectasias in acne.
- A wider distribution of lesions is noted in acne.

Seborrheic dermatitis
(Figure 1.18)
- Scale and erythema are present without acneiform lesions.
- Distribution of seborrheic dermatitis involves the nasolabial fold, eyebrows, scalp, chest, and back.
- Seborrheic dermatitis may coexist with rosacea.

Systemic lupus erythematosus
(Figure 1.19)
- Systemic lupus erythematosus lacks papules and pustules.
  - It is antinuclear antibody (ANA)–positive.
  - Other features of lupus are present.

Perioral dermatitis (Figures 1.20 and 1.21)
- Inflammatory papules and pustules appear on the lower third of the face.
- The condition may also occur in a **periorbital and paranasal** distribution.

Topical steroid–induced rosacea
- There is a history of potent topical steroid misuse on the face.
- Clinically, this condition is indistinguishable from rosacea.

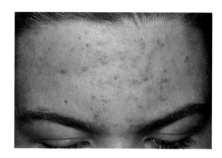

Figure 1.17.
Typical acne.

MANAGEMENT

Avoidance and elimination of precipitating factors. There is no sound evidence that avoidance of precipitating factors results in any marked improvement of rosacea; however, patients should be encouraged to find out what factors are relevant and troublesome and to understand and eliminate the environmental triggers that have been reported to exacerbate rosacea, such as:

- Excessive alcohol intake
- Sun exposure (sunblock with an sun protective factor [SPF] of 15 or higher should be applied prior to sun exposure)
- Irritating cosmetics; excessive washing of the face
- Emotional stress
- Spicy foods and caffeine intake
- Smoking

Systemic therapy
Oral antibiotics
- Treatment with **tetracycline** or **erythromycin** typically delivers a fast therapeutic response that pleases the patient and helps to confirm the diagnosis of rosacea. The mechanism of action is more likely antiinflammatory than antibacterial in nature.
  - Tetracycline is given in divided doses from 250 mg to 500 mg twice daily and then tapered when the acneiform inflammatory component has improved (usually after 3 to 4 weeks).
  - If **tetracycline** is ineffective, **minocycline or erythromycin** may be tried.
- **Isotretinoin (Accutane)** has been used in cases of severe refractory rosacea.

Topical therapy.
If possible, long-term control of rosacea should be attempted with topical therapy alone, and oral antibiotics should be used for breakthrough flares. (Patients readily learn to titrate the dosage of oral antibiotics based upon disease activity.)
- **Metronidazole 0.75%,** MetroCream, or MetroGel applied twice daily or the newer Noritate 1% (metronidazole cream) applied once daily, have been shown to decrease papules and pustules. Because it may take 6 to 8 weeks for a good therapeutic response, metronidazole may be given initially with an oral antibiotic and continued as the antibiotic is tapered or used alone in mild cases.
- Less effective, but helpful, are topical **clindamycin or erythromycin lotion,** which may be tried if metronidazole fails.
- A topical **sulfacetamide 10%, sulfur 5%** (Sulfacet-R) preparation is another treatment option that also contains a cosmetic cover-up.

Other
- **Cosmetic foundations** may be used to cover erythematous areas.
- **Electrocautery with a small needle** is employed to destroy small telangiectasias.
- **Pulse-dye lasers** are reserved for larger telangiectatic vessels.
- **Surgical reduction** is used to treat rhinophyma.

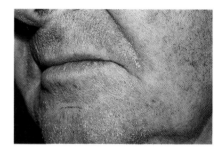

Figure 1.18.
Seborrheic dermatitis.

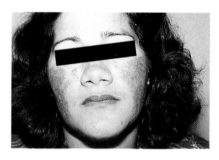

Figure 1.19.
The butterfly rash of systemic lupus erythematosus.

POINTS TO REMEMBER

- Rosacea is a chronic condition with no known cure.
- The use of potent topical steroids on the face should be avoided in treating rosacea.

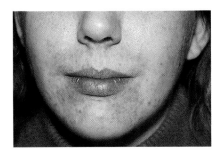

Figure 1.20.
Note perioral sparing.

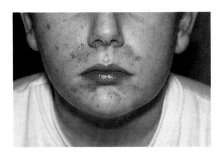

Figure 1.21.
Periorificial distribution in a child.

BASICS

- **Perioral dermatitis,** also known as **periorificial dermatitis,** is a rosacealike eruption that is seen primarily in young women and infrequently in young children of both sexes.
- The patient is usually a 15- to 40-year-old woman.
- Perioral dermatitis is usually found around the mouth but may be noted around the eyes and nose, which explains the more inclusive term, periorificial.
- As in rosacea, its etiology is unknown; potent topical steroid use and fluorinated toothpaste use have been implicated, but unproved, as possible causes.

DESCRIPTION OF LESIONS

Primary lesions are small erythematous papules or pustules.

DISTRIBUTION OF LESIONS

Characteristically, the lesions circle the mouth and spare the area bordering the lips (Figure 1.20).

CLINICAL MANIFESTATIONS

- Small erythematous papules or pustules, with occasional superimposed scaling
- Lesions generally clear in 4 to 8 weeks.

DIAGNOSIS

Acnelike papules and pustules occur in a periorificial distribution in a young woman or child (Figure 1.21).

DIFFERENTIAL DIAGNOSIS

- Acne
- Rosacea
- Steroid-induced rosacea

MANAGEMENT

Systemic antibiotics, as described for rosacea, usually bring a rapid response and often clearing.
Topical therapy with **metronidazole** is employed, as described for **rosacea.**
Short-term use of mild **topical steroids** for management of scaly lesions may be used.

POINTS TO REMEMBER

Acne, rosacea, and perioral dermatitis all share similar clinical manifestations, and overlapping management strategies, yet each has a distinctive course and prognosis; consequently, an attempt at specific diagnosis should be made.

ACNE FORMULARY

TOPICAL AGENTS

BRAND NAMES	GENERIC NAMES	PREPARATIONS
Retinoids		
PRESCRIPTION		
Retin-A Cream	Tretinoin	0.025%, 0.05%, 0.1%
Retin-A Gel	Tretinoin	0.025%, 0.01%
Avita	Tretinoin cream	0.025%
Differin Gel	Adapalene	0.1%
Benzoyl Peroxide (available in water- and alcohol-based vehicles, soaps, and washes)		
OVER-THE-COUNTER		
Oxy-5, Oxy-10	Benzoyl peroxide	5%, 10% lotion
Clear by Design	Benzoyl peroxide	2.5% gel (water)
Clearasil 10%	Benzoyl peroxide	10% lotion
Clearasil Maximum Strength	Benzoyl peroxide	10% cream (tint)
PRESCRIPTION		
Desquam-X	Benzoyl peroxide	2.5%, 5%, 10% gel (water)
Desquam-E	Benzoyl peroxide	2.5%, 5%, 10% gel (water)
Topical Antibiotics		
PRESCRIPTION		
Akne-Mycin	Erythromycin	2% ointment, solution
A/T/S	Erythromycin	2% solution, gel
Erycette	Erythromycin	2% pledgets
Cleocin T	Clindamycin	1% solution, gel, lotion
Benzoyl Peroxide plus Erythromycin		
PRESCRIPTION		
Benzamycin	3% Erythromycin plus 5% benzoyl peroxide	Gel
Other Topical Agents		
PRESCRIPTION		
Azelex	Azelaic acid	20% cream
Sulfacet-R Lotion	Sodium sulfacetamide	10% lotion (tint)
Klaron	Sodium sulfacetamide	10% lotion (water)

ORAL AGENTS

Generic Names   Dosages

Oral Antibiotics	
PRESCRIPTION	
Tetracycline	250 mg–500 mg twice daily
Erythromycin	500 mg twice daily or 333 mg twice to three times daily
Minocycline	500 mg to 100 mg twice daily

Brand Names   Generic Names   Dosages

Oral Contraceptives		
PRESCRIPTION		
Ortho Tri-Cyclen	Norgestimate/ethinyl estradiol	Ethinyl estradiol: 0.035 mg Norgestimate: 0.18, 0.21, 0.25
Demulen	Ethynodiol diacetate/	Ethinyl estradiol: 0.050 mg ethinyl estradiol

Ethynodiol diacetate: 1 mg

Oral Retinoids		
PRESCRIPTION		
Accutane	Isotretinoin	0.05 mg to 1.0 mg/kg/day

ROSACEA AND PERIORAL DERMATITIS FORMULARY

SYSTEMIC AGENTS

Systemic agents are used to treat the skin and ocular manifestations of rosacea and are tapered to the minimal required dosage.

Tetracycline	500 mg–1 g/day in divided doses
Minocycline	100 mg–200 mg/day in divided doses
Erythromycin	500 mg–1 g/day in divided doses

TOPICAL AGENTS

Topical agents are used for milder cases and for maintenance after stopping oral agents.

Metronidazole 0.075% (MetroGel, MetroCream)
Metronidazole 1% cream (Noritate)
Erythromycin 2% in a nonalcoholic base
Clindamycin 1% lotion
Sulfacetamide 10%, sulfur 5% (Sulfacet-R)

CHAPTER 2

ECZEMATOUS RASHES

Overview

BASICS

- **Eczema,** or **eczematous dermatitis (ED),** is the most common inflammatory skin disorder. The terms "eczema" and "dermatitis" are used interchangeably by dermatologists, and, although they are synonymous, it is a common convention to use the two terms together.
- ED is difficult to define because it has numerous clinical and several histologic presentations. It is best understood by seeing it repeatedly.

Etiology
ED may be caused by an outside agent (e.g., poison ivy [rhus dermatitis]), it may be endogenous as noted in some atopic patients (e.g., atopic dermatitis), or it may be idiopathic (e.g., nonspecific ED).

Histopathology
- Microscopically, epidermal inter- and intracellular fluid accumulation **(spongiosis)** and vasodilatation in the dermis account for the acute clinical manifestations of eczema: edema, erythema, vesicles, and bullae.
- Later, thickening of the epidermis **(acanthosis),** retention of nuclei in the horny layer of epidermis **(parakeratosis),** and an abundant cellular infiltrate in the dermis account for the scale and lichenification of **chronic ED.**

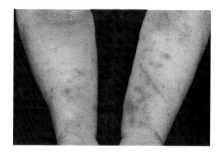

Figure 2.1.
Acute eczematous dermatitis (ED) caused by poison ivy (rhus dermatitis). Note linear configuration of vesicles.

DESCRIPTION OF LESIONS

The appearance and distribution of lesions varies with patient age and race and with the duration of the condition. The designations "acute," "subacute," and "chronic" in reference to phases of ED are part of a dynamic spectrum where any one or all may coexist on the same patient and may start at any phase and evolve into another.
- **Acute ED** is manifested by erythematous, " juicy" papules or plaques, vesicobullous lesions, or these features simultaneously (e.g., as may be seen in poison ivy; Figure 2.1).
- **Subacute** ED consists of:
  - Crusts (scabs), which are secondary lesions that arise from scratching (excoriations) or from drying papulovesicles or pustules
  - Scale and erythema (Figure 2.2)
- **Chronic** ED consists of:
  - **Lichenification,** or a plaque with an exaggeration of the normal skin markings (the hallmark lesion)
  - In addition to scale and crusting, often **postinflammatory pigmentary alterations** (hyperpigmentation and/or hypopigmentation)
  - For example, atopic dermatitis (Figure 2.3)

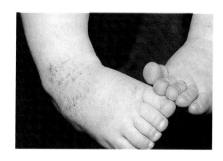

Figure 2.2.
Subacute eczematous dermatitis (ED). Crusts, scale, and early lichenification; less intense erythema than associated with acute eczema.

CLINICAL MANIFESTATIONS

The following clinical presentations of ED are discussed in this chapter:
- Atopic dermatitis (atopic eczema)
- Nonspecific ED
- Dyshidrotic eczema/chronic hand eczema
- Lichen simplex chronicus
- Neurotic excoriations
- Nummular eczema
- Asteatotic eczema
- Stasis dermatitis
- Contact dermatitis

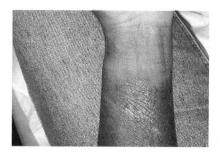

Figure 2.3.
Chronic eczematous dermatitis (ED). Note lichenification and hyperpigmentation.

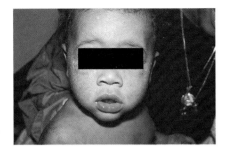

Figure 2.4.
Atopic dermatitis (AD) involving the cheeks.

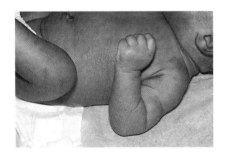

Figure 2.5.
Generalized atopic dermatitis (AD).

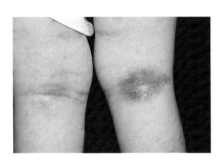

Figure 2.6.
Atopic dermatitis (AD) in flexor creases.

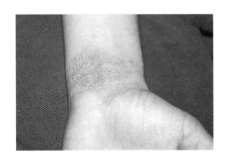

Figure 2.7.
Lichenified atopic dermatitis (AD).

BASICS

- **Atopic dermatitis (AD),** also known as atopic eczema, is a pruritic, chronic inflammatory condition. It is the most commonly seen type of eczema. It occurs in association with a personal or family history of hay fever, asthma, allergic rhinitis or sinusitis, or AD itself
- Approximately 5 to 10% of the United States population have AD.
- Course is unpredictable. AD may start at any age but most often begins in childhood and runs a course of flares and remissions. The disease frequently remits spontaneously but occasionally returns in adolescence or adulthood and may persist.
- The pattern of the skin rash tends to vary with the age of the patient.
- Severe disease in childhood portends a worse prognosis, and expected remission by puberty may be less common than previously believed.
- AD is considered to be an inherited type of hypersensitivity disorder of the skin and not a true allergic condition because AD is often outgrown and allergies are not.
- Intense itching is presumably caused by the release of vasoactive substances from sensitized mast cells and basophils in the dermis.

PHASES OF AD

The phases of AD are not always so clearly demarcated as the following descriptions may imply. Any or all phases may blend together or may be present simultaneously.

Infantile AD (age 2 months to 2 years)
Description of lesions
Lesions are scaly, red, and occasionally oozing crusted patches and plaques.

Distribution of lesions
- Lesions tend to be symmetrical.
- The face, particularly the cheeks (Figure 2.4), scalp, chest, neck, and extensor extremities, is most often affected. Lesions often spare the diaper area but may become generalized (Figure 2.5).
- As the child approaches age 2, AD begins to involve the flexor creases (Figure 2.6).

Clinical manifestations
- Pruritus may interfere with sleep.
- Scratching causes increased itching, which leads to lichenification, oozing, and secondary bacterial infection ("honey-crusted," impetiginized skin).
  - Secondary infection with *Staphylococcus aureus* may trigger relapses of AD.
  - Secondary infection with herpes simplex virus may result in eczema herpeticum (Kaposi's varicelliform eruption).
  - Secondary infections with molluscum contagiosum are found more readily on atopic skin.

Childhood AD (age 2 to 12 years)
In addition to the physical problems associated with AD, emotional problems may occur, especially in school and with peer relationships.

Description of lesions
- Inflamed lesions become lichenified because of repeated rubbing and scratching (Figure 2.7).
- Lichenification occurs more commonly in Asian and black people; however, many patients never develop lichenification.
- Lesions tend to be less acute and exudative than those seen in infancy.
- Erosions, crusts, and, later, postinflammatory pigmentary alterations become apparent.

Distribution of lesions.
Lesions in this age group are symmetrical, with the characteristic distribution in flexural folds: the antecubital (Figure 2.8), and popliteal fossae; and on the neck, wrists, and ankles on the eyelids (Figure 2.9), periorally (Figure 2.10), on the scalp, and behind the ears.

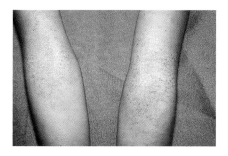

Figure 2.8.
Symmetrical atopic dermatitis (AD) with characteristic distribution in flexural folds.

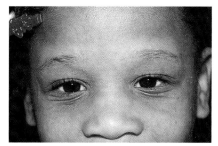

Figure 2.9.
Atopic dermatitis (AD) affecting the eyes. Note the postinflammatory hyper-pigmentation.

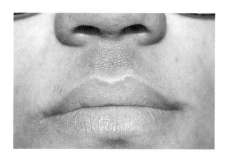

Figure 2.10.
Perioral atopic dermatitis (AD).

Adolescent and adult phase (age 13 through adulthood)

AD can present de novo in adults of any age who have an atopic history. In addition to physical symptoms, psychosocial problems, such as poor self-image, may lead to depression and social isolation.

Description of lesions

- Lichenified plaques are generally less well demarcated than those seen in psoriasis and tend to blend into the surrounding normal skin.
- Postinflammatory hyper- and hypopigmentary changes can be seen, as in the childhood pattern of AD.
- AD may change in appearance to poorly-defined, itchy erythematous papules and plaques (Figure 2.11).

Distribution of lesions

- The distribution of lesions may be similar to that seen in patients with childhood AD; however, lesions may also be on the extensor aspects of the extremities (Figure 2.12) and involve the dorsa of the hands, forearms (Figure 2.13), wrists, ankles, and feet.
- There are other clinical variants of AD noted mostly in adults:
  - Papular and/or nodular (prurigo nodularis; Figure 2.14)
  - Follicular eczema, a clinical variant of AD that tends to occur primarily on the extremities and trunk in black people (Figure 2.15)
  - Dyshidrotic eczema, or chronic hand dermatitis, which may be the only characteristic of AD that remains in some adults (see below, "Dyshidrotic Eczema/Chronic Hand Dermatitis")

DIAGNOSIS

- **Diagnosis of AD is made primarily on clinical grounds.** Criteria include:
  - Eczematous eruption
  - Itchy, dry skin
  - Flexural distribution
  - Atopic history

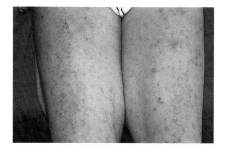

Figure 2.11.
Atopic dermatitis (AD). Poorly defined itchy erythematous papules and

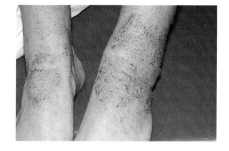

Figure 2.12.
Extensor atopic dermatitis (AD).

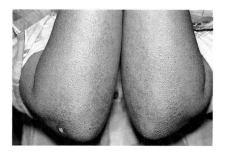

Figure 2.15.
Follicular eczema, a clinical variant of eczema that tends to occur primarily on the extremities and trunk in blacks. Note the evenly spaced "goose bump-like" papules that represent inflamed hair follicles.

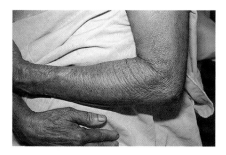

Figure 2.13.
Extensor atopic dermatitis (AD) in an elderly patient.

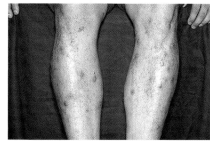

Figure 2.14.
Papular and/or nodular atopic dermatitis (AD) (prurigo nodularis).

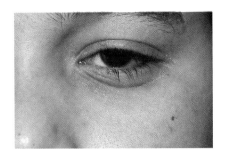

Figure 2.16.
Dennie-Morgan lines. Note the extra eyelid crease.

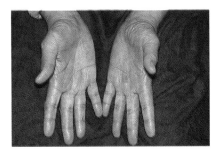

Figure 2.17.
Hyperlinear palmar creases.

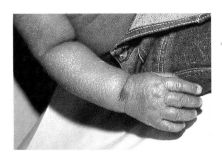

Figure 2.18.
Ichthyosis vulgaris.

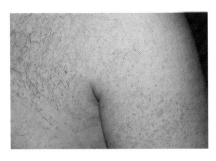

Figure 2.19.
Keratosis pilaris (KP; "allergic bumps"); tiny rough-textured whitish or red follicular papules.

- **Laboratory tests**
  - Total serum IgE levels may be elevated or normal.
  - Skin-prick tests and radioallergosorbent tests for food or environmental allergens are of little or no value.
  - A punch biopsy may be performed if the diagnosis is in doubt.
- **Other associated features and clues** to the diagnosis of AD include:
  - **Dennie-Morgan lines** (Figure 2.16), which are a characteristic double fold that extends from the inner to the outer canthus of the lower eyelid
  - **Hyperlinear palmar creases** (Figure 2.17)
  - **Ichthyosis vulgaris** (Figure 2.18)
    — Frequently associated with atopy
    — Has a fine fish-scalelike appearance, most apparent on the shins
    — Is inherited in an autosomal dominant fashion and tends to improve with age
    — Treated with 12% Lac-Hydrin Lotion and other moisturizers
  - **Keratosis pilaris (KP)** (Figure 2.19)
    — Tiny rough textured whitish or red follicular papules or pustules, which occur during adolescence
    — Most commonly occur on the deltoid and posterolateral upper arms, the upper back and thighs, and malar area of the face
    — Frequently confused with acne
    — Treatment of KP with topical Lac-Hydrin and/or Retin-A preparations, which are minimally effective
    — Essentially a cosmetic problem
  - **Xerosis, or dry skin,** is particularly dry in the winter months (See Chapter 15, "Xerosis, the Dry Patient").

DIFFERENTIAL DIAGNOSIS

Diagnosis of AD is generally not difficult, especially in the context of an atopic history and when other causes for an eczematous or eczematouslike eruption are ruled out, such as:

Contact dermatitis

A history of a clinically relevant contactant is important because contact dermatitis may otherwise be clinically indistinguishable from AD.

Scabies

- A history of exposure to scabies is important.
- The distribution of lesions may be characteristic of scabies (e.g., finger webs, flexor wrists).
- Scabies also may become secondarily eczematous in appearance.

Psoriasis

- Psoriasis is characterized by extensor distribution.
- Typical psoriatic lesions may be found elsewhere on the body.
- It is generally less pruritic than eczema.
- It may also be clinically indistinguishable from AD.
- **Tinea pedis, corporis, manum, and capitus** are associated with a positive KOH and/or fungal culture.

MANAGEMENT

In general, it is important to keep in mind that an infant or child, particularly one who is not yet in school, should not be treated aggressively for what sometimes amounts primarily to a cosmetic problem. Whenever possible, this condition should be treated for how it "feels" and not for how it "looks". (See also Appendix 2.)

Topical steroids (see General Principles of Topical Therapy)

Topical steroids usually bring a prompt improvement.

- Many patients and parents of patients are afraid of using topical steroids because of the potential side effects of systemic steroids. An explanation should be offered that the benefits far outweigh the risks when topical steroids are used appropriately.
- Topical steroids should be employed only for **short-term use**, if possible, against active disease (i.e., itching and erythema; not for prevention of eczema or for cosmetic reasons such as hyperpigmentation).
- "Stronger" is preferable to "longer" because long-term application is more often associated with side effects. Using a superpotent topical steroid to achieve a successful response is preferable to the administration of systemic steroids.
- Concomitant use of topical steroids and systemic antibiotics, such as erythromycin, cephalexin, and dicloxacillin, is sometimes helpful if there is evidence (and sometimes if there is no clinical evidence) of staphylococcal infection.

Face and intertriginous areas

- For the face and intertriginous areas, the patient should first start with a low-potency cream, such as 0.5 to 1% hydrocortisone (Cortaid). If increased potency is necessary, the patient should be prescribed desonide 0.05% cream (DesOwen). Higher potency is hydrocortisone valerate 0.2% (Westcort Cream). The drug should be applied once to twice daily, as necessary.
- When AD is under control, the frequency of application is reduced from twice daily to once daily to as necessary only, using the least-potent agent possible.

Body

- For the body, a more potent cream or ointment may be used to initiate treatment, such as triamcinolone 0.1% (Kenalog), and increased to fluocinonide 0.05% (Lidex). Even a superpotent agent, such as clobetasol 0.05% (Temovate), may be used for a limited time period (no more than 2 to 3 weeks). When control is achieved, the potency is titrated downward to weaker preparations, such as hydrocortisone valerate 0.2% (Westcort).
- A 1-lb jar of triamcinolone acetonide cream or ointment is economical.

Other measures

- Oral H_1 antihistamines may be useful in reducing itching and helping an infant sleep. However, in children and adults, the sleep-inducing characteristic of the drugs is often an unacceptable side effect.
- Topical ointments containing H_1 and H_2 blockers (e.g., doxepin) and topical anesthetic preparations (e.g., Lanacane) are potentially contact allergens and are not useful.
- **Tar baths** and **tar ointments, pastes,** and **gels** may be used in addition to topical steroids or alternated with topical steroids. They also are not very effective.
- Oozing, exudative lesions may be soothed and dried with cool to lukewarm **Burow's solution** (see Appendix 2) or by **bathing in a tub with antipruritic emollients**, such as Aveeno Shower & Bath.
- Emollients may be applied liberally on noninflamed skin.
- Measures (e.g., support groups, family psychotherapy) should be taken to help **decrease emotional stress** in the child and in the family environment.
- **Systemic steroids** or **short-term hospitalization** are sometimes necessary for the patient with severe unresponsive AD.
- Hospitalization may be required in patients with secondary herpes simplex infection (Kaposi's varicelliform eruption).
- **Sun exposure,** if possible, at times of day when it is not as hot and less likely to induce sweating (early morning and late afternoon) may improve AD in some individuals.
- **Phototherapy** with ultraviolet B (UVB) and psoralen plus ultraviolet A (PUVA) can be used in patients unresponsive to topical and systemic steroids. This is particularly helpful in treating diabetics who could have problems taking systemic steroids.
- In very severe recalcitrant cases, oral cyclosporine may be helpful

POINTS TO REMEMBER

- The chemical formula and vehicle in which a topical steroid is compounded reflects its potency; consequently, it is easy to be confused by the fact that the designated concentration of a topical steroid is a measure of its strength. For example, clobetasol (Temovate 0.05%) is extremely more potent than a 1% or even a 2.5% concentration of hydrocortisone.
- If potent topical steroids are not helping, an oral staphylocidal antibiotic for 1 week should be considered.

BASICS

There is a large group of patients who have a chronic recurrent ED, who deny any atopic history. Frequently, these patients complain of dry or sensitive skin, which tends to become drier and itchier in winter months. The eruption tends to **worsen with aging** as the skin tends to lose some of its barrier function and lubrication (asteatosis).

DESCRIPTION OF LESIONS

Nonspecific ED is an **itchy eczematous eruption without the typical distribution or atopic history** characteristic of AD.

DISTRIBUTION OF LESIONS

is random; however, nonspecific ED favors the trunk and extremities.

DIAGNOSIS AND DIFFERENTIAL DIAGNOSIS

Nonspecific ED is a diagnosis of exclusion in which no underlying cause, such as a contact allergen or scabies, is found.

MANAGEMENT

Management is by topical steroids and emollients.

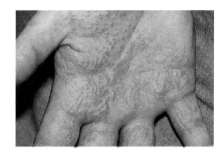

Figure 2.20.
Large palmar vesicles known as pompholyx.

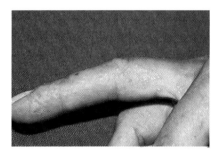

Figure 2.21.
Vesicles on the sides of the fingers.

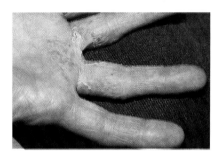

Figure 2.22.
Golden-brown color resembling tapioca pudding.

BASICS

- Dyshidrotic eczema of the hands, and less commonly, the feet, is a **chronic, recurrent pruritic eruption**, which occurs more frequently in women than in men.
- The majority of patients with dyshidrotic eczema and chronic hand dermatitis have an **atopic history**; however, a diligent history should be taken and, if necessary, patch testing may be performed to determine if it is caused by or exacerbated by a contactant.

DESCRIPTION OF LESIONS

- **Dyshidrotic vesicles**, usually symmetrical, are located on the **palms** (Figure 2.20), **sides of the fingers** (Figure 2.21), and sometimes on the **insteps (soles)** of the feet.
- Initially, the vesicles, which are small and clear, resemble tapioca pudding and later become a golden-brown color (Figure 2.22).
- The lesions dry, become scaly, and sometimes become crusted and secondarily infected (impetiginized; Figure 2.23).
- Later, chronic lesions (chronic hand eczema) may develop, forming **scaly, lichenified plaques oozing secondary bacterial infection** (honey-crusted skin), which can readily develop into **painful fissures** (Figure 2.24).
- Dyshidrotic and chronic lesions often coexist.
- **Nail dystrophy** may occur if the nail matrix (root) and nail fold become involved.

CLINICAL MANIFESTATIONS

- **Pruritus**
- **Painful fissures**
- **Patients often suffer social embarrassment.**

DIAGNOSIS

is usually made on clinical grounds or when other causes (see Differential Diagnosis) are ruled out.

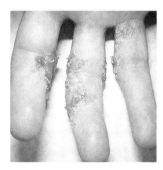

Figure 2.23.
Oozing, honey-colored, impetiginized crusts.

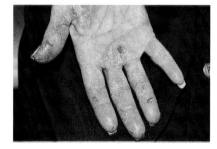

Figure 2.24.
Scaly lichenified plaques and painful fissures.

DIFFERENTIAL DIAGNOSIS

- **Contact dermatitis** is a consideration, particularly if the eruption is on the dorsa of the hands and/or feet and especially if there is a history of exposure to a suspected contactant (Figure 2.25).
- **Fungal infection,** such as tinea manum or tinea pedis, or an **id reaction** can be ruled out by KOH preparation or fungal culture.
- Well-demarcated scaly plaques on the palms (usually on one palm only) and soles suggest tinea manum or pedis, especially if there is other evidence of fungal infection, such as onychomycosis (Figure 2.26).
- **Psoriasis** or pustular psoriasis of the palms and soles may sometimes be indistinguishable from eczema (Figure 2.27).
- **Scabies** should be considered if there is an acute vesicular eruption in the web spaces of the fingers.

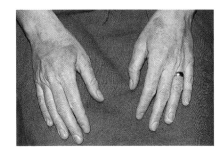

Figure 2.25.
Contact dermatitis on the dorsa of the hands.

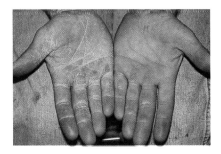

Figure 2.26.
Tinea manum. Well demarcated plaque on **one** palm.

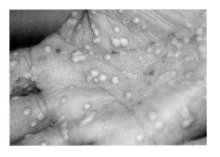

Figure 2.27.
Pustular psoriasis. Note multiple pustules.

MANAGEMENT (see also Appendix 2)

Mild cases
can be managed by:
  - Mild cleansers or soap substitutes
- Use of protective cotton-lined gloves
- Fastidious hand protection; avoidance of irritants
- Burow's solution soaks for acute oozing lesions
- Medium-potency topical steroids (e.g., triamcinolone 0.1%), with or without occlusion
- Higher-potency topical steroids (e.g., fluocinonide 0.05%), as necessary
- Lower-strength topical steroids (e.g., hydrocortisone valerate 0.2%) for long-term maintenance

Severe cases
are often difficult to manage. Treatment includes:
- Potent topical steroids under occlusion; superpotent topical steroids
- Systemic antibiotics for obvious or suspected secondary infection
- Systemic steroids used **very infrequently** for very severe flares
- Other measures, such as oral and topical psoralen plus ultraviolet A (PUVA) and oral cyclosporine, have been tried with varying degrees of improvement

---

 POINT TO REMEMBER

In stubborn, persistent cases of hand eczema, an attempt to rule out an outside cause, such as a contact dermatitis or fungal infection, should be made.

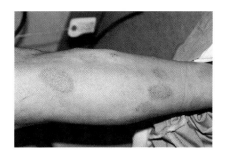

Figure 2.28.
Round (coin-shaped) eczematous patches and plaques.

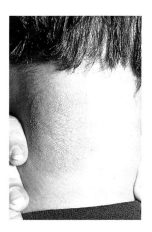

Figure 2.29.
Focal lichenified plaque.

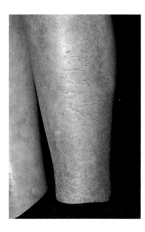

Figure 2.30.
Asteatotic eczema resembles a cracked antique vase.

BASICS

Nummular eczema, lichen simplex chronicus, and asteatotic eczema are all variants of ED. Each is more commonly noted in patients who have an atopic history; however, an atopic history is often lacking.

Nummular eczema
Description of lesions.
Round (coin-shaped) eczematous patches and plaques occur in clusters. (Figure 2.28).

Distribution of lesions
- Lesions occur mainly on legs, particularly in men.
- Nummular eczemalike lesions are sometimes seen in patients with childhood AD.

Diagnosis
- Diagnosis is made on the basis of clinical criteria.
- KOH is negative.

Differential diagnosis
- Frequently misdiagnosed as "ringworm" (tinea corporis)
- Psoriasis

Lichen simplex chronicus
Lichen simplex chronicus (also known as **neurodermatitis**; Figure 2.29) is a pruritic eruption. The lichenification is the result of repetitive rubbing and scratching. It is seen most commonly in adults.

Description of lesions
Plaques are focal and lichenified.

Distribution of lesions
- Nape of the neck
- Ankles, pretibial area
- Inner thighs
- Scrotum, vulva, anogenital area
- Wrists

Diagnosis
The lesions are easily diagnosed on clinical grounds (i.e., lichenification).

Differential diagnosis
- Psoriasis
- Cutaneous amyloidosis

Asteatotic eczema
- Asteatotic eczema is also known as winter eczema, or erythema craquelé (Figure 2.30).
- This is a common, often pruritic dermatitis, which appears in dry, cold winter months.
- It occurs exclusively in adults.

Description of lesions
Scaly patches with superficial fissures resemble a cracked, antique, porcelain vase.

Distribution of lesions
Asteatotic eczema is located most commonly on the shins, arms, hands, and trunk.

Diagnosis
is made on clinical grounds.

Differential diagnosis
- Xerosis (dry skin)
- Nummular eczema

MANAGEMENT

Lichen simplex chronicus and nummular eczema
- High-potency topical steroids; topical steroids under occlusion
- Lower-strength topical steroids used in intertriginous areas. If necessary, a dilute concentration of a corticosteroid such as Kenalog (triamcinolone acetonide) 2.0 to 4.0 mg/cc may be injected directly into the lesion (intradermally) using a very fine guage (#30) needle.

Asteatotic eczema
- Less frequent bathing
- Moisturizers, particularly Lac-Hydrin 12% Lotion
- Moderate-strength topical steroids

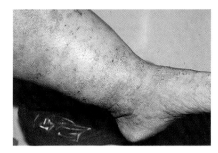

Figure 2.31.
Early-stage stasis dermatitis (SD).

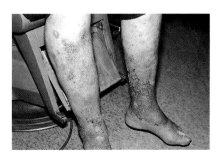

Figure 2.32.
Marked erythema, erosions, crusts, and secondary bacterial infection.

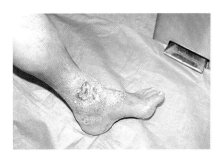

Figure 2.33.
Venous stasis ulcer.

BASICS

- Stasis dermatitis (SD) is an eczematous eruption that is located on the lower legs, particularly on the medial ankles of older patients. It is a consequence of chronic venous insufficiency ("leaky valves") and is seen more often in people with a genetic predisposition to develop varicosities.
- The following sequence of events leads to SD: varicose veins→incompetent valves→diminished venous return→increased capillary pressure→peripheral edema and relative hypoxia, which may account for the itching and the early stage of SD (Figure 2.31).

DESCRIPTION OF LESIONS

- An eczematous rash may become subacute with:
  - **Marked erythema**, erosions, crusts, and secondary bacterial infection (impetiginization; Figure 2.32), which may possibly lead to:
  - **Autoeczematization** (an idlike reaction), which is a widespread, often explosive, acute eczematous eruption presumably triggered by the secondary bacterial infection, with resulting circulating immune complexes released from the site of SD
- Features of the later stages are:
  - **Pigmentary changes** caused by extravasated red blood cells, reddish-brown coloration (because of hemosiderin), and postinflammatory hyperpigmentation (because of melanin). These colors may overlie a cyanotic background.
  - Thickened fibrotic skin (so-called lipodermatosclerosis)
  - Venous stasis ulcers, which are generally painless and can occur as a result of trauma, bacterial infection, and improper care of SD (Figure 2.33)

DISTRIBUTION OF LESIONS

SD most commonly occurs on the medial malleolus.

CLINICAL MANIFESTATIONS

- SD is pruritic and generally painless.
- There is accompanying ankle edema.
- The eruption may ulcerate and become painful.

DIFFERENTIAL DIAGNOSIS

- Typical SD is generally simple to diagnose but often is confused with **cellulitis.**
- Ulceration, particularly painful ulceration, if present, should point to other possible causes, such as **arterial disease**, **skin cancer**, and **pyoderma gangrenosum.**

MANAGEMENT

- **Help increase venous return** by:
  - Leg elevation above the level of the heart (sitting with the affected leg elevated on a stool is inadequate)
  - Ace elastic bandages and compression (Jobst-type) stockings, if there is significant edema
  - Vascular surgery, if feasible
- The **rash** should be carefully managed by:
  - Burow's solution soaks to help dry oozing and infected areas, if present
  - A mild-to-moderate–strength topical steroid (desonide 0.05% or hydrocortisone valerate applied twice daily), which is usually sufficient to treat the eczematous rash, especially if it is itching

- Long-term use of potent topical steroids, which may promote the development of atrophy, should be avoided.
- Over-the-counter preparations that contain benzocaine, lanolin, and neomycin should be avoided because patients with SD tend to easily develop contact dermatitis from these agents.
- A widespread **autoeczematized eruption** may require treatment with systemic steroids and oral antibiotics.
- Stasis ulcers are managed by measures such as: control of the underlying dermatitis, weight control, prevention of infection, compression dressings, Unna's boot, and corrective surgery, including skin grafts.

POINTS TO REMEMBER

- SD, which is generally neither warm, tender, nor painful, is often misdiagnosed as cellulitis.
- Infected SD should be considered as a cause for the sudden onset of an extensive generalized ED (autoeczematization).

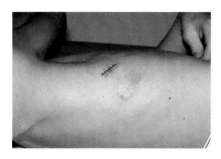

Figure 2.34.
Irritant reaction from a Band-Aid.

BASICS

There are two types of contact dermatitis.

Irritant contact dermatitis

Irritant contact dermatitis has a **nonallergic cause**. It is an erythematous, scaly, sometimes eczematous eruption, which is a reaction from rubbing, friction, maceration, exposure to a chemical, or thermal injury. The reaction:

- Is dependent on the concentration of the irritant
- Is dependent on the duration of exposure
- May occur in anyone
- Is confined only to areas of exposure (e.g., diaper rash, dishpan hands, irritation under adhesive dressing; Figure 2.34)

Allergic contact dermatitis (ACD)

- ACD is an ED caused by an allergen (antigen) that produces a delayed-type (type IV) hypersensitivity reaction.
  - It occurs only in sensitized individuals.
  - It is not dose dependent and may spread extensively beyond the site of original contact.
  - The eruption often gives clues to the contactant, suggesting an "outside job."
  - ACD is seen less commonly in young children, the elderly, and dark-skinned individuals.
- The most well-known example of ACD is **rhus dermatitis.**

RHUS DERMATITIS

BASICS

- **Poison ivy** and **poison oak** are the principal causes of rhus dermatitis in the United States. Poison oak is more commonly found in the western United States; poison ivy is found throughout the country.
- **Poison sumac** is found only in woody, swampy areas.
- The rash typically occurs 2 days after contact with the plant, but initial reactions have been noted within 12 hours and as long as 1 week after contact.
- Poison ivy, poison oak, and poison sumac all belong to the genus *Toxicodendron*, which comprises the poisonous species of the genus *Rhus.*
  - Each contains the sensitizing allergen pentadecylcatechol, which is found in the resinous oil (urushiol) of the plant. In addition to direct contact with the plant, the invisible oil may reach the skin via garden tools, the fur of pets, and the smoke of a burning plant.
  - Similar antigens are found in the resin of the Japanese lacquer tree, cashew nut shells, the dye of the India marking nut (used as a clothing dye in India), and the skin of mangoes. All cause similar skin rashes.
- Rhus dermatitis occurs mainly in the spring and summer in the eastern United States. In the western United States, where outdoor activity is prevalent all year, it may occur at any time.
- Approximately 85% of the population will develop a reaction if exposed to the plant.

DESCRIPTION OF LESIONS

Linear streaks of papules, vesicles, and blisters that appear to be artificial or look like an "outside job" (Figure 2.35)

DISTRIBUTION OF LESIONS

- **Exposed areas** of the body generally are affected first. Rhus dermatitis later spreads to other areas (e.g., the penis) that come in contact with the plant oil.
- Further dissemination, or **autoeczematization**, may occur within 5 to 7 days after the **initial exposure**. It is believed to occur through hematogenous, immune-complex deposition in the skin.

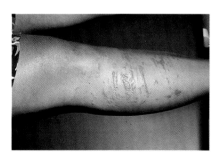

Figure 2.35.
Poison ivy. Linear streaks of papules and vesicles.

CLINICAL MANIFESTATIONS

- The rash is intensely pruritic.
- Contrary to common belief, the fluid in the blisters cannot transfer the rash to others, nor can it cause the rash to spread.
- The rash may last for 3 weeks or more.

DIAGNOSIS

- Diagnosis is based on a history of exposure.
- The distribution pattern should be suggestive of rhus dermatitis.

DIFFERENTIAL DIAGNOSIS

Scabies

- Other family members have itching.
- Distribution of lesions include the finger webs, flexor wrists, genitals, and axillae.

Contact dermatitis other than that of rhus dermatitis

MANAGEMENT

(see also Appendix 2)

Limited eruption and mild itching
may be relieved by:

- Cool showers and/or the frequent application of a water-tight plastic package of frozen peas, which prevents melting water from getting on the skin and also tends to conform to the shape of the area being treated
- Cool baths with Aveeno (colloidal oatmeal)
- Calamine lotion
- Cool compresses of Burow's solution to help dry vesicles and bullae
- Potent or super-potent topical steroids, such as clobetasol cream
- Oral antihistamines, particularly at bedtime

Widespread eruption and marked pruritus,
which may occur 5 to 7 days after exposure, may require in addition to topical steroids:

- Systemic steroids (see also Appendix 2) (usually prednisone) are administered in a tapering dosage schedule, usually starting at 1 mg/kg and decreasing by 5 mg every 2 days for at least 2 weeks and as long as 3 weeks. The dosage may be "bumped" upwards if flares occur during the tapering regimen. Medrol Dosepaks generally do not provide enough days of treatment for most cases of severe rhus dermatitis.
  - Tablets should be taken with meals.
  - Tablets may be taken once, instead of twice, daily.
  - There are advantages to consistently prescribing 5-mg-sized tablets. It is easier for the patient and the health care provide to keep track of the dosage schedule, and tablets usually do not have to be broken in half to decrease the dosage.
- Intramuscular steroids (Kenalog or Aristocort, 40 mg intramuscularly) are used if the patient has gastrointestinal intolerance to oral corticosteroids.

Side effects
possible with short-term systemic steroids include:

- Gastrointestinal upset
- Mood changes: hyperactivity, anxiety, or, possibly, depression
- Sleep disturbances

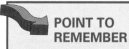

POINT TO REMEMBER

In treating severe poison ivy, it is important to continue prednisone for 2 to 3 weeks because a shorter course may be associated with a rebound dermatitis.

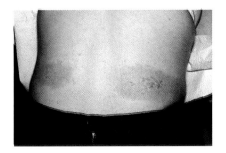

Figure 2.36.
Contact dermatitis caused by rubber elastic waistband. Note sparing at site where garment does not constantly touch skin.

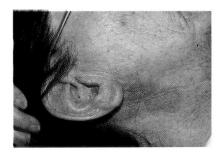

Figure 2.37.
Contact dermatitis secondary to hair dye. Note that the eruption involves the drip area and spares the scalp.

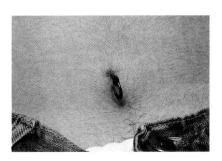

Figure 2.38.
Irritant contact dermatitis as a result of nickel in earring.

ACD OTHER THAN RHUS DERMATITIS

The characteristic patterns of distribution and the shapes of the rash may be clues to the specific allergen.

- **Dermatitis may be caused by the rubber of underpants** (Figure 2.36).
- **Dermatitis may be caused by hair dye** (Figure 2.37).
- **Latex allergy** is an occupational hazard that has recently been noted with increasing frequency in health care workers. Consequences may be serious with a urticarial type of contact dermatitis and, possibly, the following systemic symptoms may occur: shortness of breath, wheezing, and potentially fatal anaphylaxis.
- **Nickel ACD** has been common in women because the metal nickel is found in costume jewelry. An increase in its prevalence may be expected as a result of the popularity of body piercing in men and women (Figure 2.38).

DIAGNOSIS

- The patient should be questioned regarding daily habits and occupational exposures to reveal any possible contactants.
- Patch testing (see Chapter 27, "Highly Specialized Procedures") is a method used in identifying specific causative agents in patients with a history suggestive of ACD.

DIFFERENTIAL DIAGNOSIS

- Irritant dermatitis
- Other types of acute and chronic ED
- Drug reactions

DESCRIPTION OF LESIONS

Lesions may be an obvious "outside job" by virtue of shape, location, and the patient history; however, they may appear identical to the rash of acute or chronic ED.

DISTRIBUTION OF LESIONS

depends on the area of exposure; for example, an airborne contact dermatitis would involve exposed areas, especially the face.

MANAGEMENT

- Identifying and removing the inciting agent
- Educating the patient to avoid the inciting agent
- Treatment with topical and systemic steroids, if necessary

CHAPTER 3

OCCUPATIONAL SKIN DISEASE

Steven R. Cohen

Occupational Skin Disease

BASICS

- An occupational skin disease is a cutaneous disorder caused by, or otherwise expressed as the result of, factors associated primarily with the workplace.
- Three criteria may be used to define occupational dermatoses. Two of these criteria need to be positive before ascribing the problem to occupational factors.
  - The skin disorder should have developed for the first time while the worker was on a job putatively associated with the eruption.
  - The skin disorder should clearly improve when the patient is away from the work environment and/or flare while on the job.
  - There should be a plausible etiologic agent in the workplace that can be linked to the expression of the disease process.

CAUSES

In order of frequency, the direct causes of occupational dermatoses are classified as chemical, mechanical, physical, and biological in nature.

Chemical exposures
Irritants and allergens
- **Contact dermatitis** is an inflammatory condition caused by direct exposure of skin to an offending chemical.
- The term **irritant contact dermatitis** is used when the causative chemical injures the skin directly (Figure 3.1).
- Irritant chemicals include mild soaps, detergents, and solvents, which damage the skin by repeated contact (Figure 3.2), and strong alkalis and acids, which can produce blisters and ulcers after a single exposure.
- **Allergic contact dermatitis** represents a specific immunologic reaction to the etiologic chemical. The most common allergens are nickel, thimerosal (a mercurial preservative), neomycin (an antibiotic), formaldehyde, paraphenylenediamine (hair dye; Figure 3.3), and quaternium-15 (a preservative often found in cosmetics).
- A subclass of these disorders requires the presence of ultraviolet light in addition to a chemical to produce a photocontact reaction.
  - **Phototoxic reactions** are caused by direct injury to the skin (e.g., tar/pitch plus sunlight can cause injury to roofers).
  - **Photoallergic or photosensitivity reactions** depend on a worker's immunologic status (e.g., exposure to salicylanilide through the manufacture of soap plus ultraviolet exposure can adversely affect the immunocompromised).

Acnegenic agents
- **Oil acne and folliculitis** are disorders caused by mechanical blockage of the hair follicle openings by oil, which produces comedones (blackheads) and perifollicular inflammation. Chemicals that frequently provoke acne in the workplace include the insoluble cutting oils (used in metalworking operations), crude petroleum, heavy coal tar distillates (e.g., pitch, creosote), vegetable oils, and animal fat.

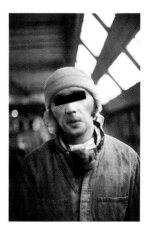

Figure 3.1.
Paint-spray operator with contaminated skin responsible for chronic facial dermatitis. Note how a respirator shields areas around mouth and nose.

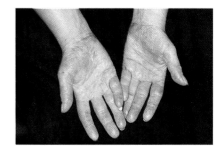

Figure 3.2.
Irritant contact dermatitis caused by unprotected exposure to soaps, detergents, waxes, and other household products.

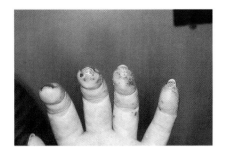

Figure 3.3.
Allergic contact dermatitis to para-phenylenediamine on fingertips of a beautician.

- **Chloracne**. Halogenated aromatic hydrocarbons, such as dibenzofurans and dioxins, cause severe cystic acne and systemic toxicity, including endocrine disturbances (loss of libido), liver toxicity (hepatitis and acute yellow atrophy), and neurologic disorders (neuritis and anxiety).

Pigment cell toxins and chemical stains

- **Staining of skin and appendages**. Chemical staining of the skin and/or hair occurs from the action of dyes (aniline: yellow; pitch: black; copper: green), which bind to keratin in the stratum corneum or hair cortex, or from the deposition of metallic substances in the dermis (tattooing).
- **Hyperpigmentation**. Increased pigmentation may result from local or systemic factors.
  - Local hyperpigmentation can be induced by a toxin that stimulates the proliferation of pigment cells (melanocytes) or by increased pigment production (melanin).
  - When systemic exposures to lead, silver, arsenic, and halogenated hydrocarbons are prolonged, hyperpigmentation is likely to develop (Figure 3.4).
- **Hypopigmentation (leukoderma)**
  - Some chemicals (hydroquinone, phenol, and catechol derivatives) induce hypopigmentation by interfering with the biochemical pathways for melanin formation or through a specific action on melanocytes or both.
  - Leukoderma is the preferred term for vitiligo caused by occupational toxins, but the terms are otherwise synonymous (Figure 3.5).

Carcinogens

- **Pitch keratoses; keratoacanthoma; basal/ squamous cell carcinoma**
  - Workers exposed to carbon black (soot), coal tar, pitch, tarry products, creosote oil, anthracene, and oil fractionation and distillation products are at increased risk for developing premalignant conditions (pitch/ tar warts) and a variety of skin cancers (squamous cell carcinoma/basal cell carcinoma).
  - Arsenic causes a wide range of toxic cutaneous effects, including hyperpigmentation, Bowen's disease, and squamous cell carcinoma.

Mechanical trauma

Friction/ pressure/pounding/penetration

- It is likely that mechanical trauma induces a continuum of skin-response patterns, including **calluses, fissures, hemorrhage, lichenification, blisters, granulomas, tattoo,** and **acne mechanica** as well as induction of **a foreign body reaction.**
- The trauma associated with particular occupations often gives rise to characteristic stigmata ("badge of the trade"). Examples include the hemorrhage from chronic pounding, which develops on the heels of athletes (**talon noir**), the telltale callous on the chin of a violinist, and the nail changes related to the repetitive trauma of laying floors, meat packing, and paint scraping (Figure 3.6).

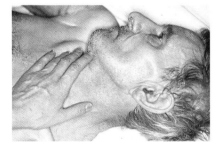

Figure 3.4.
Generalized slate-gray hyperpigmentation of argyria associated with work in a silver-plating operation for 18 years.

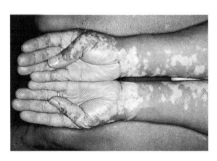

Figure 3.5.
Hands of a maintenance worker for the New York Transit Authority who cleaned subway cars with a phenolic germicide for 3 to 4 years before developing florid leukoderma (vitiligo) on the hands, palms, and volar aspect of the wrists. The condition gradually became generalized.

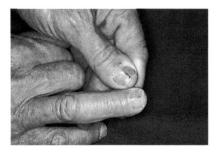

Figure 3.6.
Scraper's nails show a median dystrophy caused by repeated occupational trauma from a paint scraping tool.

Vibration

- **Raynaud's phenomenon** is a well-recognized sequela of exposure to vibrating tools (also known as **dead hand syndrome** and **white finger disease**).
- The full constellation of this syndrome (**vibration syndrome)** also includes hearing loss, musculoskeletal symptoms (neck and elbow pain, shoulder stiffness, and lumbago), and psychosensory symptoms (headaches, sleep disturbances, forgetfulness, irritability, and depression).

Physical factors

Heat

- **Erythema ab igne.** Although the most obvious consequence of local cutaneous exposure to heat is a direct burn, a less toxic variant of proximate heat exposure is the peculiar hyperpigmentation of erythema ab igne.
- **Miliaria.** Another obvious manifestation of working in a hot environment is excessive perspiration (hyperhidrosis), which may be associated with miliaria

Cold

- **Chilblains.** The persistently cold, damp environment associated with work in a refrigerated atmosphere may cause the blue, red, boggy swellings on the acral regions of the face, ears, hands, and feet known as chilblains. Street and sewer cleaners and excavation and scullery workers are typically required to stand for long periods in mud or water (Figure 3.7).
- **Immersion foot** is the term used to describe a nonfreezing injury to the tissues.
- True freezing, or **frostbite**, injury develops as a result of ice crystal formation in the tissues.

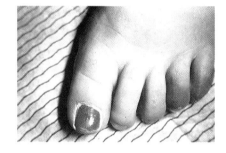

Figure 3.7.
Chilblains presented as painful swelling affecting the fourth and fifth toes of a meat packer working in a low-temperature environment.

Nonionizing and ionizing radiation

- **Ultraviolet injury** (sunburn, actinic elastosis, actinic keratosis, basal/squamous cell carcinoma). Acute and cumulative ultraviolet injury to the skin of outdoor workers is relatively common. Light-skinned individuals are at much greater risk for accelerated cutaneous aging and developing premalignant and malignant lesions.
- **Radiation injury** (radiodermatitis, atypical keratosis, squamous cell carcinoma; Figure 3.8).
  - X-rays are a prototype for ionizing radiation injury. The carcinogenic effects of x-rays follow nonlethal mutations of DNA, but clearly other factors are operative in the expression of skin cancer during a latent period, which may vary in length from 4 to 40 years.
  - Beyond the more high-risk occupational environments, such as mining, x-ray equipment manufacture, and many health care settings, the industrial applications of ionizing radiation have expanded in recent years to include food sterilization, fire alarm manufacture, curing of plastics, and the manufacture of fabricated metals, among many others.

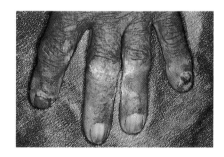

Figure 3.8.
Radiation injury affecting the hands of a radiologist with many years of unprotected exposure to fluoroscopy equipment. Premalignant radiation keratoses are present on the dorsa of the fingers. An infiltrating squamous cell carcinoma of the index finger nail bed has resulted in complete destruction of the plate.

Biological agents

Infectious diseases/infestations

Some of the wide-ranging bacterial, fungal, viral, and arthropod diseases encountered in the workplace include the following:

- **Brucellosis** is most often seen in veterinarians and abattoir workers in the meat-packing industry.
- Cutaneous **anthrax** is seen in people whose work involves imported animal products, particularly those who work in wool factories. "Woolsorters' disease" may result when spores are inhaled.
- **Leptospirosis** may occur in farmers, hunters, and abattoir workers.
- **Tularemia** may occur in hunters.
- **Milker's nodules** (paravaccinia) are seen in milkers and stockyard and slaughterhouse workers.
- **Orf** is seen in sheepherders.
- **Erysipeloid** occurs in fishermen, meat handlers, and people whose work involves meat by-products.
- **Grain itch** (a pruritic eruption caused by a mite) affects people in contact with grain or straw, and **fowl mite dermatitis** affects workers caring for pigeons or chickens.
- **Moth infestation** and **chigger** and **other bites** occur in endemic areas in people who work outdoors.

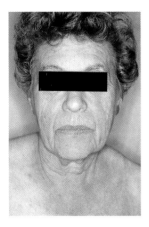

Figure 3.9.
Chrysanthemum dermatitis affecting exposed facial skin, neck, and "V" of the chest in a florist. The eruption flared most severely during the blooming season in autumn.

- **Creeping eruption** (e.g., cutaneous larva migrans) may affect farmers and gardeners.
- **Fungal infections** are seen in people whose occupations expose them to heat and moisture (e.g., soldiers in tropical areas, athletes).

Plants and plant products
- Various plants, including their leaves, bulbs, flowers, vegetables, fruit, natural resins, and woods, are capable of producing occupational sensitization.
- Biological agents that typically wreak havoc among outdoor workers are poison ivy and poison oak, primula, ragweed oil, chrysanthemum, and many species of wood. Vegetable or fruit dermatitis also affects those employed outdoors (Figure 3.9).

CHAPTER 4

PSORIASIS

The emotional toll and the personal struggle to come to terms with psoriasis is expressed in an autobiographical short story "At War with My Skin," by John Updike, who has severe psoriasis. After breaking his leg and having to undergo an operation, Updike reflects, "I chiefly remember amid my pain and helplessness being pleased that my shins, at that time, were clear and I would not offend the surgeon."

Psoriasis, General Principles

BASICS

- Psoriasis is characterized by thickened and reddened, silvery, or whitish **scaly patches** or plaques of skin, ranging from only a few small asymptomatic lesions, to larger plaques that cover extensive areas of the body, to a generalized exfoliative erythroderma. Approximately 5 to 10% of affected individuals may also develop a **psoriatic arthritis**, which may precede or follow the onset of psoriasis.
- Psoriasis is a chronic skin condition of unknown cause; however, immunologic factors have been recently shown to play an important role in its pathogenesis. Approximately 30% of patients with psoriasis have a family history of the disease.
- One to two percent of the world population is affected, and West Africans, African Americans, Native Americans, and Asians are affected to a much lesser extent than other populations. Distribution is equal between males and females. Psoriasis most frequently begins in the **second or third decade of life**; however, it can first appear in infancy or in old age.
- Most current therapies—topical corticosteroids, phototherapy, photochemotherapy, methotrexate, and cyclosporine—are directed at the **suppression of T cells.**

DESCRIPTION OF LESIONS

The classic lesion of psoriasis is the **well-demarcated, erythematous papule or plaque surmounted by a silvery (micaceous) or whitish scale** (Figures 4.1 to 4.4).

DISTRIBUTION OF LESIONS

- Psoriasis tends to be remarkably **symmetrical.** It tends to spare the face, and it is most commonly located on the:
  - Large **extensor joints** (i.e., elbows, knees, and knuckles)

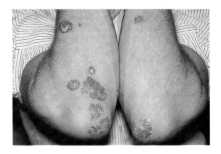

Figure 4.1.
Typical erythematous, well-demarcated plaques in psoriasis.

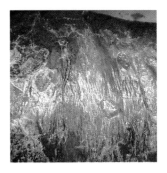

Figure 4.2.
Micaceous scale in psoriasis.

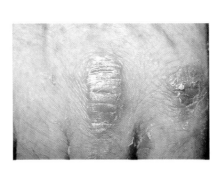

Figure 4.3.
Well-demarcated plaques over joints in psoriasis.

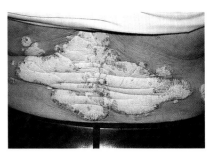

Figure 4.4.
Thick white plaques of psoriasis.

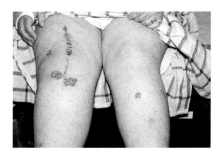

Figure 4.5.
Köebner phenomenon. Linear plaque localized to surgical scar.

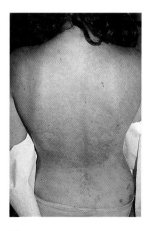

Figure 4.6.
Köebner phenomenon localized to area of sunburn.

- **Anogenital area** (i.e., perineal and perianal areas and the glans penis)
- **Palms and soles**
- **Intertriginous areas** (i.e., axillae, perineal and perianal areas, and the inguinal creases); referred to as **inverse psoriasis**
- **Trunk**, where lesions may be guttate (small, teardrop) or larger plaques
- **Scalp and ears**; when only involving the scalp and retroauricular areas, sometimes referred to as **sebopsoriasis**
- **Nails**, and often is a cause of nail deformity
- Psoriasis can also occur as **generalized, disseminated plaques.**

CLINICAL MANIFESTATIONS

- **Pruritus.** Psoriasis generally is asymptomatic but can become pruritic and uncomfortable, particularly during acute flare-ups or when it involves the scalp or intertriginous regions. It also can cause pain, functional impairment, and embarrassment when it involves the palms or soles.
- **Köebner phenomenon, or isomorphic response.** Psoriatic lesions can appear to "spread" or crop up in apparently normal areas of the skin that are traumatized by such noxious stimuli as a sunburn or by scratching and rubbing (Figures 4.5 and 4.6).

DRUGS EXACERBATING PSORIASIS

The listed drugs have been reported to worsen psoriasis; however, preexisting psoriasis is not necessarily a contraindication to their use.
- Antimalarials
- β-Blocking agents
- Systemic interferon
- Lithium carbonate
- Alcohol (abuse)
- Rapid tapering of systemic corticosteroids

DIAGNOSIS

Diagnosis is made most often on clinical grounds; however, a skin biopsy or fungal studies may be performed to rule in or rule out other possible diagnoses.

DIFFERENTIAL DIAGNOSIS

Differential diagnosis varies depending on the location and the type of psoriasis; however, in a broader sense, psoriasis most often has to be differentiated from:
- Eczematous dermatitis, which may be indistinguishable from psoriasis (e.g., lichen simplex chronicus)
- Fungal infections (e.g., tinea pedis, candidal intertrigo)
- Seborrheic dermatitis, which also may be indistinguishable from psoriasis
- Various types of parapsoriasis, whose name derives from their resemblance to psoriasis

MANAGEMENT

(See "General Principles of Topical Therapy".) Mild to relatively moderate psoriasis can be treated by primary care providers with topical steroids, topical vitamin D preparations, and tar preparations; moderate to severe psoriasis is best managed by dermatologists. **Treatment is aimed at decreasing size and thickness of plaques, relieving pruritus, and improving emotional well-being;** however, the measure of successful treatment of this chronic and unpredictable condition is often subjective and different for each patient. The health care provider should try to understand the patient's goals and help the patient to have realistic expectations.
- **Occlusive therapy** increases the potency of topical steroids. Usually, a medium-potency agent is applied and then covered with plastic wrap for several hours or overnight, if tolerated.

- **Rotational therapy/pulse therapy.** The many treatment options available, with new ones on the horizon, have generated an innovative approach to management, which consists of cycling, or rotating, the different treatment modalities. Cumulative side effects and drug tolerance (tachyphylaxis) are decreased, and often lower dosages and shorter durations of therapy in the use of each drug are possible.
- **Combination therapy.** For example, **RePUVA** combines an oral retinoid, or acitretin, with the photochemotherapy of psoralen and ultraviolet A (PUVA; Re = retinoid). By using RePUVA, it is possible to lower the dosage of both modalities and achieve better clinical responses in many patients.

NEW AGENTS IN THE TREATMENT OF PSORIASIS

- **Tazarotene** is the **first topical retinoid developed for psoriasis**.
  - Tazarotene is formulated in a gel at 0.1 and 0.05% concentrations. Psoriasis cleared with tazarotene appears to remain in remission longer than psoriasis treated with topical steroids alone. In some cases, the psoriasis has continued improvement even though the tazarotene has been stopped.
  - Tazarotene is often irritating. Topical steroids are often prescribed to counter this side effect, which allows the use of tazarotene to be continued.
- **Neoral** is a form of **cyclosporine** that offers all the advantages of the more common formulation, **Sandimmune,** with one major advantage: It is much more readily and reliably absorbed by the body than its older counterpart.
- **Calcipotriene solution** is designed specifically for scalp use.
- **Soriatane** (acitretin) is a new oral retinoid preparation.

CLINICAL PRESENTATIONS

The clinical variations of psoriasis listed here comprise a somewhat artificial classification, which is determined by the characteristics or morphology of the predominant type of lesion and its distribution. There may be combinations of different types in a given individual. Because each type is managed differently to a degree and because each has its own differential diagnosis, each will be discussed separately. Please refer to the formulary on page 68 for more detailed information about the appropriate therapy and use of each drug.

- **Localized plaque psoriasis**
- **Generalized plaque psoriasis**, including **erythrodermic psoriasis (exfoliative dermatitis secondary to psoriasis)**
- **Psoriasis in children**
- **Inverse psoriasis (affecting the groin, perianal area, penis, axillae, and inframammary area)**
- **Psoriasis of the palms and soles, including pustular psoriasis**
- **Scalp psoriasis (sebopsoriasis)**
- **Psoriatic nails**
- **Psoriatic arthritis**

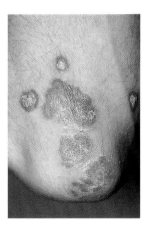

Figure 4.7.
Coin-shaped psoriasis.

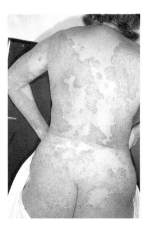

Figure 4.8.
Psoriasis. Primarily extensor distribution of well-demarcated large plaques.

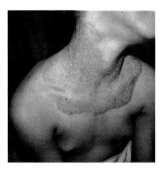

Figure 4.9.
Well-defined plaque with serpiginous border in psoriasis.

BASICS

- In its mildest manifestation, psoriasis is an incidental finding.
- The patient is frequently unaware or untroubled by the condition.

DISTRIBUTION OF LESIONS

Localized plaque psoriasis may remain limited and localized, or it may become unstable and widespread. (Figures 4.7 and 4.14 and figures 4.8 and 4.13.)

CLINICAL MANIFESTATIONS

Slightly erythematous scaly patches on the elbows or knees or nail pitting may be all that is observed.

DIAGNOSIS

- Well-demarcated whitish or silvery plaques in psoriasis-typical locations indicate the diagnosis.
- A family history of psoriasis can be helpful.
- Affected nails can be indicative.
- If necessary, a skin biopsy and fungal examination are performed to rule out other conditions.

DIFFERENTIAL DIAGNOSIS

- **Eczematous dermatitis/atopic dermatitis (atopic eczema).** There is often a history of atopy (eczema, asthma, hay fever, chronic sinusitis) in the patient or in close relatives. Flexural distribution (Figure 4.11) is seen more often than extensor distribution and is often symmetrical. Lichenification (exaggeration of normal skin markings) is the hallmark. The lesion is poorly demarcated (it blends into normal surrounding skin) and generally itches (crusts and excoriations may be seen). The skin biopsy may be "spongiotic" (ie, eczematous) or interpreted as "psoriasiform" or "psoriasiform eczematous dermatitis."
- **Nummular eczema** (Figure 4.10). There may be a history of atopy. Distribution is flexural or extensor and most often on the legs. Patches and plaques are coin-shaped. The lesions generally itch.
- **Tinea corporis** (Figure 4.12). The lesion is annular (ringlike; therefore clear in the center) (compare with Figure 4.9) and is KOH positive (potassium hydroxide mount) or there is a positive fungal culture. It usually itches.
- **Parapsoriasis** occurs as idiopathic multiple, barely elevated patches usually on the trunk and arms (similar to pityriasis rosea). There are small plaque variants. It is important to rule out mycosis fungoides from large plaque parapsoriasis.
- **Mycosis fungoides (cutaneous T-cell lymphoma;** Figure 4.15). Smudgy patches and plaques or tumors occur, particularly on the buttocks and the trunk. The lesions are often pruritic.
- **Bowen's disease (squamous cell carcinoma in situ;** Figure 4.16). The lesion is usually solitary and is a well-defined psoriasiform plaque. It is unresponsive to topical steroids.

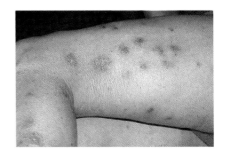

Figure 4.10.
Nummular eczema. Multiple coin-shaped eczematous plaques.

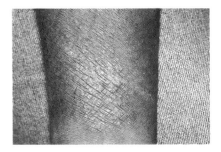

Figure 4.11.
Eczematous dermatitis (lichen simplex chronicus). Flexural distribution lichenified (note exaggeration of normal skin markings); poorly demarcated plaque.

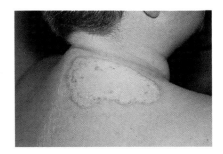

Figure 4.12.
Tinea corporis. Annular plaque; note central clearing.

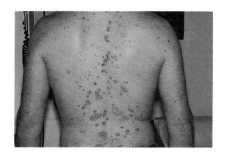

Figure 4.13.
Small papules and plaques in psoriasis.

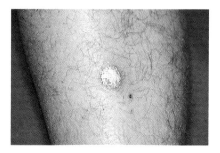

Figure 4.14.
Solitary plaque in psoriasis.

(See "General Principles of Topical Therapy".)

- **Topical steroids.** A superpotent topical steroid or a potent topical steroid under plastic occlusion is used for a limited period, followed by a less potent agent for maintenance.
  - **Advantages.** Therapy is good for short periods and has a rapid onset to decrease erythema, inflammation, and itching.
  - **Disadvantages.** Topical steroids are expensive. Tachyphylaxis often occurs. There is possible steroid rosacea, local atrophy, and telangiectasias. Hypothalamic–pituitary–adrenal suppression may occur if the drug is used incorrectly.
  - **Best bets**
    - **Rotational, or pulse, dosing** (e.g., 2 weeks use with 1 week off or weekends only using a moisturizer or topical calcipotriene on off days)
    - **Combination therapy** with other topical agents (e.g., calcipotriene may be used at bedtime and the topical steroid in the morning; after achieving control, the topical steroid is decreased, for example, to weekends only, and ultimately calcipotriene is used twice a day)
    - **Occlusive therapy** increases the potency of topical steroids. Generally, a medium-potency agent is applied and then is covered with plastic wrap for several hours or overnight, if tolerated. Cordran Tape is also very effective.
- **Intralesional steroids**
  - **Advantages.** Intralesional steroids are effective when the number of lesions is limited. They are fast acting, and the duration of remission is longer.
  - **Disadvantages.** These agents are painful, and local atrophy is possible. Office visits are necessary for injections.
  - **Best bets.** Intralesional steroids are most useful for cosmetically obvious lesions (e.g., on the dorsum of the hands) or for lesions that tend to be pruritic or difficult to treat, such as psoriatic plaques on the scalp.
- **Tar preparations**
  - **Advantages.** Tar preparations are less expensive than steroids and can be combined with topical steroids. Tar may be used before sunlight exposure or with ultraviolet B phototherapy.
  - **Disadvantages.** The onset of action is slow, and tar preparations are mildly effective.
- **Crude coal tar preparations** used alone or as an adjunct to ultraviolet therapy are messy, smelly, stain clothing and bed linen, and must be left on for long periods of time (from several hours to overnight). They also may be irritating and cause folliculitis.
  - Today, coal tars are more commonly used in psoriasis day-care centers.
  - Liquor carbonis detergens (LCD), Balnetar, and Doak Tar Oil are the least messy of the available preparations.

- **Anthralin**, a topical anthracene preparation, has been used to treat psoriasis since the nineteenth century. Anthralin is a coal tar derivative that evolved as an answer to many of the side effects of crude coal tar. It may be used for shorter periods of time (as short as 30 minutes), which is referred to as short-contact anthralin therapy (SCAT). This treatment has recently gained more popularity in Europe.
  - **Advantages**
    - There are none of the side effects of steroids.
    - The treatment is good for a limited number of lesions.
    - Remissions are longer.
    - No tolerance can build up.
    - Short-contact applications are available.
    - The treatment is less expensive than topical steroids.
  - **Disadvantages**
    - Skin irritation may occur. (Micanol Cream, 1% anthralin, is less irritating and causes less staining.)
    - There is generally a reversible brownish-purple staining of the skin.
    - It stains the bathtub.
    - The response to treatment is less predictable than with other forms of therapy.
    - Onset of action is slow.
    - It is difficult to apply.
  - **Best bets**
    - SCAT is the treatment method of choice when using anthralin.
    - Anthralin should be used when psoriasis is unresponsive to topical steroids.
    - Rotational therapy can be employed, alternating anthralin with topical steroids.
- **Calcipotriene** (Dovonex Ointment and Cream) is a vitamin D_3 preparation indicated for mild to moderate plaque psoriasis.
  - **Advantages.** The potency of calcipotriene is equivalent to that of betamethasone valerate. There is no tachyphylaxis.
  - **Disadvantages.** It is expensive. Onset of action is slower compared to other treatments. The agent is occasionally irritating, especially in intertriginous areas.
  - **Best bets.** Calcipotriene is effective alone for long-term maintenance therapy or may be used in rotational therapy with topical steroids.
- **Tazarotene**
  - **Advantages.** Longer remissions; no tachyphylaxis
  - **Disadvantage.** Expensive, irritating

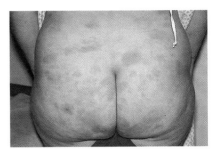

Figure 4.15.
Mycosis fungoides. "Smudgy," ill-defined, large plaques.

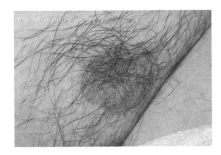

Figure 4.16.
Bowen's disease. Well-demarcated psoriasiform plaque.

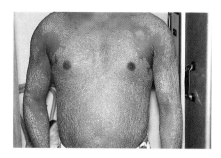

Figure 4.17.
Extensive psoriasis covering 80% of the body.

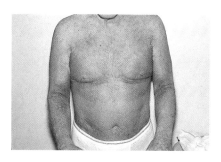

Figure 4.18.
Psoriasis. Exfoliative erythroderma.

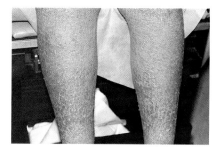

Figure 4.19.
Psoriasis. Exfoliation.

CLINICAL MANIFESTATIONS

- Psoriasis can flare quickly and unexpectedly, sometimes covering 20 to 80% of the body (Figure 4.17).
- **Exfoliative dermatitis (erythroderma;** Figures 4.18 and 4.19) is a term for the sudden or subacute appearance of generalized scaling and erythema, often with accompanying fever and chills. It **can be the presenting symptom of psoriasis** or a subsequent complication of generalized plaque psoriasis.
  - **Causes.** Some of the triggering factors that may lead to an exfoliative dermatitis in the psoriatic patient are:
    - Severe emotional stress
    - Precipitating illnesses such as severe infections
    - Major surgery
    - Withdrawal of systemic or superpotent topical steroids

MANAGEMENT

- The therapy used for more localized disease becomes less effective with generalized disease. It is also more expensive and more time-consuming and labor-intensive to administer. When available, the following measures may be tried in succession or, if necessary, in combination with one another.
  - Ultraviolet B phototherapy
  - PUVA
  - Methotrexate
  - Acetretin
  - Hydroxyurea
  - Cyclosporine
- **Management of exfoliative dermatitis (erythroderma)** ultimately may involve some of the measures used for generalized plaque psoriasis (e.g., ultraviolet therapy, oral agents) in addition to the following:
  - Bed rest
  - Cool compresses
  - Lubrication with emollients
  - Antipruritic therapy with oral antihistamines
  - Low to moderate strength topical steroids
  - Hospitalization in extreme cases

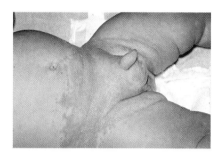

Figure 4.20.
Psoriasis.

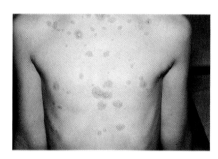

Figure 4.21.
Acute guttate psoriasis.

BASICS

- Infantile, or childhood, psoriasis deserves particular attention. It requires intensive educational guidance and counseling of the patient and family.
- In approximately 10 to 15% of patients, psoriasis begins before the age of 10 years. An early onset portends more severe disease, and there is often an associated family history of the disease.

CLINICAL MANIFESTATIONS

Psoriasis in infancy (Figure 4.20)
Clinical presentation
- In some infants, psoriasis begins as a diaper rash, which may be difficult to distinguish from:
  - Irritant dermatitis
  - Nonspecific diaper rash
  - Atopic dermatitis
  - Cutaneous candidiasis
- The rash may clear; however, the child later develops psoriasis.
- Conversely, psoriasis may present with typical plaques, such as those seen in adults.

Management
Many of the treatments that are used in adults, such as superpotent topical steroids, phototherapy, and natural sunlight, if available, are also used in children. All should be used with caution.

Acute guttate psoriasis (Figure 4.21)
Clinical presentation
- There is the sudden onset of multiple guttate (teardrop-shaped) lesions.
- This is often the initial presentation of psoriasis in children and young adults.
- Acute guttate psoriasis is occasionally preceded by group A β-hemolytic streptococcal pharyngitis.

DIFFERENTIAL DIAGNOSIS

- **Atopic dermatitis** (Figure 4.22)
- **Pityriasis rosea** (Figure 4.23)
  - Elliptical lesions with characteristic scale and typical distribution
  - Self-limiting
- **Drug eruption/viral exanthem**
  - Exanthematous
  - Self-limiting
- **Secondary syphilis**
  - Positive serology

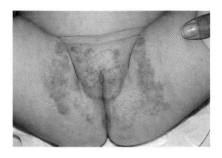

Figure 4.22.
Atopic dermatitis.

MANAGEMENT

- Low- to mid-potency topical steroids, used with caution
- SCAT
- Ultraviolet B phototherapy or natural sunlight exposure
- Appropriate antibiotic therapy (e.g., penicillin or erythromycin for group A β-hemolytic streptococcus)

POINT TO REMEMBER

Methotrexate and retinoids are generally avoided in children.

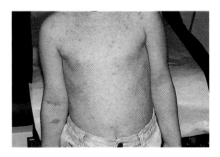

Figure 4.23.
Pityriasis rosea. Note herald patch on right forearm.

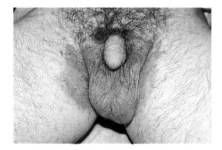

Figure 4.24.
Inverse psoriasis. Note involvement of scrotum.

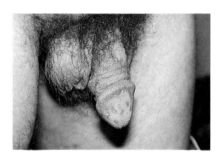

Figure 4.25.
Psoriasis of the penis. Note well-demarcated plaques.

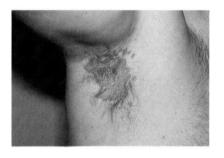

Figure 4.26.
Inverse psoriasis of the axilla.

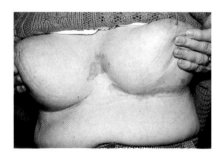

Figure 4.27.
Inverse psoriasis of the inframammary area.

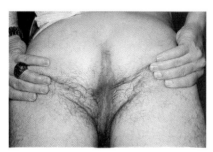

Figure 4.28.
Inverse psoriasis of the gluteal crease.

BASICS

- The well-demarcated erythematous plaques of psoriasis are generally devoid of scale when the condition occurs in a flexural distribution because of the friction and moisture of two apposed surfaces of skin rubbing together, such as occurs in the groin and axillae.
- Inverse psoriasis is a masquerader of many dermatoses.

DISTRIBUTION OF LESIONS

- **Inguinal area** (Figure 4.24)
  - Well-demarcated erythematous plaques
  - Typical scrotal involvement
- Glans penis (Figure 4.25)
- Axillae (Figure 4.26)
- Inframammary folds (Figure 4.27)
- Perianal area, gluteal fold (Figure 4.28)

CLINICAL MANIFESTATIONS

- Red, glistening, well-demarcated plaques without scale
- Fissures, which are often present in the groin and gluteal creases

DIAGNOSIS

The lesions are all KOH and fungal culture negative.

DIFFERENTIAL DIAGNOSIS

Inverse psoriasis is commonly misdiagnosed by non-dermatologists as candidiasis or "fungus" and treated accordingly.

- **Tinea cruris** (Figure 4.29)
  - KOH and fungal culture are positive for tinea.
  - Tinea has a "scalloped" shape.
  - The scrotum is usually spared.
- **Cutaneous candidiasis**
  - Cutaneous candidiasis is more common in diabetic and immune-compromised people (Figure 4.30).
  - Satellite pustules extend beyond the border of the plaque.
  - It is KOH positive for budding yeast, or culture is positive for the *Candida* genus.
  - Candidiasis typically is "beefy red" in color.
- **Contact dermatitis/irritant intertrigo of axilla and other flexor creases** is caused by contactants such as antiperspirants, or it occurs secondary to maceration and obesity.
- **Atopic dermatitis** has a positive atopic history.
- **Nonspecific balanitis**
  - Nonspecific balanitis is more common in middle-aged and elderly men.
  - Fissures can be noted.
  - Small plaques may be noted on the glans penis.
- **Candidal balanitis** (Figure 4.31)
  - "Beefy red" color is characteristic.
  - It is KOH positive for budding yeast, or culture is positive for the *Candida* genus.
- **Pruritus ani**

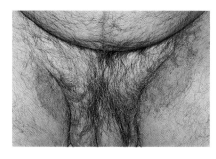

Figure 4.29.
Tinea cruris. Note scalloped border. Scrotum is spared.

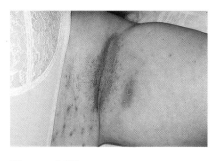

Figure 4.30.
Candidal infection of axilla in a diabetic patient. Note the "satellite" pustules.

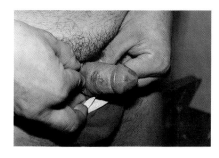

Figure 4.31.
Candidal balanitis in a diabetic patient.

MANAGEMENT

(See "General Principles of Topical Therapy".)
- **Low-potency, non-fluorinated topical steroids are used to avoid atrophy and striae.**
  - The lowest potency, such as Cortaid (over-the-counter hydrocortisone cream, 0.05 to 1%) or prescription desonide, 0.05%, should be used.
- Alternatively, Westcort Cream (0.2% hydrocortisone valerate) may be applied once or twice daily. It must be monitored regularly, and multiple refills are to be avoided.
- Treatment may begin with a higher potency steroid for several days to achieve rapid improvement, then followed by lower-potency agents.
- Dovonex Cream or **Ointment** may be used primarily, only if it is not irritating, or in rotation with a mild topical steroid.

POINTS TO REMEMBER

- Inverse psoriasis, by virtue of its location, cannot benefit from ultraviolet therapy.
- Intertriginous areas are moist and occluded; therefore, the penetration and efficacy of topical agents are increased.
- The occlusive effects of two skin surfaces in apposition means that more of the drug will be absorbed; therefore, **striae (linear atrophy)** secondary to potent topical steroids are more likely to occur in intertriginous areas.

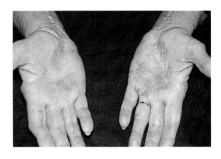

Figure 4.32.
Hyperkeratotic psoriasis of the palms. Symmetrical, well-defined plaques.

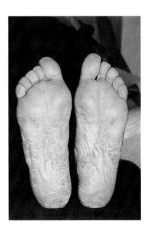

Figure 4.33.
Hyperkeratotic psoriasis of the soles. Symmetrical, well-defined plaques.

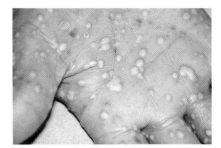

Figure 4.34.
Pustular psoriasis of the palm.

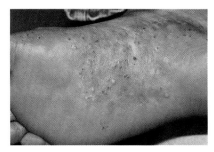

Figure 4.35.
Pustular psoriasis of the sole.

BASICS

Psoriasis of the palms and soles presents a difficult therapeutic challenge. The palms and/or soles alone may be affected, with no other evidence of psoriasis, or the condition may be part of more extensive psoriasis.

DESCRIPTION OF LESIONS

There are two variants:
- **Hyperkeratotic** (Figures 4.32 and 4.33)
  - The location of these lesions present additional problems to patients, such as pain, fissuring and bleeding, impairment of function, and embarrassment.
  - The plaques are well demarcated and scaly.
- **Pustular** (Figures 4.34 and 4.35)
  - The pustules are generally sterile.
  - The lesions favor the insteps of the feet, the heels, the thenar, or hypothenar eminences and the palms.
  - They are characteristically symmetrical.

DIFFERENTIAL DIAGNOSIS

- **Dyshidrotic eczema (eczematous dermatitis;** see Figures 4.36 and 4.38)
  - Tiny, so-called, "sago-grain" vesicles or large vesicles ("pompholyx") are characteristic (see Figure 4.38).
  - The patient often has a positive atopic history.
- **Tinea manum and pedis** (see Figure 4.37)
  - KOH and fungal culture are positive in tinea.
  - Tinea very often can involve two feet and only one hand (Figure 4.39); palm and sole psoriasis is generally symmetrical.
- **Contact dermatitis** occurs most often on the dorsum of the hands and feet.

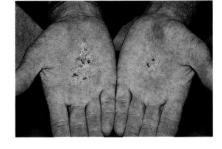

Figure 4.36.
Hand eczema. Note vesicles and crusts.

MANAGEMENT

(See "General Principles of Topical Therapy".)
- **Topical treatment is the first line of therapy.** Because the palms and soles present the greatest barrier to cutaneous penetration, the most potent topical steroids are used, even under occlusion.
  - Superpotent topical steroids, such as clobetasol propionate, initially without occlusion and subsequently with occlusion (under vinyl or rubber gloves), if necessary (this should be carefully monitored by the health-care provider)
  - **Anthralin,** overnight or SCAT
  - **Salicylic acid preparations** to remove scale, if necessary
  - **Emollients**
  - **Calcipotriene (Dovonex)** under vinyl or rubber gloves
  - **Topical retinoid (Tazorac)**
- When a patient is not responding to topical therapies, treatment options can include phototherapy and systemic treatments, such as:
  - **Systemic tetracycline/erythromycin** (for the antiinflammatory effect) to treat the pustular type of lesion
  - Oral or topical PUVA (ultraviolet B is not effective)
  - **Oral retinoids**
  - **RePUVA**
  - **Methotrexate**
  - **Cyclosporine**

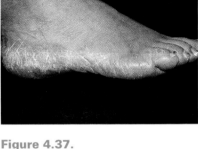

Figure 4.37.
Tinea pedis, "moccasin" type.

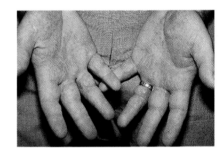

Figure 4.38.
Hand eczema. "Pompholyx"; note large vesicles.

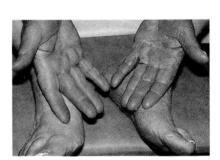

Figure 4.39.
Tinea manum, tinea pedis "two feet and only one hand" type.

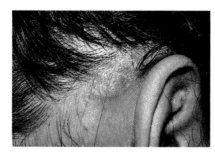

Figure 4.40.
Scalp psoriasis. Note well-demarcated plaque.

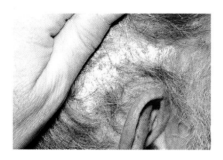

Figure 4.41.
Thick, armorlike plaque in scalp psoriasis.

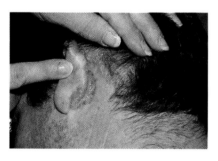

Figure 4.42.
Scalp psoriasis hidden behind the ears.

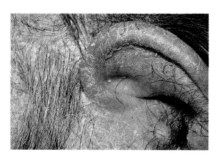

Figure 4.43.
Psoriasis involving ears and external ear canal.

BASICS

- Psoriasis may involve the scalp alone, or the scalp may be part of more extensive psoriasis.
- Pruritus and scratching may exacerbate the psoriasis **(Köebner phenomenon)**.
- When severe, it is particularly difficult to treat scalp psoriasis because hair blocks ultraviolet light and inhibits the topical application of medications.

CLINICAL MANIFESTATIONS

- Lesions range from flaky dandruff to thick, extensive, armorlike plaques (Figures 4.40 and 4.41).
- Plaques are frequently hidden by hair or behind the ears (Figure 4.42).
- The entire external ear and ear canals may be involved (Figure 4.43).
- Psoriasis **does not cause hair loss.**

DIFFERENTIAL DIAGNOSIS

- **Seborrheic dermatitis (in adults;** Figure 4.44) is often indistinguishable from scalp psoriasis.
- **Eczematous dermatitis of the scalp (in children)** must be distinguished from scalp psoriasis.
  - There is generally an **atopic history**.
  - Eczema may be present elsewhere on the body.
- **Tinea capitis** (See Chapter 10, "Superficial Fungal Infections".)
  - There should be a positive KOH and/or fungal culture.
  - Temporary hair loss is characteristic.

MANAGEMENT

- **Mild scalp psoriasis** (with minimal scaling and thin plaques; "seborrheic dermatitislike" psoriasis) can be treated with **antidandruff shampoos** and a **topical steroid,** as needed, for itching.
  - **Over-the-counter tar** (Zetar, T/Gel), **selenium sulfide** (Selsun Blue, Head & Shoulders), and **salicylic acid–containing** (T/Sal) **shampoos**
  - Prescription **Nizoral (ketoconazole)** shampoo
  - A **medium- to high-potency topical steroid** in a solution (e.g., Fluonid) or gel (e.g., Topicort) formulation every day or twice per day as needed (gel and lotion preparations more readily reach the scalp than ointments and creams)
- **Severe scalp psoriasis** (thick plaques and thick scale)
  - **Removal of scale is necessary** before treating the plaques (see Appendix 2). This is accomplished by using the following keratolytic agents:
    — A 2 to 5% salicylic acid in a petrolatum base, Hydrisalic Gel, or
    — Bakers P & S lotion, or
    — LCD in mineral oil
  - After the scale is removed, **a medium- to high-potency topical steroid** is used, such as:
    — **Fluonid Solution** or **Topicort Gel** once or twice daily as needed under shower cap occlusion overnight or for 3 to 4 hours while awake
    — A **superpotent topical steroid (clobetasol propionate lotion or gel) without occlusion**
  - **Intralesional triamcinolone** (3 to 5 mg/cc) is used in a limited amount (1 to 2 cc or less per treatment) every 4 to 8 weeks is used to target particularly itchy areas. It may bring longer remissions.
  - **Dovonex Ointment, Cream,** or **Lotion** is used as maintenance or rotational therapy.

- Anthralin is used overnight or as SCAT as maintenance or rotational therapy (avoiding contact with the eyes).
- **Maintenance therapy after control.** Topical steroids should be used in the lowest potency effective in a pulse-dosing, or rotational dosing, manner with agents such as anthralin or Dovonex, in addition to shampoos.

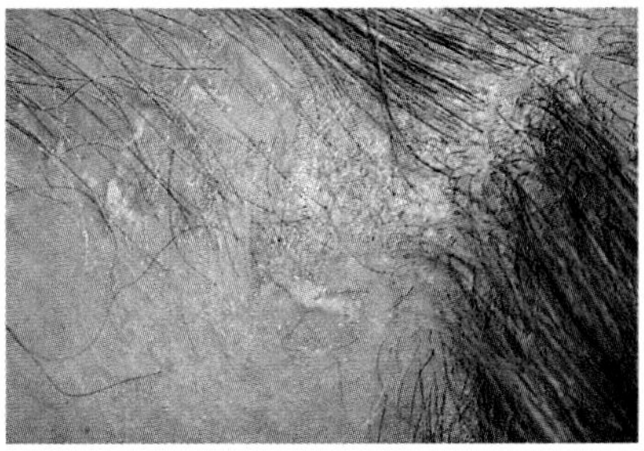

Figure 4.44.
Seborrheic dermatitis.

■ POINTS TO REMEMBER

- Scalp psoriasis, because it is inaccessible, cannot be treated by ultraviolet therapy; therefore, treatment is limited to intensive topical measures.
- When steroids are stopped, rapid relapse often occurs.
- Rotational, or pulse, treatment should be used to preclude tachyphylaxis (tolerance). The lowest-potency steroid that is effective should be used.

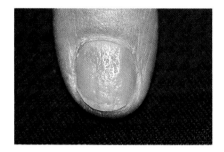

Figure 4.45.
Psoriasis of the nails with pitting.

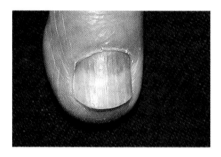

Figure 4.46.
Psoriasis of the nails with onycholysis.

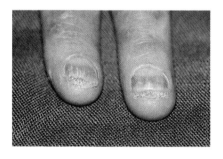

Figure 4.47.
Psoriasis of the nails with subungual hyperkeratosis.

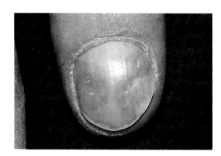

Figure 4.48.
Psoriasis of nails with "oil spots." Also note pitting and onycholysis.

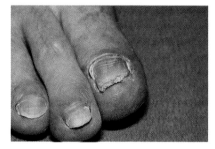

Figure 4.49.
Onychomycosis. Note subungual hyperkeratosis.

BASICS

- Nail involvement in patients with psoriasis is very common.
- Nail dystrophy is a chronic problem, the main liability of which is cosmetic; however, in some instances, thickened psoriatic toenails may become painful, and psoriatic fingernail deformity may interfere with function (e.g., picking up small objects).

CLINICAL MANIFESTATIONS

- **Pitting** (Figure 4.45) is a characteristic nail finding in psoriasis; however, it may also be seen in alopecia areata and eczematous dermatitis, and it can occur normally in some nails. It is produced by tiny punctate lesions in the nail matrix (nail root), which appear in the nail plate as it grows.
- **Onycholysis** (Figure 4.46) is separation of the nail plate from the underlying pink nail bed. The separated portion is white and opaque, in contrast to the pink translucence of the attached portion. Onycholysis is seen at the free margin of a normal nail as it grows. When involvement is more proximal, the condition can become more unsightly and can display a yellow or green tinge.
- **Subungual hyperkeratosis** (Figure 4.47) is thickening of the nail bed and is believed to represent psoriasis of the nail bed.
- **Oil spots or oil drops** (Figure 4.48) are orange–brown colored areas under the nail plate. Oil spots are believed to represent psoriasis of the nail bed as well.

DIFFERENTIAL DIAGNOSIS

- **Onychomycosis** (Figure 4.49) may be indistinguishable clinically from psoriatic nails; however, the lesions are positive for KOH, the fungal culture is positive, or both. Onychomycosis responds to systemic fungal therapy.
- **Eczematous dermatitis with secondary nail dystrophy** (see Figure 13.1) is inflammation of the matrix, or root of the nail, resulting in dystrophy of the nail plate.
- **Onycholysis** (see Figure 13.2), separation of the nail plate from the underlying pink nail bed, is also associated with thyroid disease as well as onychomycosis. It can occur secondary to trauma and as a drug reaction.

MANAGEMENT

Management is generally unrewarding but the following measures may be helpful:
- Careful trimming and paring of the nails
- Potent topical steroids applied, with plastic wrap or plastic glove occlusion
- Injection of steroids into the nail matrix, which is painful

PSORIATIC ARTHRITIS

BASICS

- Psoriatic arthritis can occur at any age, but onset is most often between ages 35 and 45 years (Figures 4.50 and 4.51).
- It may occur before or, more often, following the outbreak of skin disease.
- **Early onset often portends a poor prognosis;** frequently, destructive arthropathy results.

DESCRIPTION OF LESIONS

There are five clinical patterns:
- **Asymmetric,** small and medium-size joint involvement, which is most common, with "sausage finger" deformity
- **Distal interphalangeal joint (DIP) disease (classic type),** which is milder and often associated with nail disease
- **Rheumatoid arthritis–type,** which is symmetric and rheumatoid factor negative
- **Ankylosing spondylitis**
- **Mutilating,** grossly deforming arthritis mutilans

CLINICAL MANIFESTATIONS

- **Rheumatoid factor is usually negative.**
- **Onset usually follows skin manifestations of psoriasis.**
- Psoriatic arthritis is seen in approximately 5 to 10% of patients with psoriasis; however, many patients without arthritis have symptoms of **chronic arthralgias.**
- It is more likely seen in patients with more severe cutaneous disease.
- **Nail pathology** is more common in patients with psoriatic arthritis.

DIFFERENTIAL DIAGNOSIS

Peripheral psoriatic arthritis may be indistinguishable from:
- **Reiter's disease**
- **Rheumatoid arthritis,** latex-negative

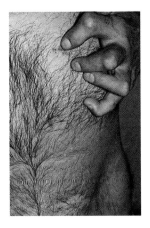

Figure 4.50.
Psoriatic arthritis. Note psoriatic plaque on the abdomen.

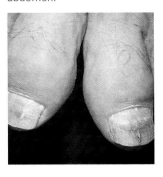

Figure 4.51.
Psoriatic arthritis with distal interphalangeal joint (DIP) involvement.

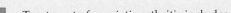

MANAGEMENT

Treatment of psoriatic arthritis includes:
- Nonsteroidal anti-inflammatory drugs (NSAIDs)
- Gold
- Methotrexate
- Cyclosporine
- Retinoids
- PUVA
- RePUVA
- Physical therapy

FORMULARY FOR THE TOPICAL TREATMENT OF PSORIASIS

NOTE. The formulary that follows is not comprehensive. It lists proprietary names and attempts to designate generic equivalents, whenever possible. It is intended to provide more than enough treatment options; it contains more agents than most dermatologists use on a regular basis.

BRAND NAMES	GENERIC NAMES
Keratolytic Agents	
Baker's P & S Lotion	Salicylic acid, 2 to 5%, in a petrolatum base
Hydrisalic Gel	Salicylic acid, 5% in a gel base
Keralyt Gel	Salicylic acid, 6% gel
Moisturizers	
Eucerin Cream	
Aquaphor	
Moisturel Lotion	
Complex 15 Cream	
Topical Vitamin D3	
Dovonex Cream, Ointment, Lotion 0.005%	Calcipotriene cream, ointment, lotion
Anthralin Preparations	
Dritho-Creme, 0.1%, 0.25%, 0.5%	
Dritho-Creme, 1% HP	
Dritho-Scalp, 0.25%, 0.5%	
Micanol (1% anthralin) Cream	

Topical Steroids (listed in order of decreasing potency)

GROUP I, SUPERPOTENT

Temovate Cream, Ointment	Clobetasol propionate cream, ointment,0.05%
Temovate Gel	Clobetasol propionate gel, 0.05%
Psorcon Ointment	Diflorasone diacetate ointment, 0.05%
Cordran Tape	Flurandrenolide tape
Diprolene Lotion	Betamethasone dipropionate lotion, 0.05%

GROUP II, VERY HIGH POTENCY

Lidex Cream, Ointment, Gel	Fluocinonide cream, ointment, gel, 0.05%
Topicort Gel	Desoximetasone gel, 0.05%

GROUP III, HIGH POTENCY

Valisone Ointment	Betamethasone valerate ointment, 0.1%

GROUP IV, MEDIUM TO HIGH POTENCY

Kenalog, Aristocort Ointment	Triamcinolone acetonide ointment, 0.1% Westcort Ointment
	Hydrocortisone valerate ointment, 0.2%

GROUP V, MEDIUM POTENCY

Valisone Cream, Lotion	Betamethasone valerate cream, lotion 0.1%
Desowen Ointment	Desonide ointment, 0.05%
Westcort Cream	Hydrocortisone valerate cream, 0.2%
Kenalog, Artistocort Cream, Lotion	Triamcinolone acetonide cream, lotion, 0.1%

GROUP VI, LOW TO MEDIUM POTENCY

Tridesilon, Desowen Cream	Desonide cream, 0.05%
Fluonid Solution	Fluocinolone acetonide solution, 0.01%

GROUP VII, LOW POTENCY

Cortaid, Cortizone-5 (over-the-counter)	Hydrocortisone cream, lotion 1.0%, 0.5%

Tar Preparations	
Estar	
Psorigel	
T/Derm Tar Emollient	
Balnetar	
Doak Tar Oil	
Liquor carbonis detergens (LCD)	
Retinoids	
Tazorac	Tazarotne gel 0.05, 0.1%

CHAPTER 5

ERUPTIONS OF UNKNOWN CAUSE

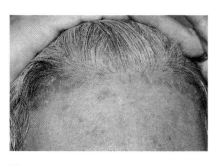

Figure 5.1.
Typical seborrheic dermatitis (SD) on scalp.

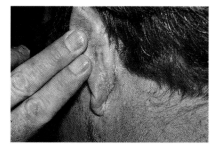

Figure 5.2.
Seborrheic dermatitis (SD) behind the ear.

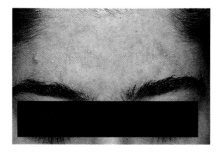

Figure 5.3.
Seborrheic dermatitis (SD) on the forehead.

ADULT SEBORRHEIC DERMATITIS (SD)

BASICS

- Adult SD is a very common chronic inflammatory dermatitis with a characteristic distribution involving areas that have the greatest concentration of sebaceous glands, such as the scalp and face or in body folds (intertriginous areas).
- It usually flares in the winter and improves in the summer.
- Many people experience some degree of **dandruff,** a whitish scaling of the scalp, which is sometimes itchy and fairly easily controlled with dandruff shampoos. When the dandruff is **accompanied by erythema,** which is a sign of inflammation, it is then referred to as **SD.**
- SD is seen more commonly in men and often begins after puberty. There appears to be a **hereditary predisposition** to its development. When it presents in patients who are HIV-positive, SD may serve as an early marker of AIDS. It is also seen commonly in patients with Parkinson's disease and in patients taking phenothiazines.
- The condition has traditionally been described as being idiopathic; however, there is some evidence that *Pityrosporon ovale,* a small yeast, may play a part in its pathogenesis because SD occasionally responds to antifungal medications such as ketoconazole.

DESCRIPTION OF LESIONS

Lesions are erythematous patches with a whitish or light-brown scale; they may also appear as orange–yellow greasy patches.

DISTRIBUTION OF LESIONS

- The eruption tends to be **bilaterally symmetric** in its distribution.
- In the posterior auricular, inguinal, and intergluteal creases, the eruption may consist of sharply defined, bright-red plaques, often with **fissures.** In these areas, SD is often referred to as **intertrigo,** or **intertriginous SD,** when other causes for the rash, such as candidiasis or psoriasis, are ruled out.

Scalp, ears, face
- **Scalp** (Figure 5.1). SD may range in severity from a mild erythema and scaling to thick armorlike plaques that are indistinguishable from **psoriasis** ("sebopsoriasis").
- **Ears.** SD is seen behind the ears and in the external ear canal (Figure 5.2).
- **Face.** SD is seen on the forehead, in the eyebrows, in the eyelashes, on the cheeks, in the beard, and in the nasolabial folds (Figures 5.3 and 5.4).

Trunk
SD affects the trunk in the presternal area and the umbilicus.

Body folds (intertrigo)
SD affects the inframammary areas, axillae, inguinal creases, and intergluteal crease and perianal area (Figures 5.5 and 5.6).

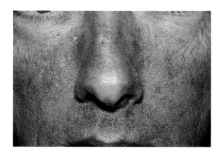

Figure 5.4.
Seborrheic dermatitis (SD) on cheeks and in nasolabial folds.

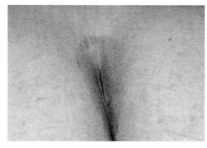

Figure 5.5.
Fissured plaque of intergluteal crease.

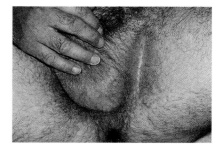

Figure 5.6.
Seborrheic dermatitis (SD) (intertrigo); KOH-negative.

DIFFERENTIAL DIAGNOSIS

Scalp and ears
- **Psoriasis** present only on the scalp may be indistinguishable from SD ("sebopsoriasis"; Figure 5.7).
- **Lichen simplex chronicus** of scalp (eczematous dermatitis)
  - There may be an atopic history.
  - Lichen simplex chronicus is exacerbated by shampoos and soaps.

Face
- **Early, or "pre-rosacea"** (Figure 5.8), lacks scale.
  - **Telangiectasia** acneiform papules and pustules develop later.
- **Tinea faciale** (Figure 5.9)
  - The lesions are generally annular with asymmetric distribution.
  - Tinea faciale is KOH positive.
- **Systemic lupus erythematosus** (SLE) butterfly rash
  - SLE is antinuclear antibody positive.
  - The patient may have other features of lupus.

Body folds
- **Inverse psoriasis** (Figure 5.10)
  - Inverse psoriasis is KOH negative.
  - It may be indistinguishable from SD.
  - There may be other evidence of psoriasis.

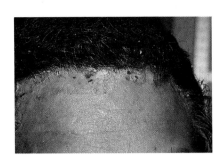

Figure 5.7.
Psoriasis. Note well-defined psoriatic plaque with white scale.

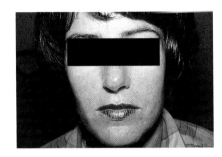

Figure 5.8.
Pre-rosacea.

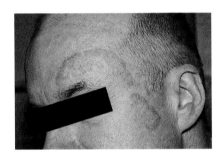

Figure 5.9.
Tinea faciale; KOH-positive.

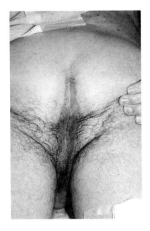

Figure 5.10.
Inverse psoriasis of "keyhole area."

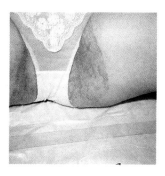

Figure 5.11.
Tinea cruris.

• **Tinea cruris** (Figure 5.11)
  ■ Tinea cruris is KOH positive.
  ■ There is an arcuate shape with an advancing active border and central clearing.

Also to be considered in the differential diagnosis:
• **Candidiasis** (body folds, especially in diabetics)
• **Lichen simplex chronicus** (scrotal involvement)
• **Nonspecific balanitis, irritant dermatitis, atopic dermatitis**

MANAGEMENT

• **SD of the scalp**
  ■ Mild SD of the scalp generally responds to antidandruff shampoos or ketoconazole shampoo 2%; for itching and inflammation, a medium-strength topical steroid in a gel or solution formulation may be used.
  ■ **Severe SD of the scalp (sebopsoriasis)** is managed the same way as psoriasis in this location; that is, **potent topical steroids**, frequently preceded by **keratolytic agents** to remove thick scale (see Appendix 2).
• **SD of the face**
  ■ SD of the face quickly responds to **low-potency topical steroids;** long-term maintenance and vigilance are required to avoid atrophy, telangiectasias, and rosacealike side effects.
  ■ **Low-potency topical steroids** may be alternated with **ketoconazole cream 2%** to minimize unwanted side effects; occasionally, ketoconazole cream alone affords control.
  ■ **Very low–potency topical steroids** should be used with caution when treating eyelid SD.
• **SD involving other areas of the body,** including **body folds (intertrigo)** and **genital areas,** are similarly treated with **low-potency topical steroids**.
• **Prevention**
  ■ The area should be kept dry by using a hair dryer after bathing.
  ■ Liberal use of drying powders, such as **Zeasorb Powder**, help to prevent maceration and secondary bacterial infection.

BASICS

- SD in infancy probably represents a different condition than adult SD. It is **self-limiting,** generally disappearing by 8 months of age.
- It may be impossible to distinguish infant SD from atopic dermatitis or diaper rash.
- **Leiner's disease** is a rare form of an SD-like eruption manifested by an erythroderma, diarrhea, and a failure to thrive.

DISTRIBUTION OF LESIONS

- **Scalp.** "Cradle cap" (Figure 5.12) is a common buildup of a scaly, greasy adherent plaque on the vertex of the scalp in newborns.
- **Body folds**. SD of body folds generally consists of erythematous patches when it involves the diaper area or axillae.

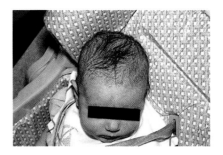

Figure 5.12.
Seborrheic dermatitis (SD). Cradle cap.

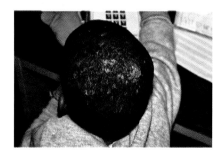

Figure 5.13.
Tinea capitis.

DIFFERENTIAL DIAGNOSIS

Scalp
- **Tinea capitis** should be suspected in urban black infants, especially after the age of 1 (Figure 5.13).
- **Atopic dermatitis** is considered if there is an atopic history, especially if the child is older than 1 year and is itching

Body folds
- **Diaper rash** characteristically spares the folds.
- **Candidiasis** sometimes appears as a secondary infection of diaper rash.
- **Atopic dermatitis**

MANAGEMENT

- **Scalp SD "cradle cap"**
  - Minor amounts of scale can be removed with **antiseborrheic shampoos** that contain sulfur and salicylic acid such as Sebulex.
  - Stronger keratolytic agents, such as 2 to 6% salicylic acid in petrolatum are used for thick, dense, adherent scale. Mineral oil or olive oil also helps to remove scale.
  - Hydrisalic acid, an over-the-counter 5% salicylic acid gel preparation, can also be used.
  - Mild topical steroids may be applied to reduce inflammation and itching.
- **Body folds**
  - Very mild topical steroids can be used.
  - Topical antifungal creams, if indicated, may be combined with topical steroids.
  - Maceration should be prevented with the liberal use of baby powders.

POINTS TO REMEMBER

- **Adult.** Antiseborrheic shampoos should be left on for at least 5 minutes after lathering.
- **Adult and infant**
SD is not seen in preadolescent children; therefore, excessive use of shampoos should not be used in this age-group because the child may have atopic dermatitis.
- **Topical steroids should be used for brief periods only.**

DANDRUFF AND SEBORRHEIC DERMATITIS (SD) FORMULARY

ANTISEBORRHEIC SHAMPOOS/ LOTIONS
Antiseborrheic shampoos contain alone, or in combination: zinc pyrithione, coal tar, salicylic acid, selenium sulfide, ketoconazole, and sulfur.

Over-the-counter
Head & Shoulders Shampoo
Zincon Shampoo
Neutrogena T/Gel
Zetar Shampoo and Emulsion

Prescription	
Selsun Lotion	2.5% selenium sulfide

ANTIFUNGAL SHAMPOO

Prescription
Nizoral Shampoo

KERATOLYTICS (AGENTS THAT REMOVE EXCESSIVE SCALE)

Over-the-counter	
Sebulex Shampoo	Sulfur 2%, salicylic acid 2%
Neutrogena T/Sal Shampoo	Tar plus salicylic acid
Hydrisalic gel	5% salicylic acid
Keratyt gel	6% salicylic acid

Prescription
Salicylic acid 2 to 6% in petrolatum

MODERATE- AND HIGH-STRENGTH TOPICAL CORTICOSTEROIDS (SCALP)

Prescription	
Medium potency	Betamethasone valerate 0.1% gel or lotion
High potency	Fluocinonide (Lidex 0.05%) gel or lotion

LOW-STRENGTH TOPICAL STEROIDS (FACE AND INTERTRIGINOUS AREAS)

Over-the-counter	
Very low potency	Hydrocortisone 0.5 to 1% cream or ointment

Prescription	
Low potency	Desonide 0.05% cream
Medium potency	Hydrocortisone valerate (Westcort) 0.2%

Topical Antifungal Cream

Prescription	
Nizoral Cream 2%	Ketoconazole

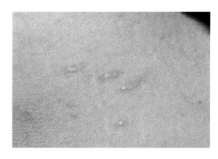

Figure 5.14.
Pityriasis rosea primary lesion with fine scale. Note elliptical shapes.

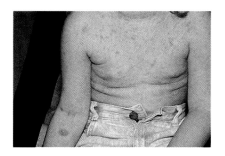

Figure 5.15.
"Herald patch" on flexor forearm.

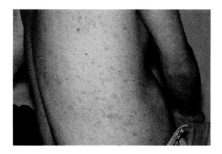

Figure 5.16.
Pityriasis rosea "Christmas tree" pattern following lines of cleavage.

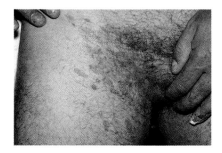

Figure 5.17.
Atypical (inverse) pityriasis rosea in inguinal distribution.

BASICS

Pityriasis rosea is an acute, benign, self-limiting eruption of unknown cause, which has a characteristic course. It tends to occur in the spring and fall and is seen mostly in young adults and older children, although it may occur at any age.

DESCRIPTION OF LESIONS

- **Primary lesions of pityriasis rosea** are generally papulosquamous, consisting of fine scaly erythematous patches with fine, thin scale (Figure 5.14).
- The **typical course** of pityriasis rosea begins with the larger "**herald patch**" (Figure 5.15), which is followed in several days to 2 weeks by multiple smaller oval or elliptically shaped scaly patches.
- In dark-skinned people, the eruption may be papular or vesicular with little or no scaling.
- Itching is usually mild but may be severe; recurrences are rare.
- **Less typical presentations (atypical pityriasis rosea)** are seen, including those in which the herald patch is not noted by the patient or clinician, or the lesions may be vesicular and uncharacteristically pruritic (which is noted more commonly in dark-skinned patients).

DISTRIBUTION OF LESIONS

- The lesions appear on the trunk, neck, arms, and legs in an "old-fashioned bathing suit" distribution.
- Often a "Christmas tree" pattern is noted on the trunk, where the lesions follow the skin folds (Figure 5.16).
- In **atypical pityriasis rosea**, the eruption may be limited in its distribution or it may present in an inverse fashion involving the groin, axillae, or distal extremities (**inverse pityriasis rosea;** Figure 5.17)

DIFFERENTIAL DIAGNOSIS

- **Secondary syphilis**
  - Lesions are often seen on the palms, soles, and face as well as the trunk (Figure 5.18).
  - Serology is positive. (In all cases of atypical pityriasis rosea, it is good to obtain a serology to rule out secondary syphilis.)
- **Tinea versicolor** (Figure 5.19)
  - KOH is positive.
  - Tinea versicolor is a chronic condition.
- **Drug eruption or viral exanthem** (Figure 5.20)
  - The lesions are more acute than that of pityriasis rosea.
  - The lesions are redder, less scaly, and itchier.
  - There may be other symptoms (e.g., fever).
  - Resolution is speedier than that of pityriasis rosea.
- **Guttate psoriasis** (Figure 5.21)
  - Abrupt onset is easily confused with pityriasis rosea.
  - The scale is silvery and thicker than that of pityriasis rosea.
- **Parapsoriasis** is uncommon.

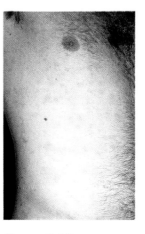

Figure 5.18.
Lesions of secondary syphilis.

MANAGEMENT

- Because pityriasis rosea is self-limiting and often asymptomatic, all that is usually necessary is to advise the patient and family about the usual course of the rash and its noncontagious nature and to suggest follow-up or referral to a dermatologist if the rash persists beyond the typical 8 to 12 weeks.
- Itching, if present, is treated with oral antihistamines.
- Topical steroids are of minimal benefit.
- Sunlight exposure or ultraviolet light therapy may speed resolution.

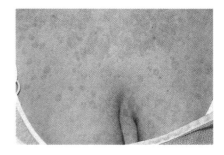

Figure 5.19.
Tinea versicolor.

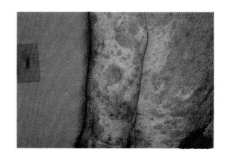

Figure 5.20.
Drug eruption.

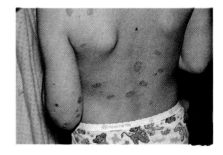

Figure 5.21.
Guttate psoriasis.

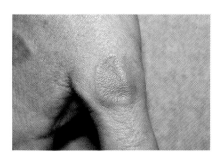

Figure 5.22.
Granuloma annulare (GA) in annular plaques with central clearing.

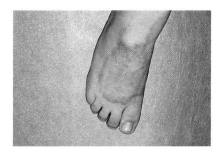

Figure 5.23.
Granuloma annulare (GA) lesions are often symmetrically distributed on the dorsa of the hands and feet.

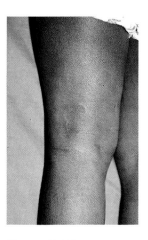

Figure 5.24.
Granuloma annulare (GA) may appear on the arms and legs.

BASICS

- **Granuloma annulare (GA)** is an idiopathic, generally asymptomatic, ring-shaped grouping of dermal papules. The papules are comprised of focal granulomas that coalesce to form curious circles or semicircular plaques, which are often misdiagnosed as "ringworm."
- GA is seen most frequently in very young children in whom it is usually self-limiting.
- It is also seen in women by a 2.5:1 female:male ratio. In adults, GA tends to be more chronic.
- There is also an adult form of disseminated GA, which may be associated with diabetes.

DESCRIPTION OF LESIONS

- There are skin-colored or red firm papules, with no epidermal change (scale).
- The lesions may be individual, isolated papules or may be joined in annular or semi-annular (arciform) plaques with central clearing (Figure 5.22).
- Occasionally, subcutaneous nodules are seen.

DISTRIBUTION OF LESIONS

- Lesions are often **symmetrically distributed** on dorsa of hands, fingers, and feet (Figure 5.23).
- Lesions may appear on arms and legs (Figure 5.24).
- Subcutaneous nodules may be seen on arms and legs.

CLINICAL MANIFESTATIONS

- GA is generally asymptomatic and generally only a cosmetic problem.

DIAGNOSIS

- Diagnosis is most often made on clinical grounds.
- GA has a **characteristic histopathology**. It consists of foci of altered collagen and mucin surrounded by histiocytic and lymphocytic cells referred to as **necrobiosis.**

DIFFERENTIAL DIAGNOSIS

- **Tinea corporis** (Figure 5.25)
  - There is scale (an "active border") associated with tinea corporis.
  - The lesion is KOH positive.
  - Distribution is asymmetrical.
  - Lesions generally itch.
- **Erythema migrans rash of Lyme disease** (Figure 5.26)
  - Lesions associated with erythema migrans are generally larger than those associated with GA.
  - The duration of the rash is self-limited.
  - Lesions generally are not firm.
- **Sarcoidosis of the skin**
  - Sarcoidosis most often is seen in adult blacks and Scandinavians.
  - Lesions often appear periorificially or develop in scars.
  - Other clinical features of sarcoidosis are usually present.
  - Sarcoid lesions are sometimes annular.
- **Necrobiosis lipoidica diabeticorum**
- **Rheumatoid nodules,** which resemble subcutaneous nodules of GA

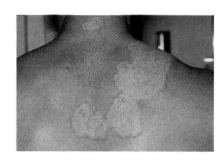

Figure 5.25.
Tinea corporis.

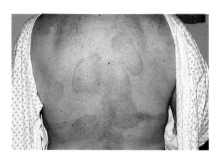

Figure 5.26.
Erythema migrans of Lyme disease.

MANAGEMENT

- The patient should be reassured about the benign nature of this condition.
- Localized lesions in children are best left untreated.
- Potent topical steroids, if necessary, should be used under plastic occlusion.
- Intralesional triamcinolone acetonide (2 mg/cc to 4 mg/cc) is injected directly into the elevated border of the lesions.

POINT TO REMEMBER

Diabetes mellitus may be associated with the generalized form of GA.

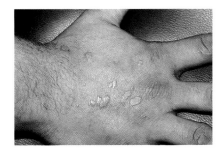

Figure 5.27.
Lichen planus (LP). Flat-topped, violaceous, polygonal papules.

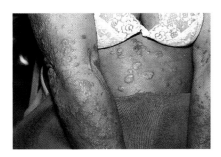

Figure 5.28.
Lichen planus (LP). Flat-topped, violaceous papules and plaques

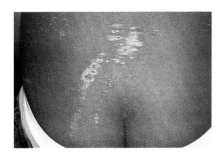

Figure 5.29.
Lichen planus (LP). Linear lesions.

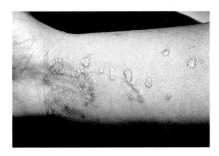

Figure 5.30.
Lichen planus (LP). Active and resolving lesions. Note postinflammatory hyperpigmentation.

BASICS

- Lichen planus (LP) is an **idiopathic eruption** with characteristic shiny, flat-topped papules on the skin, often accompanied by mucous membrane lesions.
- LP is a unique skin disorder, associated with a spectrum of lesions, which can involve the hair and nails in addition to the skin.
- Other **LP-like eruptions** are seen in:
  - Drug-induced LP associated with gold, thiazides, captopril, and antimalarial agents
  - Lichenoid reactions associated with graft-versus-host disease
  - Association with hepatitis C
- LP is relatively uncommon. It is seen more frequently in adults and more often in women than men

DESCRIPTION OF LESIONS

- **Seven "Ps"** of LP (Figure 5.27)
  - Lesions are often **pruritic**, although they may be asymptomatic.
  - Lesions are often **purple** (actually violaceous) in color.
  - Lesions tend to be **planar** (flat-topped).
  - Lesions form **papules** or **plaques** (Figure 5.28).
  - Lesions may be **polygonal,** or
  - Lesions may be **pleomorphic** in shape and configuration (i.e., oval, annular, linear, confluent [plaquelike], large, and small—even on the same person [Figure 5.29]).
  - Lesions tend to heal with residual **postinflammatory hyperpigmentation** (Figure 5.30).
- In addition, lesions may be atrophic, hypertrophic (Figure 5.31), or vesicobullous.
- The **Köebner phenomenon** (isomorphic response) is seen as a reaction to trauma such as scratching (Figure 5.32). (See also Chapter 4, "Psoriasis".)
- **Wickham's striae** are white streaks that are best visualized on the surface of lesions after mineral oil is applied (Figure 5.33).
- Mucous membrane lesions are characterized by white lacy streaks in a netlike pattern or by atrophic erosions or ulcers (Figure 5.34). (See also Chapter 12, "Disorders of the Mouth, Lips, and Tongue")
- The patient may exhibit mild nail dystrophy to total loss of the nails.
- A scarring follicular alopecia (lichen planopilaris) may occur.

DISTRIBUTION OF LESIONS

- Flexor areas such as the wrists, pretibial shafts, scalp, trunk, and glans penis
- On the buccal mucosa, tongue, and lips

CLINICAL MANIFESTATIONS

- Pruritus occurs in the majority of patients.
- Lesions may persist for months and then spontaneously disappear. In some instances, the problem can last for years, or even a lifetime.
- Oral lesions may become ulcerative and painful. Rare malignant transformation to squamous cell carcinoma has been documented.

DIAGNOSIS

LP is often easy to diagnose by its appearance, despite its range of clinical presentations.

- Presence of **Wickham's striae**
- Characteristic oral lesions
- Biopsy of skin, if necessary

DIFFERENTIAL DIAGNOSIS

- **Pityriasis rosea**
  - Elliptical lesions with fine scale
  - "Christmas tree" pattern on trunk (see Figure 5.16)
- **Psoriasis**
  - Extensor distribution over large joints
  - White or silvery scale
- **Lichen simplex chronicus**
  - Lichenification
  - Excoriations, crusts
- **Lichenoid (LP-like) eruptions**
  - Lesions that are indistinguishable from classic LP
  - No oral lesions
  - History of drug ingestion, bone marrow transplantation, etc.

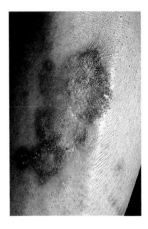

Figure 5.31.
Lichen planus (LP). Hypertrophic lesions on pretibial shaft.

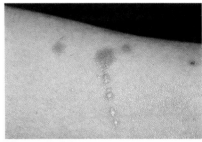

Figure 5.32.
Lichen planus (LP). The Köebner phenomenon (isomorphic response) caused by scratching.

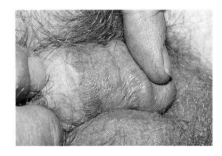

Figure 5.33.
Lichen planus (LP). Wickham's striae. White streaks on the surface of a lesion on the penis after application of mineral oil.

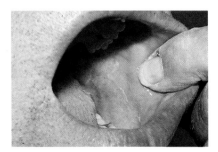

Figure 5.34.
Lichen planus (LP). Oral lesions, white lacy pattern on buccal mucosa.

MANAGEMENT

- Potent topical steroids under occlusion
- Systemic steroids in short tapering courses
- Psoralen plus ultraviolet A (PUVA)

POINT TO REMEMBER

LP is seen frequently enough and has such an unusual array of features so as to be recognizable to the non-dermatologist.

CHAPTER 6

DIAPER DERMATITIS (RASH)

BASICS

- The term **diaper dermatitis** refers to all eruptions that occur in the area covered by a diaper.
- **Irritant diaper dermatitis (IDD)** is, by far, the **most common rash in infancy**. It is caused by chafing, irritation by soaps and detergents, and, possibly, contact with ammonia, which is produced as a breakdown product of urea by bacteria in feces.
- Added to this wet, excrement-laden milieu is the occlusive effect of rubber or plastic diapers or diaper covers and the constant contact of moisture from cloth diapers when diapers are not immediately changed.
- Diaper dermatitis may also be caused, or exacerbated, by atopic dermatitis, seborrheic dermatitis, and secondary *Candida* infection.

DESCRIPTION OF LESIONS

- **Erythema, scale,** and possibly **papules** and **plaques**
- Occasionally, **vesicles** and **bullae**
- With neglect, possible erosion and ulceration

DISTRIBUTION OF LESIONS

- Typically **spares the creases**
- May conform to the shape of the diaper (Figure 6.1)

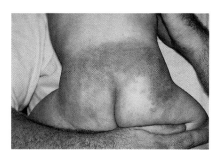

Figure 6.1.
Diaper rash with eruption conforming to the shape of a diaper.

CLINICAL VARIANTS

Candidal diaper dermatitis
Description of lesions
Beefy redness and **satellite pustules** suggest secondary infection of IDD with *Candida*.

Distribution of lesions
Creases are involved.

Diagnosis
is confirmed by a positive KOH.

Atopic diaper dermatitis (Figure 6.2)
Basics
- In general, patients with atopic dermatitis are more likely to experience **irritant contact dermatitis;** nonetheless, the diaper area is often remarkably spared in atopic dermatitis.
- If present, the rash may be similar to IDD, or it may be characteristically eczematous in appearance.

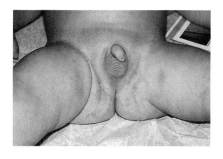

Figure 6.2.
Atopic dermatitis.

Diagnosis
- The creases are involved.
- There is other evidence of atopic dermatitis and a family history of atopy.
- Occasionally, there is secondary infection with *Staphylococcus aureus.*

Seborrheic dermatitis (Figure 6.3)
Diagnosis
- Creases are involved.
- Similar lesions are found elsewhere.
- The patient may exhibit "cradle cap".

DIFFERENTIAL DIAGNOSIS

- **Tinea cruris** (Figure 6.4)
- **Impetigo**
- **Kawasaki's disease**
- **Psoriasis,** particularly if there is a positive family history or other evidence of psoriasis
- **Rare diseases** should be considered in recalcitrant cases, such as:
  - Letterer-Siwe disease (a form of histiocytosis X)
  - Acrodermatitis enteropathica (because of zinc deficiency)

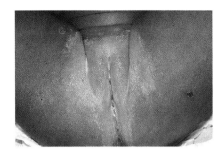

Figure 6.3.
Seborrheic dermatitis. Note involvement of inguinal creases.

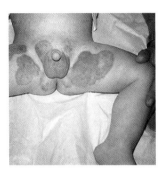

Figure 6.4.
Tinea cruris; positive KOH.

MANAGEMENT

- **General measures** to minimize friction, absorb moisture, and protect the skin from urine and feces include the following:
  - Disposable or super-absorbent diapers that hold moisture in and keep it away from the skin.
  - Diaper changing promptly after voiding or soiling.
  - Use of rubber and plastic pants should be avoided.
  - Soap-free cleansers such as Cetaphil
  - Emollients, such as Balmex ointment, and barrier creams, such as zinc oxide preparations, should be applied frequently.
  - Absorbant baby powders should be used.
- **Specific measures of treatment**
  - Low-potency hydrocortisone 1% or 0.5% is often all that is necessary for uncomplicated IDD.
  - Stronger topical steroids such as desonide 0.05% or hydrocortisone valerate 0.02% creams may be used for short periods, as necessary.
  - Potent topical steroids combined with an antifungal agent, such as contained in Lotrisone or Mycolog II, should be avoided in the diaper area.
  - If candidiasis is suspected, particularly if there is no improvement after several days, a topical antifungal preparation, such as the over-the-counter preparations Lotrimin and Micatin or prescription ketoconazole, can be applied.
  - The addition of nonabsorbable oral nystatin in recalcitrant cases should be considered.

POINTS TO REMEMBER

- The use of potent topical steroids is to be avoided.
- Fever, crankiness, and a scaly eruption in the diaper area (especially perianal) may be an early clue to Kawasaki's disease.
- Child abuse should be considered when the dermatitis does not fit any of the diagnoses discussed above.

CHAPTER 7

SUPERFICIAL VIRAL INFECTIONS

BASICS

- **Herpes simplex virus (HSV)** infections are caused by two types of virus, HSV-1 and HSV-2. HSV-1 causes mostly nongenital infections, while HSV-2 is the leading cause of genital ulcer disease. HSV is highly contagious and is spread by direct contact with the skin or mucous membranes. After the primary infection, the HSV virus retreats to a dorsal root ganglion, where it remains latent until it becomes reactivated by precipitating factors or triggers, such as sunlight exposure, menses, fever, common colds, and possibly stress.
- Primary infections are acquired in infancy and early childhood; the majority are subclinical. Patients with AIDS and patients taking immunosuppressant therapy for organ transplantation or cancer chemotherapy are at greatest risk for severe recalcitrant infections.

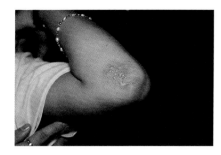

Figure 7.1.
The classic grouped vesicles of herpes simplex virus (HSV) on an erythematous base.

DESCRIPTION OF LESIONS

Sequence of events:
- Grouped vesicles with an umbilicated center (Figure 7.1) later may become pustules (Figure 7.2).
- Lesions dry and become crusts or erosions (Figure 7.3).
- The lesions heal with no scars.

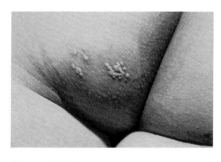

Figure 7.2.
Pustular lesions of herpes simplex virus (HSV).

DISTRIBUTION OF LESIONS

- **Primary HSV** (Figure 7.4)
  - The oral cavity is affected (gingivostomatitis): lips, gums, buccal mucosa, fauces, tongue, and hard palate.
  - Lesions may be extensive over the lips and lower face.
- **Recurrent HSV**
  - Recurrence occurs at the site innervated by the dorsal root ganglion in which the virus resides.
  - The face and hands may be affected, or recurrent HSV may occur anywhere on body.
  - Recurrence is seen most often on the vermilion border of the lip (herpes labialis) and on the presacral area in women.
  - Rarely is it seen inside the mouth.

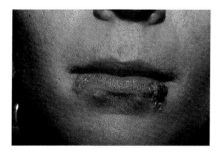

Figure 7.3.
Vesicular and crusted lesions of herpes simplex virus (HSV).

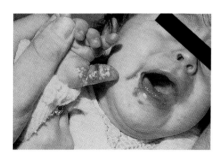

Figure 7.4.
Primary herpes simplex virus (HSV) in an infant.

CLINICAL MANIFESTATIONS

- **Primary HSV**
  - The vast majority of cases are subclinical.
  - It may be difficult to distinguish primary HSV from severe recurrent HSV.
  - Symptoms of primary HSV tend to be more severe than those of recurrent HSV and include gingivostomatitis, fever, lymphadenitis, and sore throat.
  - Encephalitis is a rare complication.
- **Recurrent HSV**
  - There is a prodrome of itching, pain or numbness.
  - Symptoms are generally milder than those of symptomatic primary HSV.
  - The number of lesions is fewer than those associated with primary HSV.
  - Usually, only nonspecific crusted lesions are seen (Figure 7.5).
  - Occasional regional lymphadenopathy occurs.
  - The majority of cases of recurrent erythema multiforme minor are related to recurrent (clinical and subclinical) HSV episodes (see Chapter 18, "Diseases of Vasculature").
  - Over time, recurrences decrease in frequency and often stop altogether.
  - Persistent ulcerative or verrucous keratotic lesions may be seen in patients with AIDS (see Chapter 24, "The Cutaneous Manifestations of HIV Infection").

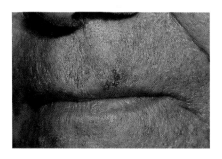

Figure 7.5.
Typical crust at vermilion border of lip in recurrent herpes simplex virus (HSV).

DIAGNOSIS

- Diagnosis is usually made by clinical appearance.
- Tzanck preparation, if positive, suggests **HSV or varicella-zoster virus (VZV)** infection. (See Chapter 26, Basic Procedures.)
- Viral cultures may be positive within 2 to 3 days because the virus grows rapidly.
- HSV tissue culture using monoclonal antibodies requires only 24 hours; the test is 90% sensitive, but it is expensive.
- Polymerase chain reaction can be conducted but is expensive.
- Serologic tests for HSV are generally not useful because there is such a high incidence of antibodies to herpes simplex in the general population.

DIFFERENTIAL DIAGNOSIS

- **Herpes zoster**
  - Herpes zoster is unilateral, dermatomal, and often painful.
  - It may be impossible to distinguish clinically from HSV.
  - It also has a positive Tzanck smear.
  - In time, recurrent disease (as seen with HSV) distinguishes the two.

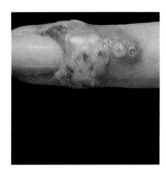

Figure 7.6.
Herpetic whitlow.

Intraoral, or Primary HSV:

- **Aphthous stomatitis** (See Chapter 12, "Disorders of the Mouth, Lips, and Tongue").
  - There is no fever or lymphadenopathy.
  - The Tzanck smear is negative, and there is no HSV on culture.
- **Hand, foot, and mouth disease** (caused by Coxsackie A16 virus)
  - There are oval, erythematous erosions, which are more often seen on the soft palate and uvula.
  - There may be symmetrical lesions on the hands and feet.
  - The lesions are asymptomatic because they are shallower than the lesions of primary HSV.

CLINICAL VARIANTS

- **Herpetic whitlow** (Figure 7.6)
  - Herpetic whitlow is an HSV infection of the fingertip.
  - It can be very painful.
  - It is an occupational hazard among dental and medical health care workers, whose fingertips may come in contact with patients infected with HSV. It is also seen in infants, in whom it is spread from the mouth to the thumb by thumb-sucking (Figure 7.4).
- **Eczema herpeticum (Kaposi's varicelliform eruption)**
  - This is an uncommon disseminated form of HSV.
  - It occurs mainly in children with severe atopic dermatitis.

MANAGEMENT

- • **Topical therapy**
  - ■ Oral discomfort may be lessened with viscous lidocaine applications, oral analgesics, and sucking on ice cubes.
  - ■ Skin symptoms may be eased with Burow's soaks or other moist soaks with water or saline to help dry the eruption and prevent secondary infection.
- ■ Topical acyclovir ointment and penciclovir cream have not been proven to be very effective.
- • **Systemic therapy**
  - ■ **Primary HSV**
    - — **Children.** Oral elixir acyclovir 5 mg/kg per day (five times per day for 7 days)
    - — **Adults**
      Valacyclovir 500 mg twice daily for 10 days or acyclovir 200 mg 5 times/day or 400 mg three times daily for 10 days or
      Famciclovir 250 mg three times daily for 10 days
  - ■ **Recurrent HSV.** Treatment should be initiated at the first sign or prodrome of HSV.
    - — Valacyclovir 500 mg five times daily for 5 days or
    - — Acyclovir 200 mg twice daily or 400 mg three times daily for 5 days or
    - — Famciclovir 125 mg twice daily for 5 days
  - ■ **Frequent recurrences**. Long-term suppressive oral therapy may be used for frequent recurrences (more than six recurrences per year), **persistent HSV,** or **recurrent erythema multiforme minor.**
    - — Valacyclovir 500 mg once per day for 6 to 12 months, then an attempt to taper or discontinue
    - — Acyclovir 400 mg twice daily, or
    - — Famciclovir 200 mg twice daily
  - ■ **Immunocompromised hosts,** those with **Kaposi's varicelliform eruption,** or those with **HSV encephalitis** often require intravenous acyclovir therapy.

POINTS TO REMEMBER

- • Recurrent HSV infections should be treated in the prodromal stage, if possible.
- • Valacyclovir should not be used in HIV patients, allogenic bone marrow recipients, and renal transplant recipients.

BASICS

- **Herpes zoster ("shingles")** is caused by the same herpesvirus that causes varicella (chickenpox). The VZV first occurs as varicella (see Chapter 8, "Exanthems"), a primary infection that usually is seen in childhood; subsequently, its second episode as herpes zoster is the result of a reactivation of the same latent virus.
- After resolution of the primary infection, the virus retreats to the dorsal root ganglion where it remains in a dormant state. Reactivation into dermatomal "shingles" may be caused by severe illness or infection with HIV, or it may occur spontaneously, without an obvious precipitating cause. This reemergence as a local vesicobullous eruption derives from the migration of virions through the axon to the skin of a single dermatome or several adjacent dermatomes.
- The pain of herpes zoster is thought to be associated with the nerve damage caused by the virus spreading to the skin through the peripheral nerves. An inflammatory reaction then occurs and leads to scarring of the peripheral nerves and dorsal root ganglia, resulting in hyperexcitability of neurons, which tend to discharge spontaneously, and may lead to postherpetic neuralgia **(PHN).**
- Herpes zoster is seen more commonly in the elderly and in immunocompromised people, such as patients who are HIV-positive, transplant recipients, and people with malignancies, particularly lymphoproliferative malignancies (e.g., Hodgkin's disease). These populations also tend to have more severe herpes zoster, with complications such as PHN, disseminated herpes zoster, and chronic herpes zoster.

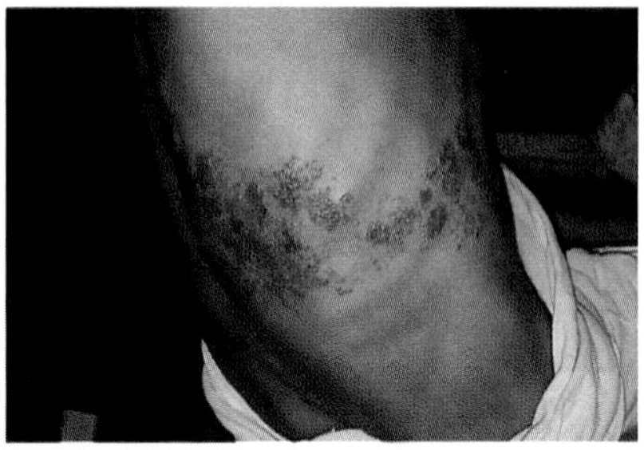

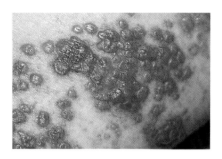

Figure 7.7.
Vesicles and bullae in a zosteriform distribution.

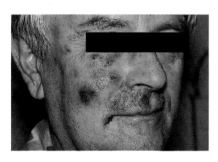

Figure 7.8.
Umbilicated, hemorrhagic blisters.

DESCRIPTION OF LESIONS

- Vesicles or bullae or both occur in a dermatomal ("zosteriform") distribution (Figure 7.7).
- Lesions begin as erythematous papules that usually become clustered vesicles or bullae, which are sometimes umbilicated and pustular and possibly hemorrhagic (Figure 7.8).
- Lesions then rupture or dry, forming erosions and crusts.
- Infrequently, dermatomal neuralgia may be accompanied by nonbullous or urticarial lesions, and rarely, there is a total absence of skin lesions ("zoster sine herpete").

DISTRIBUTION OF LESIONS

- Lesions are characteristically distributed in a unilateral dermatomal ("zosteriform") manner.
- Lesions may involve contiguous dermatomes.
- Most common sites are the thoracic, trigeminal (Figure 7.9), lumbosacral, and cervical areas.
- Immunocompromised patients have a higher risk of multidermatomal zoster, recurrent zoster, and dissemination beyond the skin (e.g., into the eyes or lungs).

Figure 7.9.
Ophthalmic herpes zoster.

CLINICAL MANIFESTATIONS

- Localized acute pain is described as boring, burning, or lancinating.
- Pain and paresthesia in the affected dermatome may accompany the eruption or precede it by 1 to 2 weeks. The pain may mimic a myocardial infarction or pleurisy until the characteristic eruption occurs.
- Herpes zoster may be preceded by a prodrome of headache, malaise, and fever.
- Duration of the eruption is from 2 to 5 weeks in patients with normal immunity.
- Lesions frequently heal with postinflammatory hyper- or hypopigmentation and occasional scarring.
- Acute and chronic pain is significantly increased in patients more than 50 years old.
- Herpes zoster in children is often asymptomatic.

Complications

- **PHN** is defined as pain persisting for more than 1 month after the eruption of herpes zoster lesions. The pain may also develop after a pain-free interval.
- **PHN** occurs more commonly in people with compromised immunity, such as patients with HIV, as well as in elderly people.

DIAGNOSIS

- Herpes zoster can be diagnosed on the basis of clinical appearance.
- Pain is present in the affected dermatome.
- Tzanck smear is positive in HSV and VZV. (See Chapter 26, "Basic Procedures".)
- Skin biopsy can help confirm the diagnosis.
- The following studies are conducted only under special circumstances (e.g., pregnancy):
  - Immunofluorescent antibody stains of vesicle fluid
  - Culture of vesicle fluid
  - Polymerase chain reaction

DIFFERENTIAL DIAGNOSIS

- **HSV**
  - HSV may be indistinguishable from herpes zoster.
  - It is less painful or may be painless.
  - HSV tends to recur.
- **Poison ivy** presenting as linear vesicles or bullae
  - It itches and is painless.
  - The patient often has a history of contact with poison ivy.

MANAGEMENT

- **Acute herpes zoster**
  - **Oral medication**
    - — Oral acyclovir 800 mg every 4 hours, five times per day for 7 to 10 days (immunocompromised patients may require intravenous acyclovir) or
  - — Oral valacyclovir two 500-mg caplets three times daily for 7 days or
  - — Famciclovir 500 mg three times daily for 7 days
  - **Intravenous foscarnet** is used for acyclovir-resistant VZV infection.
  - **Topical therapy** with Burow's solution or other moist soaks with water or saline is soothing.
- **Acute pain.** Pain control is generally the paramount concern in herpes zoster.
  - **Oral analgesics,** such as aspirin, acetaminophen, other nonsteroidal anti-inflammatory drugs (NSAIDs), and mild narcotics are helpful in mild, self-limited cases.
  - Combination of systemic steroids and oral acyclovir, valacyclovir, or famciclovir in patients within 72 hours of the zoster rash may result in faster resolution of acute pain; however, there appears to be no decrease in the subsequent incidence of PHN in these patients.
- **Chronic pain (PHN).** Treatment of PHN has been more problematic. The following measures have met with varying degrees of success:
  - Topical agents, such as lidocaine, capsaicin (Zostrix)
  - Low-dose tricyclic antidepressants, such as amitriptyline
  - Tricyclic antidepressants alone, or combined with phenothiazines
  - Neurosurgical procedures; nerve blocks with local anesthetics
  - Transcutaneous electrical nerve stimulation (TENS)
  - Acupuncture
  - Intralesional corticosteroids
  - Systemic steroids
  - Oral acyclovir, famciclovir, and valacyclovir
  - Combination of systemic steroids and oral acyclovir

 POINTS TO REMEMBER

- Herpes zoster, particularly recurrent or disseminated herpes zoster, may be an early indicator of HIV infection.
- Chickenpox, in susceptible individuals, may be caused by contact with VZV from vesicles of herpes zoster.
- Herpes zoster during pregnancy appears to have no harmful effect on the mother or the infant.
- Ophthalmic zoster warrants an ophthalmologic consultation.
- Nonhealing ulcers and resistant VZV have been reported in patients with AIDS.
- Valacyclovir should not be used in patients infected with HIV.

ANTIVIRAL FORMULARY

ORAL AGENTS

Oral acyclovir	Zovirax 200-mg capsule; 800-mg tablet
Valacyclovir	Valtrex 500-mg caplet; 1-g caplet
Famciclovir	Famvir 125-mg tablet; 500-mg tablet

TOPICAL AGENTS

Topical acyclovir	Zovirax Ointment
Penciclovir cream	Denavir

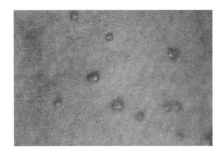

Figure 7.10.
Dome-shaped, waxy papules with central white core.

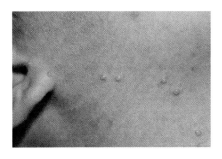

Figure 7.11.
Autoinoculation of lesions ("pseudo-Köebner phenomenon").

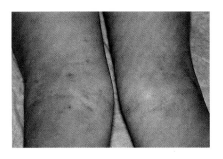

Figure 7.12.
Molluscum contagiosum on lesions of atopic dermatitis.

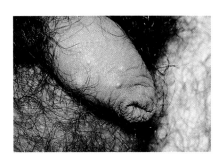

Figure 7.13.
Molluscum contagiosum on penis.

BASICS

- **Molluscum contagiosum** is a common superficial viral infection of the epidermis. It is spread by skin-to-skin contact and is caused by a large DNA-containing poxvirus. It is seen most often in three clinical contexts:
  - Young healthy children (infants and preschoolers), in whom the incidence decreases after the age of 6 or 7 years
  - Patients who are HIV-positive, who are susceptible to and commonly infected by molluscum contagiosum
  - Young adults who are sexually active and non-HIV–positive, in whom molluscum contagiosum is uncommon, but when it occurs, is usually spread by sexual transmission to the external genitalia

DESCRIPTION OF LESIONS

- The lesions are dome-shaped, waxy or pearly white papules with a central white core (Figure 7.10). Less frequently, the papules are flesh-colored.
- Lesions are generally 1 mm to 3 mm in diameter.
- Frequently, the lesions are grouped.

DISTRIBUTION OF LESIONS

- Usually lesions are asymmetric, depending on sites of initial inoculation.
- They are spread by autoinoculation ("pseudo-Köebner" phenomenon; Figure 7.11) by picking and rubbing. They are also spread in men who are HIV-positive by shaving of the beard.
- Lesions can appear in areas of the skin that are traumatized or inflamed, as seen in the flexural creases in children who have underlying atopic dermatitis at these sites (Figure 7.12).
- They may be seen on the external genitalia (Figure 7.13).
- They can also appear on the face, trunk, axilla, extremities, and eyelids (Figure 7.14).

CLINICAL MANIFESTATIONS

- Generally asymptomatic, molluscum contagiosum may itch slightly, be scratched, and become secondarily infected.
- The course is self-limiting, and recurrences are rare in immunocompetent individuals.
- Molluscum contagiosum in patients with HIV is common (see Chapter 24, "The Cutaneous Manifestations of HIV Infection").
  - More than 100 lesions may be seen.
  - They appear most commonly on the face (Figure 7.15).
  - The "giant" molluscum, or coalescent double or triple lesions are frequently seen in these patients.
  - The lesions are often chronic and disfiguring and are difficult to eradicate.

DIAGNOSIS

- Typical papules are easily recognized.

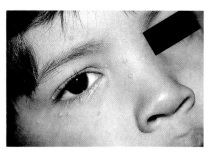

Figure 7.14.
Molluscum contagiosum on face and eyelids.

- Inspection with a hand-held magnifier often reveals the central core.
- A short application of cryotherapy with liquid nitrogen (LN_2) accentuates the central core (Figure 7.16).
- A direct microscopic smear of a lesion (crush preparation) demonstrates characteristic "molluscum bodies" (Figure 7.17).
- A shave biopsy is performed, if necessary.

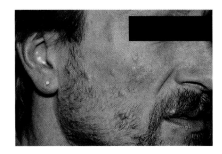

Figure 7.15.
Molluscum contagiosum on face of patient with AIDS.

DIFFERENTIAL DIAGNOSIS

- **Warts**, especially small flat warts (Figure 7.18)
  - Warts are not waxy.
  - They are tan or brown in color.
  - They have no central white core.
- **Condylomata acuminata** on the penis (Figure 7.19)
  - There is no central core.
  - A biopsy may be necessary to differentiate from molluscum contagiosum.
- **Disseminated cryptococcosis, toxoplasmosis,** and **histoplasmosis in AIDS patients**, which may need biopsy to differentiate from molluscum contagiosum (see Chapter 24, "The Cutaneous Manifestations of HIV Infection")

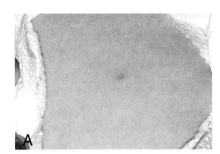

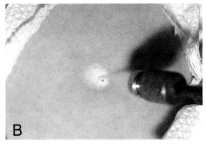

Figure 7.16.
(*A*) Short application of liquid nitrogen (LN_2); (*B*) LN_2 accentuates the central core.

MANAGEMENT

- Lesions on an infant or young preschool child should not be treated aggressively.
- **Lesions may be ignored** until they resolve spontaneously, or
- They may be treated with a **topical antiwart preparation**, such as **Duofilm**, applied daily to the core of each lesion with a toothpick or
- They may be **frozen lightly with LN_2** applied with a Q-Tip or a CRY-Ac or Cryogun spray apparatus.
- A **topical vesicant (blistering agent)**, such as cantharidin, may be applied carefully to each lesion or
- Lesions may also be flicked off with a sharp curette while using manual traction on the skin, or
- **Electrodesiccation and curettage** may be necessary for patients with refractory lesions.
- **Trichloroacetic acid peels** have been performed with some success in patients with HIV with extensive lesions.

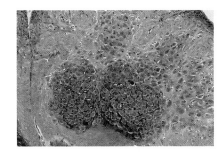

Figure 7.17.
"Molluscum bodies."

POINTS TO REMEMBER

- Molluscum contagiosum in an adult should alert the clinician to the possibility of HIV infection.
- For anxious children, a topical anesthetic, such as EMLA Cream, may be applied 1 hour before treatment with LN_2.

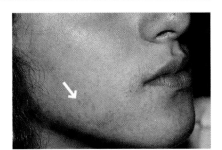

Figure 7.18.
Flat warts (*arrow*).

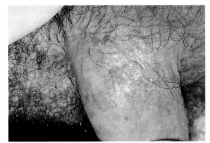

Figure 7.19.
Condyloma acuminatum.

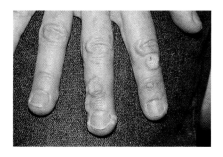

Figure 7.20.
Multiple warts

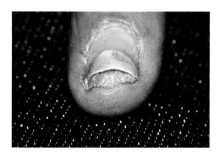

Figure 7.21.
Subungual wart, easily mistaken for onychomycosis.

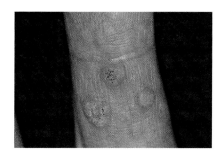

Figure 7.22.
Finger verrucae with "black dots."

BASICS

- Warts are extremely common, particularly in the pediatric age group. It has been estimated that 20% of school-age children will at some time have one or more warts.
- Warts are easy to diagnose and tend to regress spontaneously, particularly in children. In some adults and in immunocompromised individuals, they often prove difficult to eradicate.
- All warts are caused by the **human papilloma virus (HPV)**, of which there are more than 70 different subtypes.
- The virus infects keratinocytes, which stimulate epidermal proliferation.
- Transmission is primarily through skin-to-skin contact.
- The different names for warts generally reflect their clinical appearance, location, or both.

DESCRIPTION OF LESIONS

Warts are papillomatous, corrugated, hyperkeratotic growths confined to the epidermis. They may be found on any area of the body, but they have distinct regional predilections, particularly at sites subject to frequent trauma.

COMMON WARTS (VERRUCAE VULGARIS)

DISTRIBUTION OF LESIONS

- Common warts occur most often on the hands and fingers (Figure 7.20); they also can be found around (periungual) and beneath (subungual) nails (Figure 7.21).
- They occur as well on the knees and elbows, especially in children.
- Distribution is generally asymmetrical.

CLINICAL MANIFESTATIONS

- Common warts have a verrucous, or vegetative, appearance.
- Lesions show loss of normal skin markings (e.g., finger and hand prints).
- "Black dots," or thrombosed capillaries, are pathognomonic (Figure 7.22).

DIFFERENTIAL DIAGNOSIS

There is usually little difficulty in diagnosing warts; however, it is important to keep in mind the following in the appropriate clinical setting:

- Seborrheic keratosis (benign; Figure 7.23)
- Solar keratosis
- Squamous cell carcinoma

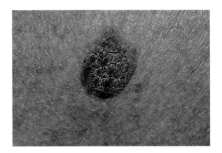

Figure 7.23.
Typical seborrheic keratosis.

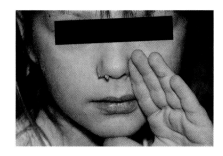

Figure 7.24.
Filiform wart.

Filiform warts are another variation of common warts, which are more common in children.

DISTRIBUTION OF LESIONS

Filiform warts are most commonly seen on the face, usually around the ala nasi, mouth, and eyelids, and on the neck.

CLINICAL MANIFESTATIONS

There are tan, fingerlike projections that emanate from the skin (Figure 7.24).

DIFFERENTIAL DIAGNOSIS

See "Common Warts."

PLANTAR WARTS

DISTRIBUTION OF LESIONS

- Plantar warts are usually seen on the metatarsal area, heels, and toes.
- Distribution is asymmetrical.

CLINICAL MANIFESTATIONS

- The warts may be painful upon pressure from footwear or from walking.
- They may occur as a solitary lesion, multiple lesions, or clustered lesions (mosaic warts; Figure 7.25).
- Black dots, or thrombosed capillaries, can be demonstrated after paring with a #15 blade (Figure 7.26).
- There is loss of normal skin markings (i.e., footprints).

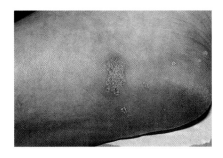

Figure 7.25.
Clustering (mosaic) warts.

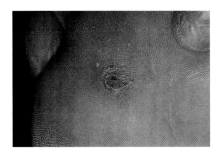

Figure 7.26.
Plantar wart. Punctate bleeding after paring.

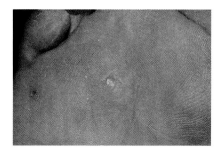

Figure 7.27.
Corn.

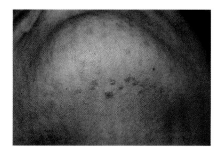

Figure 7.28.
Verruca plana. Note subtle skin-colored flat papules on chin.

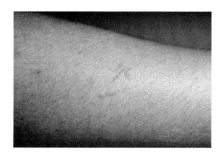

Figure 7.29.
Flat warts showing linear configuration due to autoinoculation.

DIFFERENTIAL DIAGNOSIS

- **Corn** (clavus; Figure 7.27)
  - Corns tend to be painful on direct pressure.
  - Corns occur at sites of repeated friction and pressure.
  - Skin markings are retained.
  - There is a central translucent core.
  - Corns do not have black dots.

FLAT WARTS (VERRUCA PLANA)

Figure 7.28

DISTRIBUTION OF LESIONS

- Flat warts occur on the forehead, cheeks, chin, arms, and dorsa of the hands.
- They are also commonly found in the beard area in men and on the shins in women, where the lesions are spread by shaving.

CLINICAL MANIFESTATIONS

- The lesions are comprised of flat, well-defined skin-colored or brown papules that are 1 mm to 5 mm in size.
- Sometimes flat warts show a linear configuration because of autoinoculation (Figure 7.29).

DIFFERENTIAL DIAGNOSIS

- Molluscum contagiosum (Figure 7.30), which occurs as shiny, waxy, dome-shaped papules with a central white core
- **Genital warts** are discussed in Chapter 19, Sexually Transmitted Disease.

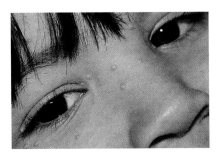

Figure 7.30.
Molluscum contagiosum.

MANAGEMENT

The hero of successful wart treatment is usually the last person to treat the wart or the last person to recommend a treatment before the wart regresses. The **wart hero** may have been a wart charmer, a dermatologist, or an application of garlic. More often than not, warts tend to cure themselves over the passage of time, especially in immunocompetent individuals. This should be borne in mind and explained to patients early in the course of therapy.

- The method of treatment chosen depends on the age of the patient, the patient's pain threshold, and the location of the lesions.
- Social factors are also important. For example, a 2-year-old child with a filiform wart located near the ala nasi, or with multiple hand warts, should warrant less aggressive treatment than a 6-year-old kindergartner with similar lesions who may suffer from the needling of other children.
- The abundant treatment modalities available are a reflection of the fact that none of them is uniformly effective.

TREATMENT OF COMMON WARTS (VERRUCAE VULGARIS)

Painful aggressive therapy should be avoided initially, especially in children. Unless there is a pressing need to eliminate the wart, the following suggestions are given in a stepwise fashion so as to begin with methods that are the least painful:

- **Topical salicylic acid preparations**
  - There are many over-the-counter preparations that can be self-administered, such as Compound W, Duofilm, and Occlusal-HP.
  - Mediplast is a 40% salicylic acid plaster, which is cut to fit the size of the wart.
  - **Advantages**
    - Best treatment for small children (especially because warts are self-limiting)
    - Can be used on periungual warts
    - Nonscarring
    - Painless application
    - Relatively inexpensive
    - Do not require office visits
  - **Disadvantages**
    - Slower response
    - Time-consuming daily application

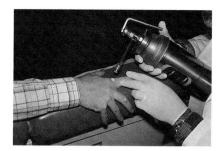

Figure 7.31.
Cryotherapy with liquid nitrogen (LN₂).

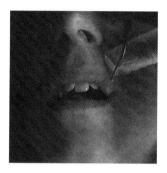

Figure 7.32.
Electrodesiccation.

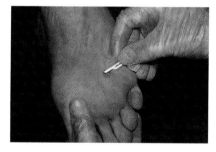

Figure 7.33.
Paring plantar wart.

- LN$_2$ (See Chapter 26, "Cryotherapy," Basic Procedures, for technique; Figure 7.31)
  - **Advantages**
  - Best for warts on hands
    — Fast; can treat many lesions per visit
  - **Disadvantages**
    — Availability of LN$_2$ unit and storage of holding tank
    — Painful; must be used cautiously on fingertips and on periungual lesions
    — Scarring if treatment is overly aggressive
    — Often requires multiple office visits
- **Light electrocautery, blunt dissection, or both** (Figure 7.32)
  - **Advantages**
    — Best for warts on knees, elbows, dorsa of hands
    — Good for filiform warts
    — Tolerable in most adults
  - **Disadvantages**
    — Can be very painful, especially on fingers and soles of feet
    — Requires local anesthesia, sometimes digital block
    — Potentially scarring

TREATMENT OF PLANTAR WARTS

- **Simple paring** with a **#15** blade parallel to the skin surface (Figure 7.33) often affords immediate relief of pain upon walking.
- **Self-application of salicylic acid preparations or sanding** with an emery board often keeps the wart flat, and, thus, pain free.
- **Mediplast** (40% salicylic plaster) is useful for large mosaic warts.
- LN$_2$, blunt dissection, electrodesiccation, and curettage are reserved for the more recalcitrant warts or when patients insist upon aggressive therapy.

OTHER TREATMENTS

- **Chemical applications**, such as cantharidin, a blistering agent, bi- and trichloroacetic acids, and formalin
- **Laser ablation, intralesional bleomycin, immunotherapy with topical sensitizing agents, and oral immunomodulating techniques** such as high-dose oral cimetidine have been used with varying degrees of success. These methods often require multiple office visits and may be expensive; some have potential side effects.

POINTS TO REMEMBER

- For small filiform warts in children and adults, a quick snip with sharp iris scissors may be done without local anesthesia (pressure is applied for 5 to 10 minutes to obtain hemostasis.) Similarly, light LN$_2$ and electrocautery may be used without anesthesia.
- Multiple filiform warts may be seen in the beard area and are difficult to eliminate.
- For anxious children and adults, a topical anesthetic, EMLA, may be applied 1 hour before potentially painful treatment. Two percent lidocaine jelly is often helpful before treating mucous membranes.
- Topical cantharidin may be used on periungual warts if salicylic acid fails.
- Flat warts may be treated initially with a tretinoin cream such as Retin-A. Cautious application of LN$_2$ or light electrodesiccation may also be effective.

CHAPTER 8

EXANTHEMS

Kenneth Howe

Basics

- Viral exanthems are the **cutaneous manifestation of an acute viral infection**. In most exanthems, viral particles are present within the visible lesions, having reached the skin through the bloodstream. It is unclear whether the observed exanthem results from active viral infection of the skin, the immune response to the virus, or a combination of these two.
- Most common in children, viral exanthems may be seen as distinct, clinically recognizable illnesses such as measles or chickenpox. More frequently, however, a nonspecific eruption is seen, making an exact diagnosis elusive. More than 50 viral agents are known to cause exanthems, and many of these rashes are indistinguishable from one another. A specific diagnosis is often not made because **most viral illnesses are benign and self-limited.**
- In some situations, however, determining the precise cause may be of vital importance. Examples include the appearance of a viral exanthem in a pregnant woman or in an immunocompromised patient. It is also important to distinguish viral exanthems from rashes caused by treatable bacterial or rickettsial infections and from hypersensitivity reactions to medications.

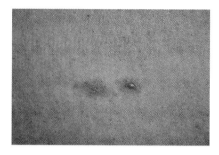

Figure 8.1.
Varicella. "Dew drops on rose petals."

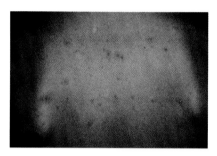

Figure 8.2.
Varicella. Lesions in various stages of development.

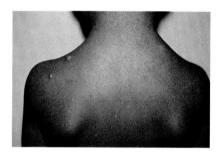

Figure 8.3.
Varicella. Hypertrophic scars on trunk.

BASICS

- Varicella, or chickenpox, is an infection caused by the **varicella-zoster virus** (VZV). Transmission occurs by aerosolized droplet spread, with initial infection occurring in the mucosa of the upper respiratory tract. Traveling through the blood and lymphatics (primary viremia), a small amount of virus reaches cells of the reticuloendothelial system, where the virus replicates during the remainder of the incubation period. Nonspecific host defenses contain the incubating infection at this point, but, in most cases, these defenses are eventually overwhelmed, resulting in a large secondary viremia. It is through this secondary viremia that VZV reaches the skin. The viremia occurs cyclically over a period of approximately 3 days, resulting in successive crops of lesions.
- Most cases occur during childhood, and half of the patients are younger than 5 years old.
- Epidemics have a peak incidence during late winter and spring.

DESCRIPTION OF LESIONS

- The characteristic lesions begin as **red macules** and progress rapidly from **papules** to **vesicles** to **pustules** to **crusts.** The entire cycle may occur within 8 to 12 hours. The typical vesicles are superficial, thin-walled, and surrounded by an irregular area of erythema, giving them the appearance of a "dew drop on a rose petal" (Figure 8.1).
- The lesions are usually pruritic.
- Involvement of the oral mucous membranes also occurs, most commonly on the palate. As vesicles in these sites quickly rupture, it is more common to observe shallow erosions.
- As the lesions appear in successive crops, a characteristic feature of varicella is the simultaneous presence of **lesions in varying stages of development** (Figure 8.2). In any given area, macules, vesicles, pustules, and crusts may be seen.
- Crusts usually fall off within 1 to 3 weeks, depending on the depth of involvement. Extensive scarring is unusual in uncomplicated varicella; however, facial punched-out scars are fairly common, as are raised scars on the trunk (Figure 8.3).
- Large blisters (superimposed bullous impetigo) can also be seen in varicella, often as a result of superinfection with *Staphylococcus aureus*.

DISTRIBUTION OF LESIONS

The eruption typically begins on the face, scalp, and trunk and then spreads to involve the extremities. Successive crops appear during a 3- to 5-day period, resulting in a diffuse, widespread eruption of discrete lesions.

CLINICAL MANIFESTATIONS

- **Incubation period**
  - Duration of incubation is typically 14 days (a range of 10 to 21 days).
  - During this period, children are usually asymptomatic, with onset of the rash being the first sign of illness.
  - In older children and adults, symptoms are typically more severe. The rash is frequently preceded by 2 to 3 days of fever and flulike symptoms, which often persist during the acute illness.
- **Complications of varicella**
  - Complications in healthy children are rare and occur more commonly in infected adults.
  - Varicella pneumonia is a relatively uncommon complication, which usually occurs in adults. It begins 1 to 6 days after onset of the rash, with pulmonary symptoms such as cough, dyspnea, and pleuritic chest pain. The severity of the symptoms is out of proportion to the findings on physical examination. Chest radiographs typically reveal diffuse nodular densities.

DIAGNOSIS

The diagnosis of varicella is usually straightforward **based on the characteristic presentation and clinical findings**.
- A **Tzanck smear** can be helpful in confirming the diagnosis (see Chapter 26, "Basic Procedures"). It reveals characteristic multinucleated giant cells. Identical findings are seen in herpes zoster and herpes simplex virus (HSV) infections.
- Smears obtained from active lesions can be tested by the direct immunofluorescence technique, which uses fluorescent-labeled antibodies to detect the presence of VZV. This technique has a sensitivity and specificity nearly equal to that of culture, with the advantage of providing rapid results.
- Active lesions can also be cultured for VZV.

DIFFERENTIAL DIAGNOSIS

- **Other viral exanthems**
  - Vesicular exanthems of **coxsackievirus** and **echovirus** may be mistaken for varicella.
  - These exanthems may show a characteristic distribution, as in **hand-foot-and-mouth disease** (HFMD).
- **Disseminated herpes zoster**
  - Patients have a previous history of primary varicella.
  - There is a typical zosteriform dermatomal eruption in addition to a widespread rash indistinguishable from varicella.
  - The patient is generally immunocompromised, secondary to medications, malignancy, or HIV.
- **Eczema herpeticum** (Kaposi's varicelliform eruption)
  - Preexisting skin disease, such as atopic dermatitis, becomes secondarily infected with HSV.
  - Direct immunofluorescence or culture results are indicative of HSV infection.
- **Atypical measles** occurs in adults who received killed measles virus vaccine from 1963 to 1967.
  - Eruption begins on palms and soles, then spreads proximally.
  - Pneumonia is a common feature.
  - Diagnosis can be confirmed by a rise in measles antibody titers.
- **Impetigo**
  - The patient generally feels well.
  - Moist, honey-colored crusts are characteristic and are often periorificial.
  - Lesions are fewer and distribution is less symmetrical than in chickenpox.
  - Bacterial cultures reveal the presence of *S. aureus* and, less commonly, *Streptococcus pyogenes*.

MANAGEMENT

- Acute varicella
  - Uncomplicated varicella in otherwise healthy children is generally managed with **supportive care** in the form of antipruritics and antipyretics. **Aspirin should be avoided because of the risk of Reye's syndrome.**
  - **Oral acyclovir** is warranted in patients at increased risk for the development of complications and, in general, should be started within 24 hours of the onset of the rash. These patients include:
    — Otherwise healthy, nonpregnant individuals 13 years old and older
    — Children older than 12 months with chronic skin or pulmonary conditions or who are receiving long-term salicylate therapy
    — Children receiving short, intermittent or aerosolized courses of corticosteroids.
  - **Intravenous acyclovir.** Treatment with intravenous acyclovir is indicated in immunocompromised patients or patients with virally mediated complications of varicella.
  - **Varicella vaccine**. The VZV vaccine (Varivax) is recommended as universal immunization in all children.
    — It is optimally given between age 12 and 18 months and may be administered in a single dose at any time before 13 years of age.
    — In older adolescents or adults, two doses of vaccine should be administered 4 to 8 weeks apart.
- **Varicella and pregnancy**
  - Peripartum maternal varicella poses a particular risk to the newborn. Neonates born 2 days before or 5 days after the onset of maternal varicella should be given varicella-zoster immune globulin (VZIG). Those newborns who develop varicella should be treated with intravenous acyclovir.
  - Pregnant patients in whom varicella develops in the first trimester have a 2.3 to 4.9% risk of delivering a child with the **fetal varicella syndrome**.
    — This syndrome is a congenital malformation complex with features such as intrauterine growth retardation, prematurity, cicatricial lesions in a dermatomal distribution, limb paresis and hypoplasia, chorioretinitis, and cataracts.
    — It is not known whether the administration of acyclovir will prevent these complications.

POINT TO REMEMBER

Patients remain contagious until all cutaneous lesions are crusted.

HAND-FOOT-AND-MOUTH DISEASE

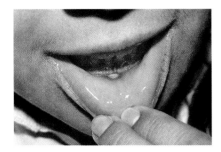

Figure 8.4.
Hand-foot-and-mouth disease (HFMD).
Oral lesion.

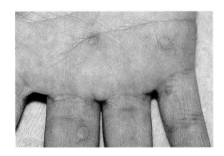

Figure 8.5.
Hand-foot-and-mouth disease (HFMD).
Oval vesicles on the palm.

BASICS

- HFMD is an acute viral infection that manifests as a vesicular eruption with a characteristic distribution. The infection is caused by enteroviruses, most commonly **coxsackievirus A16.** The virus is spread from person to person by the fecal–oral route.
- Outbreaks are typically in the summer or early fall, and epidemics may occur. Transmission is more likely in crowded environments.
- Young children (ages 1 to 5 years) are most commonly infected.
- The incubation period ranges from 4 to 6 days.

DESCRIPTION OF LESIONS

- Oral lesions are the first manifestation of HFMD. Although lesions are initially vesicular, it is more common to see **multiple shallow erosions** because the vesicles are fragile.
- Individual lesions may range in size from **1 to 5 mm in diameter,** and they may exhibit a rim of erythema. These oral lesions may be painful, and they frequently interfere with eating (Figure 8.4).
- The **exanthem** consists of round or angulated, grayish-white vesicles typically **3 to 7 mm in diameter.** These **vesicles,** which are located **on the palms and soles,** have a characteristic oval or linear shape and tend not to rupture (Figure 8.5).

DISTRIBUTION OF LESIONS

- The oral lesions appear most commonly on the **tongue** and **buccal mucosa** and occasionally on the lips, palate, and gums.
- The exanthem is characteristically present on the **hands** and **feet.** Lesions occur on the dorsal or lateral aspects of the fingers and toes and on the palms and soles.
- All sites may not be involved at the time of presentation.

CLINICAL MANIFESTATIONS

- The illness most frequently begins as a **sore throat** or mouth. In young children, **refusal to eat** is often a presenting sign.
- Occasionally, a 1- to 2-day prodrome of fever and abdominal pain may be seen.
- The acral eruption follows the development of oral lesions. It is usually not pruritic, although it may be painful.
- In contrast to most viral illnesses, **lymphadenopathy is absent to minimal.**

DIAGNOSIS

- Diagnosis is made on the basis of the characteristic **clinical presentation.**
- Although not routinely indicated, **laboratory testing** can confirm the diagnosis.
  - Virus can be cultured from throat washings or stool, with the latter giving a higher yield.
  - Acute and convalescent sera show an increase in antibody titer to the causative virus.

DIFFERENTIAL DIAGNOSIS

- **Primary oral HSV infection**
  - Usually the lips and gingiva are affected, and the back of the throat is spared.
  - There are recurrent outbreaks.
  - Tzanck smear and culture are positive for HSV.
- **Aphthous ulcers**
  - Lesions are painful.
  - As with HSV, the lips and gingiva are usually affected and the back of the throat is spared.

MANAGEMENT

Treatment is with **supportive care**. Antipyretics and a clear liquid diet while the throat is sore is typically all that is necessary.

POINTS TO REMEMBER

- The course of the illness is self-limited, lasting less than 1 week in most cases.
- Although in general complications are rare, the one seen most frequently is **aseptic meningitis.**

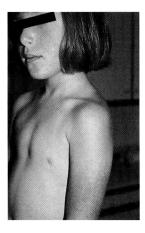

Figure 8.6.
Erythema infectiosum (EI). "Slapped cheek" appearance and reticulate erythema on the arm.

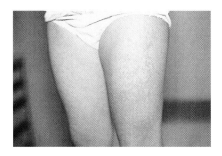

Figure 8.7.
Erythema infectiosum (EI). Reticulate erythema on the legs.

BASICS

- Erythema infectiosum (EI) is a common viral illness caused by infection with **parvovirus B19**. Transmission is person-to-person, probably through respiratory secretions.
- EI occurs most commonly in the late winter and spring. Epidemics are frequently seen, particularly among school-age children.
- The incubation period is 4 to 14 days but may be as long as 3 weeks.
- By the time the characteristic exanthem appears, the patient is unlikely to be infectious.

DESCRIPTION OF LESIONS

- EI is most commonly identified in children by characteristic facial erythema. Bright red, macular, and tending to involve the malar surfaces, this eruption has a **slapped cheek appearance** (Figure 8.6).
- An exanthem also appears on the extremities and trunk (Figure 8.7). This develops 1 to 4 days after the facial erythema and begins as a macular or macular and papular erythema, which then clears centrally to produce a characteristic **reticular (lacy) pattern.**
- Although the exanthem usually resolves in 1 to 2 weeks, the reticular erythema may have a recrudescent course in some patients, which is often exacerbated by sunlight.

DISTRIBUTION OF LESIONS

- The **facial erythema** favors the malar surfaces. The slapped cheek appearance is further accentuated by a tendency to spare the nasal bridge and the periorbital and perioral areas.
- The reticular erythema most commonly affects the **extensor surfaces of the extremities and the buttocks.** The palms and soles are usually spared.

CLINICAL MANIFESTATIONS

- Although **facial erythema** is the most common initial presentation, some patients experience a mild prodrome of low-grade fever, malaise, upper respiratory or gastrointestinal symptoms, and myalgias.
- EI can be associated with **joint symptoms** in adults, particularly in women. A symmetrical polyarthropathy develops, involving the hands, feet, elbows, and knees.
- The illness is benign and self-limited, with the exanthem resolving within 1 to 2 weeks.
- Although joint symptoms generally resolve within 2 to 3 weeks, it is not uncommon for them to persist for several months.
- EI during pregnancy may result in **fetal death** resulting from the development of **hydrops fetalis.** Infection with parvovirus B19 can lead to **aplastic crisis** in patients with chronic anemias such as sickle cell disease, hereditary spherocytosis, and thalassemia intermedia.
- Immunocompromised patients in whom chronic parvovirus B19 infection develops are at risk for **chronic red cell aplasia** or more generalized **bone marrow failure.**

DIAGNOSIS

- The diagnosis is based on the characteristic **clinical presentation**.
- Although usually unnecessary, **serologic testing** is the most accurate method of confirming infection. The presence of IgM antibodies to parvovirus B19 is indicative of recent infection. These antibodies appear approximately 3 days after the onset of the exanthem and begin to decline 1 to 2 months later.

DIFFERENTIAL DIAGNOSIS

- **Erysipelas** is distinguished by high fever and pain.
- **Systemic lupus erythematosus**
  - Difficult to differentiate from EI with associated joint symptoms
  - Positive antinuclear antibodies
  - Other signs of systemic involvement, such as serositis, renal disease, and central nervous system involvement

MANAGEMENT

Supportive care is all that is required for uncomplicated cases. No effective antiviral therapy exists for parvovirus B19.

POINTS TO REMEMBER

- Facial erythema is often absent in infected adults.
- Because they are at risk for aplastic crisis, all EI patients with a chronic anemia should have a complete blood cell count evaluated.

BASICS

- Roseola infantum (RI), or **exanthem subitum,** is an acute viral illness marked by a high fever, which characteristically resolves with the onset of the rash.
- RI is caused by infection with **human herpesvirus 6** (HHV-6).
- Although the exact route of transmission is unknown, it is probably spread through oral or respiratory secretions.
- Following HHV-6 exposure, there is an incubation period of 7 to 15 days before onset of symptoms.
- As with other herpesvirus infections, it is likely that HHV-6 establishes a latent infection after the acute illness. The isolation of HHV-6 from the saliva of healthy adults lends support to this view.

DESCRIPTION OF LESIONS

- The exanthem appears 1 day before to 1 day after defervescence.
- It consists of **discrete macules** or **papules, 1 to 5 mm in diameter,** often with a surrounding rim of pallor. The color of these lesions has been described as **rose pink.** Frequently, the individual lesions coalesce to form areas of confluent erythema.
- The exanthem typically clears within 1 to 2 days, although it may persist for up to 10 days.

DISTRIBUTION

Distribution is **widespread**, with lesions appearing on the trunk, buttocks, neck, and, occasionally, the face and limbs.

CLINICAL MANIFESTATIONS

- A **febrile illness** typically precedes the exanthem by 3 to 5 days. Characteristically, this prodrome is marked by a high fever in an otherwise well child.
- On occasion, the fever is accompanied by coryza, cough, headache, or abdominal pain.
- Occipital, cervical, and postauricular **lymphadenopathy** are commonly present.
- **Complications** are uncommon and include **seizures, encephalitis,** and **thrombocytopenia.**

DIAGNOSIS

- The characteristic **clinical presentation** is usually sufficient for diagnosis.
- Although rarely necessary, the diagnosis can be confirmed by **laboratory studies** demonstrating either the presence of IgM to HHV-6 or a fourfold increase in IgG titers to the virus.

DIFFERENTIAL DIAGNOSIS

- **Febrile viral exanthems** must be ruled out.
- **Scarlet fever** has severe constitutional symptoms and characteristic oral changes. It resolves with acral desquamation.
- **Measles** are distinguished by Koplik's spots, severe upper respiratory tract infection symptoms, and the long duration of the rash.
- **Rubella** tends to occur in older children and lacks a high fever.

MANAGEMENT

During the prodromal phase of illness, **antipyretics** are often useful, particularly because they may reduce the risk of febrile seizures.

POINT TO REMEMBER

Infection with HHV-6 is one of the most common causes of febrile illness in young children.

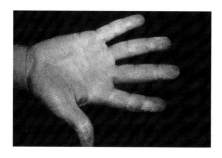

Figure 8.8.
Kawasaki's syndrome. Peeling off of skin from the fingertips.

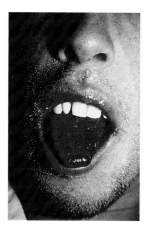

Figure 8.9.
Kawasaki's syndrome. "Strawberry tongue."

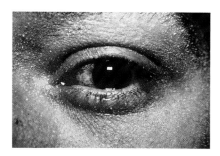

Figure 8.10.
Kawasaki's syndrome. Ocular involvement.

BASICS

- Kawasaki syndrome (KS), also known as **mucocutaneous lymph node syndrome,** is an acute, febrile, multisystem illness that primarily affects young children. Its most serious complications are the result of a **systemic vasculopathy.**
- The **peak incidence** of KS is **between 1 and 2 years of age**. It is more common in boys.
- In the United States, children of Asian ancestry are affected 6 times more often than whites, whereas African American children are affected 1.5 times more often than whites.
- KS occurs sporadically and in epidemics. A seasonal predilection has been observed, with more cases occurring in the winter and spring.
- Although the exact cause of KS is unknown, it is most likely the result of a superantigen produced by an infectious agent such as *S. aureus*, resulting in massive cytokine release.

DESCRIPTION OF LESIONS

- The **truncal rash** of KS is polymorphous and may be scarlatiniform, morbilliform, or targetoid in appearance.
- **Changes of the hands and feet** are distinctive. An intense erythema appears on the palms and soles on days 3 to 5 of the illness, followed by an indurated edema. A sharp demarcation may be seen at the wrists and the sides of the hands and feet. During the convalescent phase of the illness, the **skin of the fingertips and toes peels off in sheets** (Figure 8.8).
- The presence of a **scarlatiniform erythema in the perineal area** may be a useful diagnostic sign. The rash in this area progresses to desquamation before the palms and soles begin to peel.
- Characteristic findings are present in the mouth, lips, and tongue. The earliest manifestations are seen on the **lips,** with **bright red erythema** accompanied by **cracking and swelling**. Prominent papillae create the appearance of a **"strawberry tongue"** (Figure 8.9). Examination of the oropharynx reveals a diffuse erythema without vesicles, erosions, or ulcers.
- **Eye involvement** (Figure 8.10) consists of bilateral, nonpurulent conjunctival infection. Patients may exhibit signs of photophobia.

DISTRIBUTION OF LESIONS

The **polymorphous eruption** favors the **trunk** and proximal **extremities** but may be generalized.

CLINICAL MANIFESTATIONS

- **Fever** usually marks the onset of KS. Elevated temperature shows a remittent pattern, with spikes to 103°F to 105°F. The average duration of the fever is 11 days.
- Seen in 75% of patients, **cervical lymphadenopathy** is the least common of the diagnostic features of KS. It usually manifests as a single, enlarged, nonsuppurative node on one side of the neck.
- **Cardiac involvement** is the most worrisome complication of KS. During the acute phase of the illness, tachycardia may develop, with gallop rhythm, subtle electrocardiographic changes, pericardial effusion, tricuspid insufficiency, or mitral regurgitation. Coronary artery aneurisms may result in thrombosis with subsequent infarction.

DIAGNOSIS

- The diagnosis of KS is based on recognition of its **clinical features**, supported by compatible laboratory findings.
- **Laboratory findings** in KS are **nonspecific but consistent.** None of these findings are in themselves diagnostic, but the pattern can be used to include or exclude KS.
- Diagnostic guidelines for KS include the following **principal signs**:
  - Fever persisting 5 days or more
  - Polymorphous rash
  - Bilateral conjunctival infection
  - Oral mucous membrane changes
  - Cervical lymphadenopathy
  - Changes of peripheral extremities: erythema of palms and soles, indurative edema of hands and feet, desquamation of fingertips

DIFFERENTIAL DIAGNOSIS

- **Staphylococcal or streptococcal toxic shock syndrome**
- **Scarlet fever**
- **Measles**
- **Febrile viral exanthems**
- **Hypersensitivity reactions (including Stevens-Johnson syndrome)**

MANAGEMENT

- Most children with KS are **hospitalized** for a complete workup and **supportive care**. Because high temperature and irritability make feeding difficult, **intravenous fluids** are often needed for hydration.
- Children with evidence of cardiac disease may require intensive support.
- Once the diagnosis of KS has been established, therapy with **intravenous γ-globulin** and **aspirin** should be started.

POINTS TO REMEMBER

- All patients with KS should have an echocardiogram during the acute illness and 3 to 6 weeks after onset of fever.
- Prompt treatment with aspirin and intravenous γ-globulin significantly lowers the risk of cardiac complications.
- KS should be considered in children with an unexplained fever lasting more than 5 days, who have a polymorphous rash that may look like scarlet fever or measles, and a conjunctival infection without pus.

BASICS

- Rubella is a **mild viral illness**, which, because of its **devastating effects on the developing human fetus,** is recognized as a major public health issue.
  - **Maternal infection** may lead to **fetal death** or **permanent damage.** The consequences are more severe when the infection occurs during the first 8 weeks of gestation. Fetal damage is rare after 5 months gestation.
  - **Sensory neural hearing loss, cataracts,** and **cardiac anomalies** are the most common defects of congenital rubella.
- The rubella virus is an RNA virus of the Togaviridae family. Humans are the only known natural host. The initial infection occurs in the nasopharyngeal mucosa.
- The incidence of rubella has declined markedly since **mass immunization for rubella began in 1969.**

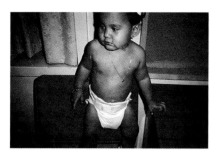

Figure 8.11.
Rubella. Exanthem on trunk (second day). (Courtesy of Steven R. Cohen)

DESCRIPTION OF LESIONS

- The eruption consists of **pink to red macules** with faint pinpoint papules.
- Initially discrete, the lesions may coalesce to form an **erythematous rash similar to that of scarlet fever** (Figure 8.11).
- The eruption may be pruritic, particularly in adults.

DISTRIBUTION OF LESIONS

- The **eruption begins on the face** and spreads within 24 hours to the trunk and extremities.
- The exanthem of rubella is characteristically short-lived, with resolution beginning on the first or second day of the rash. Resolution proceeds in a cephalocaudad direction and may be accompanied by a fine desquamation.

CLINICAL MANIFESTATIONS

- A mild prodromal illness is the earliest clinical feature of infection.
  - A **mild fever** develops, accompanied by **lymphadenopathy**. The lymphadenopathy most commonly affects the postauricular, suboccipital, and posterior cervical nodes and may be impressive.
  - In older patients, the prodrome may be longer and more severe.
- Constitutional symptoms usually resolve within 24 hours of the onset of the rash. In some cases, however, the lymphadenopathy persists for weeks.
- **Complications are rare**.

DIAGNOSIS

- The clinical features of rubella are not distinctive enough to allow one to make the diagnosis with certainty based on clinical presentation alone.
- Acute and convalescent **antibody titers can confirm the diagnosis**. Although unnecessary in most cases, these tests are important in pregnant women exposed to rubella.

DIFFERENTIAL DIAGNOSIS

- **Measles**
  - Prodromal symptoms of greater severity
  - Koplik's spots
  - Longer duration of rash
- **Roseola**
  - High prodromal temperature in absence of other symptoms
  - Morphologic appearance and duration of the exanthem similar to those of rubella
- **Mononucleosis**
  - Prominent lymphadenopathy, hepatosplenomegaly, and exudative pharyngitis
  - Atypical lymphocytes and heterophil antibodies in blood
- **EI**
  - Distinctive slapped cheek erythema
  - Lacy, reticular eruption on extremities
  - Longer lasting exanthem in comparison to rubella
- **Enterovirus infection**, which is distinguished by a prominent enanthem
- **Scarlet fever**
  - Severe constitutional symptoms and pharyngitis
  - Strawberry tongue
  - "Sandpapery" exanthem
  - Marked desquamation associated with resolution
- **Drug reaction**
  - Marked pruritus
  - Longer duration than rubella exanthem

MANAGEMENT

- **No specific therapy** is available. When necessary, **supportive care** should be provided (e.g., **antipyretics** or **antiinflammatory medications** for arthralgias).
- Infected patients should be **isolated from susceptible individuals**.

POINTS TO REMEMBER

- Patients are contagious from 5 to 7 days before and until 7 days after the onset of the rash.
- Rubella immunization should be well-documented in young women; if anti-rubella antibiotic titers are negative, rubella immunization should be given.

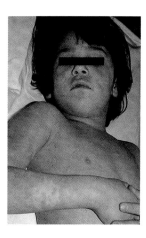

Figure 8.12.
Rubeola (measles).
Exanthem.

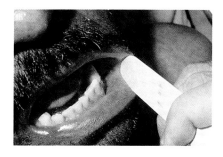

Figure 8.13.
Rubeola (measles). Koplik's spots.
Bluish-white macules on a background
of erythema.

BASICS

- Measles is a viral illness characterized by a distinctive exanthem and enanthem. The **primary site of infection is the respiratory epithelium of the oropharynx.**
- The measles virus is a single-stranded RNA virus of the Paramyxoviridae family. Humans are the natural host for the virus, although other primates may be infected as well.
  - Transmission occurs via the respiratory aerosol route. The incubation period lasts from 9 to 11 days.
  - The incidence of measles in the United States has decreased dramatically since the introduction of the measles vaccine.

DESCRIPTION OF LESIONS

The exanthem appears 3 to 5 days after the onset of the prodromal illness. Lesions begin as **discrete erythematous macules and papules**, which soon coalesce into areas of **confluent erythema** (Figure 8.12). Pruritus is usually absent.

The rash lasts 4 to 7 days before resolving, often with fine desquamation.

A characteristic enanthem known as **Koplik's spots** (Figure 8.13) appears 2 days before the onset of the exanthem. The lesions are **1-mm bluish-white macules**, which develop on a background of erythematous oral mucosa. These lesions are **pathognomonic for measles**, and, because they develop before the rash, they provide an opportunity for early diagnosis.

DISTRIBUTION OF LESIONS

- The **rash** most characteristically **begins on the forehead or behind the ears**, then spreads to involve the remainder of the face, the trunk, and the arms and legs during a 2- to 3-day period. It follows a cephalocaudad order in its development and later resolves in the same direction.
- Koplik's spots are most prominent on the buccal mucosa opposite the molars, although they may appear on the labial and gingival mucosa as well.

CLINICAL MANIFESTATIONS

In most cases, measles is a benign and self-limited infection. Recovery is usually complete within 14 days of the onset of the prodrome.
- The illness begins with a **2- to 4-day prodrome** of fever, hacking, barklike cough, coryza, conjunctivitis, and photophobia. These patients appear acutely ill and often have **cervical** and **preauricular lymphadenopathy** on examination.

- **Pneumonia** is the most common complication. In children, this is most frequently a primary measles pneumonitis, whereas in adults, secondary bacterial pneumonias are more common. Measles pneumonia is particularly **severe in immunosuppressed patients**.
- **Encephalitis** occurs in 1 to 2 per 1000 measles patients.
- Patients vaccinated with the killed virus vaccine, which was in use from 1963 to 1967, are at risk for the development of **atypical measles.** Following a 2- to 3-day prodrome of fever, dry cough, headache, and abdominal pain, a macular and papular exanthem appears. In contrast to classic measles, this eruption begins on the palms and soles, and then spreads proximally. Pneumonia is often present in these patients as well.

DIAGNOSIS

- The diagnosis of measles is usually made on **clinical grounds**.
- Although usually unnecessary, **serologic testing** is available. A fourfold, or greater, increase in antibody titers between acute and convalescent sera confirms the diagnosis.

DIFFERENTIAL DIAGNOSIS

- **Atypical measles**
  - Centripetally spread exanthem
  - No Koplik's spots
- **Rubella**
  - Mild prodromal symptoms
  - No Koplik's spots
  - Shorter duration of exanthem
- **EI**
  - Mild or absent prodrome
  - Rash with characteristic slapped cheek appearance
  - Reticular erythema on extremities
- **Scarlet fever**
  - Prominent pharyngitis
  - Strawberry tongue and circumoral pallor
  - Characteristic "sandpapery" exanthem, which is often accentuated in the skin folds
- **Roseola**
- **Drug hypersensitivity reaction**

MANAGEMENT

- **No specific therapy** for measles virus infection exists.
- **Supportive care** should be provided, and patients should be **isolated from susceptible individuals**.
- **Oral vitamin A,** 400,000 U, may decrease the morbidity and mortality rate in patients with severe infections.
- **Passive immunization** should be given to pregnant women, infants younger than 1 year of age, and immunocompromised patients who lack antibodies to the measles virus. Immune globulin preparations containing a high antimeasles titer should be administered within 6 days of exposure.
- **Routine immunization** is recommended for all children 15 months of age or older.

POINTS TO REMEMBER

- A patient with measles becomes contagious 3 days before onset of the rash and remains so until desquamation of the rash.
- **All cases should be reported to local public health officials.**

CHAPTER 9

SUPERFICIAL BACTERIAL INFECTIONS

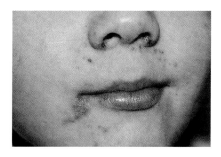

Figure 9.1.
Impetigo. Dried, stuck-on appearance of "honey-crusted" lesions.

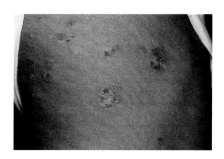

Figure 9.2.
Impetigo. A collarette of scale and dark, crusted borders.

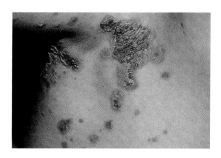

Figure 9.3.
Impetigo. Intact bullae and drying crusts of impetigo.

BASICS

- Impetigo is a primary superficial bacterial infection of the skin. It is a common, contagious finding in preschoolers. Impetigo has traditionally been divided into **bullous (staphylococcal impetigo)** and **nonbullous (impetigo contagiosa)**. Because the two varieties are clinically difficult to differentiate, the term **"impetigo" is used herein to describe both**.
- The causative organism of impetigo is most often *Staphylococcus aureus,* but mixed infections with *S. aureus* and group A β-hemolytic streptococcus also occur.
- *S. aureus* can also colonize preexisting dermatoses, resulting in **secondary impetiginization**; for example:
  - Impetiginized eczema
  - Impetiginized stasis dermatitis
  - Impetiginized herpes simplex and varicella infections
  - Impetiginized scabies and insect bites
  - Infected lacerations and burns

DESCRIPTION OF LESIONS

- Impetigo begins as a thin-roofed vesicle or bulla that ruptures; oozing serum dries and gives rise to the classic golden-yellow, **"honey-crusted"** lesion.
- Lesions appear to be **stuck-on** (Figure 9.1).
- The residual bulla may leave a **collarette of scale** or a darker hemorrhagic crusted border (Figures 9.2 and 9.3).

DISTRIBUTION OF LESIONS

- The **head** (particularly around the nose and mouth in children) and extremities are most commonly involved.
- Lesions may occur anywhere on the body.

CLINICAL MANIFESTATIONS

- Spread of lesions is by **autoinoculation**.
- Patients are usually asymptomatic but may have mild itching.
- Disease is **self-limiting**, even without treatment.
- Lesions usually heal **without scarring**.
- Impetigo may cause a **temporary postinflammatory hyperpigmentation** in dark-skinned individuals.
- Recurrent impetigo may indicate a carrier state of *S. aureus* in the patient or the patient's family.

DIAGNOSIS

- Diagnosis is usually made on **clinical grounds** (typical honey-colored crusts; Figure 9.4).
- **Gram's stain** and **culture** may be needed for confirmation.

DIFFERENTIAL DIAGNOSIS

- **Tinea corporis**
  - KOH positive
  - Central clearing of lesions
- **Primary bullous diseases,** although much less common, such as **bullous dermatosis of childhood** and **bullous pemphigoid**

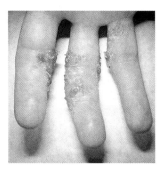

Figure 9.4.
Hand eczema, impetiginized.

MANAGEMENT

- **Antibacterial soaps**, such as Betadine Skin Cleanser or Hibiclens, are used twice daily.
- **Mupirocin ointment (Bactroban)** applied topically three times daily until all lesions are clear may be used alone to treat very limited cases of impetigo.
- For widespread involvement, an **oral staphylocidal penicillinase-resistant antibiotic** (e.g., cephalosporin, dicloxacillin, erythromycin) may be used alone or in conjunction with topical antibiotics.
- For recurrent impetigo with suspicion or evidence of nasal carriage, mupirocin (Bactroban) ointment is applied to the nares twice daily.

POINTS TO REMEMBER

- Rarely, **poststreptococcal glomerulonephritis** (but not rheumatic fever) has been reported to occur secondary to impetigo caused by certain strains of streptococcus.
- Family members should be evaluated as potential nasal carriers of *S. aureus*, and they should receive treatment, if necessary.
- Chronic or recurrent impetigo should alert the clinician to the possibility of an **impaired immune status**.

BASICS

Folliculitis and furunculosis are more common in **diabetics** and **obese individuals**.

Folliculitis

- Folliculitis refers to a **pustular infection or inflammation of a hair follicle**.
- Folliculitis may evolve into a furuncle **(boil)**, which represents a deep folliculitis.
- *S. aureus* is the most common pathogenic bacterium found in folliculitis and furunculosis.
- Folliculitis may occur as a **secondary infection** in conditions such as eczema, scabies, and excoriated insect bites.

Furunculosis

- Furuncles are painful nodules or **abscesses** (a walled-off collection of pus) in an infected hair follicle; they are more common in **boys and young adults**.
- **Chronic**, or **recurrent, furunculosis**, is a difficult therapeutic problem, which is often caused by nasal carriage of *S. aureus*.

DESCRIPTION OF LESIONS

Folliculitis

- A pustule or **papule with a central hair** is the primary lesion (Figure 9.5).
- Rupture of pustules leads to erosions and crusts.

Furuncle

- A furuncle is a **tender, painful nodule** with overlying erythema (Figure 9.6).
- As the lesion evolves, a fluctuant **abscess** may form.
- If untreated, the furuncle may rupture and drain spontaneously.

DISTRIBUTION OF LESIONS

- **Hair-bearing areas** are the primary areas of distribution, and body folds are the common sites.
- Distribution on scalp, face, buttocks, thighs, axillae, and inguinal areas is common.
- Folliculitis may involve the eyelashes, causing a **hordeolum** (stye).
- Folliculitis may involve the axillae, groin, and legs in women who shave these areas.
- Furuncles are often seen in the axillae, groin, posterior neck, thighs, and buttocks. When they occur in a contiguous cluster on the occipital scalp, it is referred to as a **carbuncle**.

CLINICAL MANIFESTATIONS

- **Folliculitis generally elicits a mild discomfort** and cosmetic concern.
- **Furuncles can cause a throbbing pain** and be tender.

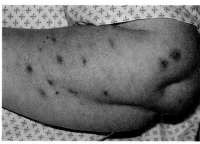

Figure 9.5.
Folliculitis. Pustules and papules in a follicular distribution.

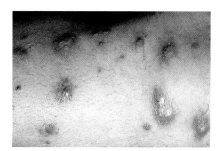

Figure 9.6.
Multiple furuncles and folliculitis.

CLINICAL VARIANTS

- **Variants of folliculitis** (nonstaphylococcal folliculitis) may be seen as the following:
  - **Pseudomonas folliculitis** may be acquired from communal hot tubs **(hot tub folliculitis)** and tends to be pruritic.
  - **Eosinophilic pustular folliculitis (EPF)** is a sterile, intensely pruritic folliculitis seen in some HIV patients (see Chapter 24, "Cutaneous Manifestions of HIV Infection"). A rare non-HIV variant of EPF may be seen in infancy.
  - **Pityrosporum folliculitis** is a pruritic, acnelike eruption seen on the trunk and caused by yeast forms of *Pityrosporum ovale*.

DIAGNOSIS

Diagnosis is based on **clinical presentation**; however, confirmation may be necessary.

- **Staphylococcal folliculitis**
  - **Gram's stain** generally reveals gram-positive cocci.
  - **Culture** grows *S. aureus*.
- **Nonstaphylococcal folliculitis**
  - **Pseudomonas folliculitis**. Diagnosis is based on history, symptoms, and bacterial culture, if necessary.
  - **EPF**. Diagnosis based on history (HIV) and skin biopsy.
  - **Pityrosporum** folliculitis. Yeast forms of *P. ovale* may be seen on biopsy.
  - **Furunculosis**. *S. aureus* may be cultured or found on Gram's stain.

DIFFERENTIAL DIAGNOSIS

Folliculitis
- **Acne**
  - Generally no hairs are seen in acne pustules.
  - Comedones are common.

Furunculosis
- **Hidradenitis suppurativa (Figure 9.7)**
  - Hidradenitis suppurativa is a chronic, scarring inflammatory disease of the apocrine gland regions.
  - There are furunclelike abscesses.
  - There are comedones and sinus tracts.
  - Secondary invasion with bacteria occurs.
  - It is more common in women.
  - It may be indistinguishable from furunculosis in its early stages.

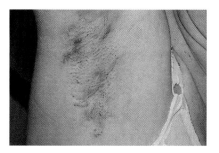

Figure 9.7.
Hidradenitis suppurativa. Note scars and comedones.

MANAGEMENT

Folliculitis

- Mild cases of folliculitis can sometimes be prevented or controlled with **antibacterial soaps**, such as Betadine Skin Cleanser and Hibiclens.
- **Topical antibiotics,** such as erythromycin 2% solution and clindamycin 1% solution, may be applied twice daily.
- **Systemic antibiotics** may be given if necessary.

Pseudomonas folliculitis

Pseudomonas folliculitis (hot tub folliculitis) may resolve spontaneously or be treated with **oral ciprofloxacin**.

EPF

EPF associated with HIV is a difficult therapeutic problem; many agents have been used to combat the intense pruritus, including ultraviolet B, itraconazole, and systemic steroids, with varying degrees of success.

Pityrosporum folliculitis

Pityrosporum folliculitis is treated with topical broad-spectrum antifungal agents or systemic antifungals such as itraconazole or terbinafine.

Furunculosis

- Furuncles may come to a head with **warm compresses**, or they may be **incised and drained**.
- Systemic **staphylocidal antibiotics** (e.g., dicloxacillin, erythromycin, cephalosporin) may be added. Minocycline is sometimes used for methicillin-resistant *S. aureus*.

Recurrent furunculosis and/or folliculitis

present difficult therapeutic problems.
- **Mupirocin ointment** may be applied intranasally.
- Family members should be evaluated as potential nasal carriers of *S. aureus* and be given treatment, if necessary.
- **Rifampin** has been used to treat the carrier state.

POINTS TO REMEMBER

- Bacterial, fungal, or viral **cultures** should be considered in cases that are resistant to therapy.
- Culturing and **treatment of family members** may be needed in cases of chronic bacterial folliculitis or furunculosis.

CHAPTER 10

SUPERFICIAL FUNGAL INFECTIONS

BASICS

- Superficial fungi live on the dead outer horny layer of skin. They produce enzymes (keratinases), which allow them to digest keratin, resulting in epidermal scale, thickened crumbly nails, or hair loss. In the dermis, an inflammatory reaction may result in erythema, vesicles, and possibly a more widespread "id" reaction.
- Infection may be acquired:
  - By person-to-person contact
  - From animals, especially kittens and puppies
  - From inanimate objects (fomites)
- Environmental and hereditary factors leading to fungal infections are:
  - **Warm, moist, occluded environments,** such as the groin, axillae and feet
  - **Family history** of fungal infections
  - **Lowered immune status** of the host, as occurs in **patients with AIDS, diabetes, collagen vascular diseases,** and long-term **systemic steroid therapy**

DIAGNOSIS

- Diagnosis can often (but not always) be made on clinical grounds.
- Diagnostic tests include:
  - **KOH** or **fungal culture** (the gold standard of diagnosis) (see Chapter 26, "KOH Examination and Fungal Culture.")
  - **Periodic acid–Schiff (PAS)** stain on biopsy specimens
  - **Wood's light** examination, which may be useful in some cases of **tinea capitis** and **tinea versicolor (TV)**

CLINICAL PRESENTATIONS OF SUPERFICIAL FUNGAL INFECTIONS

- The term "**tinea**" refers to an infection by dermatophytes. Tinea is named according to location on the body:
  - **Tinea pedis** and **tinea manum** (feet and hands)
  - **Tinea cruris** (inguinal folds)
  - **Tinea capitis** (scalp)
  - **Tinea corporis** and **tinea faciale** (body and face)
  - **Tinea unguium (onychomycosis)** (nails)
- **TV** is an exception; in fact, it **is not caused by a dermatophyte** but rather a yeastlike organism. **TV** is referred to as pityriasis versicolor by many authors.
- **Cutaneous candidiasis**

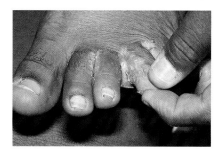

Figure 10.1.
Interdigital tinea pedis (toe web infection). Note fissuring and maceration.

BASICS

- Tinea pedis is a common problem seen mainly in young men. Ubiquitous media advertising for athlete's foot sprays and creams are testimony to the commonplace occurrence of this annoying dermatosis. Most cases are caused by *Trichophyton rubrum*, which evokes a minimal inflammatory response, and less often by *T. mentagrophytes*, which may produce vesicles and bullae.
- The **major causes of tinea pedis** or more broadly, "athlete's foot," are:
  - The dermatophytes *Epidermophyton floccosum, T. rubrum, T. mentagrophytes*, and *T. tonsurans* (in children)
  - The yeast *Candida albicans*
  - Saprophytic fungi *Hendersonula toruloidea* and *Scytalidium hyalinum*
- There are **three clinical types of tinea pedis**.

TYPE 1 INTERDIGITAL TINEA PEDIS

Figure 10.1

BASICS

- Most common type of tinea pedis
- Male predominance

DESCRIPTION OF LESIONS

Scale, maceration, and fissures are characteristic.

CLINICAL MANIFESTATIONS

- Itching and burning, marked inflammation, and fissures suggest bacterial superinfection.
- There may be coexistent yeast or saprophytic fungal involvement.

DISTRIBUTION OF LESIONS

Toe web involvement is seen, especially between the third, fourth, and fifth toes.

DIAGNOSIS

A positive KOH examination and/or fungal culture is diagnostic.

DIFFERENTIAL DIAGNOSIS

Conditions listed in the differential diagnosis are KOH negative, in contrast to tinea pedis.

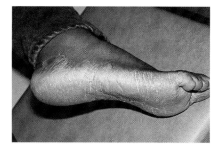

Figure 10.2.
Tinea pedis. Chronic scaly infection of the plantar surface of the foot.

- **Atopic dermatitis** (Figure 10.3)
  - Atopic dermatitis may be clinically indistinguishable from tinea pedis.
  - There is a positive atopic history.
  - It is seen especially in children on the dorsal or plantar surface of the feet (tinea pedis is unusual in preteens).
- **Contact dermatitis** caused by footwear occurs generally on the dorsum of the feet.

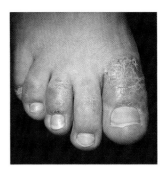

Figure 10.3.
Atopic dermatitis versus contact dermatitis.

MANAGEMENT

- For acute oozing and maceration, Burow's solution compresses are used two to three times daily.
- Broad-spectrum topical antifungal agents are applied once or twice daily.
- **Prevention** consists of maintaining dryness in the area:
  - Drying the area after bathing with a hair dryer
  - Powders, such as Zeasorb-AF and talcum powder

TYPE 2 CHRONIC PLANTAR TINEA PEDIS

BASICS

Tinea pedis ("moccasin" type) is relatively common (Figure 10.2).

DESCRIPTION OF LESIONS

Lesions are usually "dry" diffuse scaling of the soles.

DISTRIBUTION OF LESIONS

- The entire plantar surface of the foot is usually involved. Borders are distinct.
- There is often nail involvement.

CLINICAL MANIFESTATIONS

Symptoms are minimal, if any.

DIAGNOSIS

Lesions are KOH positive.

DIFFERENTIAL DIAGNOSIS

Psoriasis (Figure 10.4)
- Psoriasis has sharply demarcated plaques.
- **Or**
- It can occur in the form of sterile pustules of pustular psoriasis (rare).

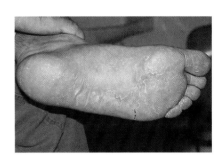

Figure 10.4.
Psoriasis. Note well-demarcated plaque.

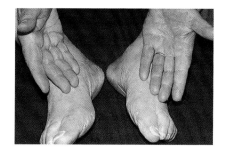

Figure 10.5.
"Two feet, one hand" variant of tinea pedis. Note the scale on one hand only and nail involvement.

CLINICAL VARIANT CHRONIC PALMO-PLANTAR TINEA PEDIS

Figure 10.5
- The "two feet, one hand" variant is pathognomonic for tinea.
- It is the same as type 2 tinea pedis, but it also involves the palms (tinea manum), soles, and, more often, only one palm, the soles, and often the nails.

MANAGEMENT

- **This is the most difficult type of tinea pedis to cure**
- **Treatment generally requires oral antifungal agents as well as broad-spectrum topical agents**

TYPE 3 ACUTE VESICULAR TINEA PEDIS

BASICS

Acute vesicular tinea pedis (Figure 10.6) is uncommon.

DESCRIPTION OF LESIONS

There are blisters on the sole or instep.

CLINICAL MANIFESTATIONS

- Acute vesicular tinea pedis is pruritic.
- An id reaction (dermatophytid) may occur.

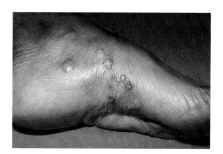

Figure 10.6.
Acute vesicular tinea pedis.

DIAGNOSIS

For diagnosis, the specimen should be taken from the inner part of the roof of the blister for KOH examination or culture.

DIFFERENTIAL DIAGNOSIS

Dyshidrotic eczema (Figure 10.7) is easily confused with acute tinea pedis.
* Patients often have a positive atopic history.
* It is KOH negative.

MANAGEMENT

* **General principles**
  * Over-the-counter preparations, such as Micatin and Lotrimin, applied once or twice daily, are often effective in controlling localized infections.
  * For symptomatic relief of severe inflammation and itching, a potent topical steroid, such as triamcinolone acetonide cream, may be used for 4 to 5 days.
  * Systemic antifungal therapy may be necessary in cases in which topical therapy fails:
    — Griseofulvin 330 mg twice daily for 30 to 45 days
    — Itraconazole 200 mg daily for 7 to 14 days or longer
    — Terbinafine 250 mg daily for 14 days or longer
* **Prevention** involves decreasing wetness, friction, and maceration:
  * Absorbent powders, such as Zeasorb-AF or talcum powder
  * Drying the area with a hair dryer after bathing
* Management of acute vesicular tinea pedis is similar to that of interdigital tinea pedis, although systemic antifungals are sometimes necessary.

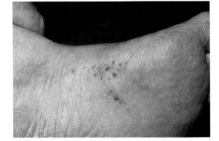

Figure 10.7.
Dyshidrotic eczema. Note the small vesicles.

POINTS TO REMEMBER

* Not all rashes of the feet are fungal in etiology. In fact, if a child under the age of 12 has what appears to be tinea pedis, it is probably another skin condition, such as eczema.
* Positive results of KOH and fungal cultures are not necessarily proof of pathogenesis because some organisms, especially yeasts and molds, may be saprophytes, or "contaminants."
* Be aware of coexistent bacterial infection.
* Recurrence is common after therapy and can lead to chronic infection.

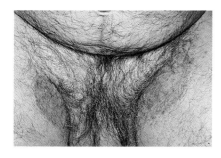

Figure 10.8.
Tinea cruris. Note the scalloped shape with "active border."

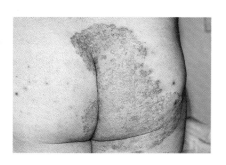

Figure 10.9.
Tinea cruris extending to the buttocks.

BASICS

- Tinea cruris ("jock itch") is a common infection of the upper inner thighs, most often occurring in postpubertal males and generally caused by the dermatophytes *T. rubrum* and *E. floccosum*.
- In contrast to candidiasis and lichen simplex chronicus, it **rarely involves the scrotum**.

DESCRIPTION OF LESIONS

Lesions are **bilateral** fan-shaped or **annular plaques** (plaques with central clearing) with a slightly elevated **"active border"** (Figure 10.8).

DISTRIBUTION OF LESIONS

- Tinea cruris involves the **upper thighs**, **crural folds**, and sometimes extends to the **pubic area** and **buttocks** (Figure 10.9).
- The scrotum and penis are spared.

CLINICAL MANIFESTATIONS

- Generally, the lesions are **pruritic** or **irritating**.
- Frequently, the patient has **tinea pedis** as well.
- The condition may be chronic or recurrent, depending on environmental factors, exercise, etc.
- The likelihood of the spread of tinea cruris between sexual partners appears to be small.

DIAGNOSIS

A positive KOH examination and/or fungal culture is found most easily at the border of lesions.

DIFFERENTIAL DIAGNOSIS

Lichen simplex chronicus (eczematous dermatitis; Figure 10.11)
Lichen simplex chronicus is KOH negative.
It involves the scrotum or vulva.
Lichenification occurs as the conditions becomes chronic.
The patient often has an atopic history.
Inverse psoriasis (Figure 10.10)
Inverse psoriasis is KOH negative.
There may be evidence of psoriasis elsewhere.
Intertrigo/seborrheic dermatitis (see Chapter 5, "Eruptions of Unknown Cause")
Irritant intertrigo and intertriginous seborrheic dermatitis primarily involve the creases.
There is possible fissuring.
The lesions are KOH negative.
Candidal intertrigo (See Figures 10.34 to 10.36.)
Candidal intertrigo is beefy red in color.
There is often scrotal or vulvar involvement.
There may be satellite pustules.
The lesions are confluent (i.e., they have no central clearing).
The lesions are KOH positive for pseudo-hyphae or hyphae or positive culture for *candida* is obtained.

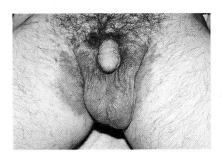

Figure 10.10.
Psoriasis. Well-demarcated plaques with no "active border." (Note scrotal and inguinal involvement.)

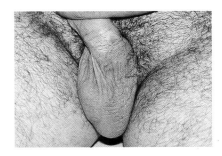

Figure 10.11.
Lichen simplex chronicus. Note lichenification.

MANAGEMENT

- Topical antifungal creams applied once or twice daily are often effective in controlling and often curing uncomplicated, localized infections. Over-the-counter preparations, such as Micatin and Lotrimin, are effective
- For severe inflammation and itching, a mild hydrocortisone (1%) preparation or moderate-strength Westcort (hydrocortisone valerate, 0.2%) may be used for 4 to 5 days for symptomatic relief.
- **Systemic antifungal therapy** may be necessary in cases that do not respond to topical therapy or for extensive chronic recurrent tinea cruris, particularly in immunocompromised patients:
  - Griseofulvin 330 mg twice daily for 30 to 45 days
  - Itraconazole 200 mg daily for 7 days or longer
  - Terbinafine 250 mg daily for 14 days or longer
- **Prevention** involves decreasing wetness, friction, and maceration:
  - Absorbent powders such as Zeasorb-AF or talcum powder
  - Drying the area with a hair dryer after bathing

POINTS TO REMEMBER

- A common error by many health care providers is to assume automatically that a rash in the genital area, commonly referred to as "jock itch," and itchy scaly rashes of the feet, or "athlete's foot," are fungal in origin. Often these are treated with topical antifungal preparations alone or in combination with topical steroids in a "shotgun" approach. Careful observation and a positive KOH examination or fungal culture reveal the true nature of the problem.
- Tinea pedis, if present concurrently with tinea cruris, should also be treated to minimize reinfection.

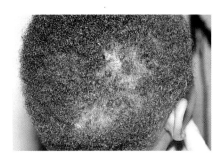

Figure 10.12.
Tinea capitis (TC). Scaly alopecic patches mimic seborrheic dermatitis.

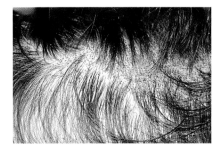

Figure 10.13.
Tinea capitis (TC). "Black dot" ringworm.

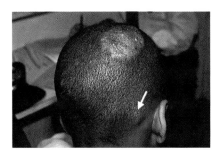

Figure 10.14.
Kerion of tinea capitis (TC). There is also a palpable asymptomatic nontender right occipital lymph node (see *arrow*).

BASICS

- Tinea capitis (TC), or "ringworm," most commonly occurs in prepubertal children. In the United States, African American children are disproportionately affected by this superficial fungal infection of the hair shaft.
- The incidence of TC has been increasing and presents a growing public heath concern, especially in overcrowded, impoverished inner-city communities.
- *T. tonsurans* is, by far, the most common etiologic agent; more than 90% of cases are caused by it.
- TC is contagious and is generally spread by person-to-person contact. Recent studies have demonstrated a 30% carrier state of adults exposed to a child with *T. tonsurans.*
- It has also been shown that the organism could be isolated from such inanimate objects as hairbrushes and pillows.
- Other species, such as *Microsporum audouinii*, which is spread from human to human, and *M. canis,* which is spread from animals (cats and dogs), are more often seen in Caucasian children. There is frequently a family member, pet, or playmate with tinea.

DESCRIPTION OF LESIONS

Clinical types. There are essentially four clinical expressions of TC, with some overlapping physical presentations:

Inflamed, scaly, often alopecic patches, which mimic seborrheic dermatitis, are especially common in infancy until age 6 to 8 months (Figure 10.12).

A diffuse scaling often is seen with multiple round areas, characterized by an alopecia that occurs secondary to broken hair shafts, leaving residual black stumps ("black dot" ringworm; Figure 10.13). It is seen uncommonly and is often mistaken for alopecia areata.

Painful pustular nodules or plaques called **kerions** (Figure 10.14) may occur.

A kerion is a boggy, pustular, indurated, tumorlike mass, which represents an inflammatory hypersensitivity reaction to the fungus, which can result in scarring.

Secondary bacterial invaders such as *Staphylococcus aureus* and some gram-negative organisms may sometimes be recovered from a kerion. Often there is an accompanying nontender regional adenopathy.

Occasionally a pustular variety, with or without alopecia, can mimic a bacterial infection.

DIAGNOSIS

- A KOH preparation or fungal culture confirms the diagnosis; however, a KOH examination may be falsely negative because of the marked inflammation that accompanies a kerion.
  - When in doubt, or when a KOH preparation is negative, a fungal culture placed on Sabouraud's agar should be done. This can easily be performed by obtaining broken hairs and scale by stroking the affected area with a sterile toothbrush, a familiar object to a child, which is less frightening than a surgical blade or forceps (see Chapter 26, "KOH Examination and Fungal Culture"). The collected material is then tapped onto the surface of Sabouraud's agar.
  - An alternative method of harvesting broken hairs is by rubbing a moistened gauze pad on the involved area of scalp and then using forceps to place the hairs on the culture medium or slide. Pustules generally are sterile or grow bacterial contaminants.
- A biopsy is rarely necessary.
- In the past, Wood's light examination was a valuable screening tool to diagnose TC easily (because *Microsporum* species are usually fluorescent), but it has lost its usefulness because most cases are caused by the nonfluorescing *T. tonsurans.*

DIFFERENTIAL DIAGNOSIS

Each diagnosis considered in the differential is **KOH and/or fungal-culture negative.**

- **Alopecia areata** (Figure 10.15)
  - Well-demarcated symmetrical patch of alopecia
  - Scale-free, smooth
- **Seborrheic dermatitis**
  - Often thickened scale
  - "Cradle cap"
- **Atopic dermatitis**
- **Psoriasis**
- **Tinea amiantacea** is a probable variant of seborrheic dermatitis, which is a KOH-negative local patch or plaque of adherent scale. "Tinea" is a misnomer.
- **Trichotillomania** (a self-induced cause of hair loss)
- **Also to be considered:**
  - Bacterial scalp infection
  - Secondary syphilis
  - Acute and chronic cutaneous discoid lupus erythematosus

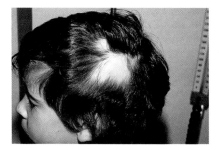

Figure 10.15.
Alopecia areata, with smooth, well-demarcated, noninflammatory patches of alopecia.

MANAGEMENT

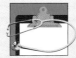

- **Topical therapy is of little or no value** in treating TC, although an adjunctive antifungal shampoo that contains ketoconazole or 2.5% selenium sulfide (over-the-counter 1% selenium sulfide is less expensive and equally effective) may be used by the infected person and contacts to prevent reinfection and spread.
- **Systemic therapy with a liquid suspension of microsized griseofulvin** has been the mainstay of therapy.
  - The dosage is from 10 to 15 mg/kg per day and sometimes as high as 25 mg/kg per day in divided doses.
  - It should be given with milk or food, which increases its absorption, and continued until the patient is clinically cured, which generally takes from 6 to 8 weeks. Some cases may require longer therapy.
  - Occasionally, an id reaction occurs shortly after the initiation of griseofulvin therapy. This consists of multiple small sterile papules on the face or body, which probably represents a hypersensitivity response.
  - Treatment failure, which is uncommon with griseofulvin, may indicate inadequate dosing or duration of therapy, drug resistance, reinfection from another family member, poor compliance, or immune incompetence.
  - Itraconazole, terbinafine, and fluconazole are new and potentially more efficacious agents and have been used in some instances of griseofulvin failures, but these drugs have not as yet been approved for this indication in the United States.
- In many instances, therapy may have to be initiated in the face of negative KOH and fungal cultures and based solely upon clinical appearance.
- Occasionally, concomitant systemic steroid therapy is warranted in addition to griseofulvin, when the patient is experiencing a severe, tender, or painful kerion. A short course (usually 3 or 4 days) of oral prednisone, 1 mg/kg per day, is sufficient.

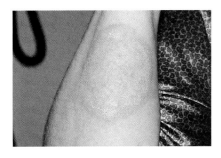

Figure 10.16.
Annular, scaly plaque of tinea corporis.

BASICS

- Commonly referred to as "ringworm," tinea corporis is the name used by the lay and, frequently, the health care community to describe almost any annular, or ring-like, eruption on the body.
- There are many conditions that assume an annular configuration: granuloma annulare, erythema multiforme, erythema migrans (seen in acute Lyme disease), as well as annular erythemas, such as urticaria. All are **KOH negative**.
- **Tinea corporis** (referred to as **tinea faciale** if it is located on the face) is most often acquired by contact with an infected animal, usually kittens and occasionally dogs. It may also spread from infected humans, or it may be autoinoculated from other areas of the body that are infected by tinea (e.g., tinea pedis or TC).
- *M. canis, T. rubrum,* and *T. mentagrophytes* are the usual pathogens.

DESCRIPTION OF LESIONS

- Lesion are generally **annular,** with peripheral enlargement and central clearing. Odd gyrate or concentric rings can often be found (Figures 10.16–10.18).
- There is a scaly, or "active border," which can sometimes be **vesicular** or **pustular**.
- Lesions are **single** or **multiple** (see Figure 10.17).

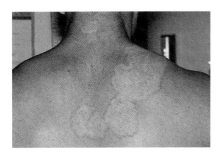

Figure 10.17.
Multiple lesions of tinea corporis.

DISTRIBUTION OF LESIONS

- Lesions are asymmetric.
- They are seen most often on the extremities and face (see Figure 10.18).

CLINICAL MANIFESTATIONS

- Lesions may be pruritic or asymptomatic.
- Majocchi's granuloma is a deep form of tinea corporis. It may result when inappropriate therapy (primarily topical steroids) or shaving drives fungi into the hair follicles.

DIAGNOSIS

- Diagnosis is confirmed by a positive KOH or fungal culture (it is especially easy to find hyphae in those patients who have been previously treated with topical steroids.)
- A history of **a newly adopted kitten,** or another infected contact, is helpful.

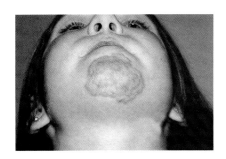

Figure 10.18.
Tinea faciale.

DIFFERENTIAL DIAGNOSIS

- **Urticaria** (Figure 10.19). No scale is present.
- **Acute Lyme disease** (erythema migrans; Figure 10.20). There is no scale.

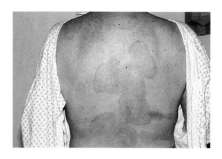

Figure 10.19.
Urticaria.

MANAGEMENT

- **Topical antifungal agents** (see Formulary at end of this chapter)
- **Systemic antifungal agents** (including **griseofulvin**) are sometimes necessary when multiple lesions are present. They are also used when treating areas that are repeatedly shaven (e.g., men's beards, or, especially, women legs where granulomatous lesions [Majocchi's granuloma] occur).
- Treatment of other coexisting sites of tinea infection on the body

POINTS TO REMEMBER

- If pets appear to be the source of infection, they may also need antifungal treatment after evaluation by a veterinarian.
- **Tinea corporis is often misdiagnosed** and treated with topical steroids **("tinea incognito").**

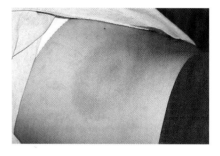

Figure 10.20.
Acute Lyme disease (erythema migrans). Note the concentric rings with no scale.

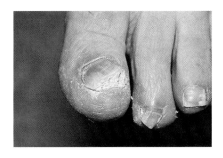

Figure 10.21.
Distal subungual onychomycosis (DSO).

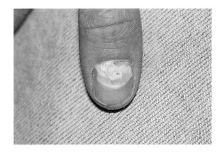

Figure 10.22.
Superficial white onychomycosis (SWO).

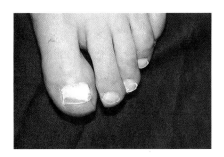

Figure 10.23.
Proximal white subungual onychomycosis (PWSO).

BASICS

- **Onychomycosis** is an infection of the fingernails or toenails caused by various fungi, yeasts, and molds.
- **Tinea unguium** refers to infections of the nail that are caused specifically by dermatophytes.
- Recent media attention has brought scores of patients to their health-care providers to have their unsightly nails treated with the newer antifungal agents, terbinafine, itraconazole, and fluconazole. These drugs have replaced griseofulvin, which is less effective and is associated with a high recurrence rate, and ketoconazole, which may be associated with the rare occurrence of idiosyncratic hepatitis.
- Onychomycosis is uncommon in children but increases in prevalence with advancing age. Aside from footwear causing occasional physical discomfort and the psychosocial liability of unsightly nails, it is usually asymptomatic. Left untreated, onychomycotic nails can act as a portal of entry for more serious bacterial infections of the lower leg, particularly in diabetics.
- The **major causes of onychomycosis** are:
  - The dermatophytes *E. floccosum, T. rubrum,* and *T. mentagrophytes*
  - Yeasts, mainly *C. albicans*
  - Molds *Aspergillus, Fusarium,* and *Scopulariopsis*

DESCRIPTION OF LESIONS

- **Distal subungual onychomycosis** (**DSO**; Figure 10.21)
  - Nail thickening and subungual hyperkeratosis (scale buildup under the nail)
  - Nail discoloration (yellow, yellow–green, white, or brown)
  - Nail dystrophy
  - Nail plate elevation from nail bed (onycholysis)

CLINICAL VARIANTS

- **Superficial white onychomycosis** (**SWO**; Figure 10.22). The fungus is superficial, and material for scraping may be obtained from the dorsal surface of the nail.
- **Proximal white subungual onychomycosis** (**PWSO**; Figure 10.23) occurs commonly in individuals with HIV disease.

CLINICAL MANIFESTATIONS

- DSO is by far the most common type (> 90%).

- Susceptibility is inherited as an autosomal dominant trait.
- DSO is generally asymptomatic.
- DSO is sometimes associated with chronic palmo–plantar tinea (i.e., "two feet, one hand" variant of tinea) (Figure 10.5).

DIAGNOSIS

Positive KOH and/or growth of dermatophyte, yeast, or mold on culture is diagnostic.

DIFFERENTIAL DIAGNOSIS (See Chapter 13, "Diseases and Abnormalities of Nails.")

- **Psoriasis of the nails** (Figure 10.24)
  - Usually, psoriasis is found elsewhere on the body as well as on the nails.
  - KOH examination is generally negative.
  - There may be nail pitting.
  - There may be nail discoloration (oil spots; yellowish-brown pigmentation).
  - Nail thickening, subungual hyperkeratosis, nail dystrophy, and onycholysis associated with psoriasis may be indistinguishable from onychomycosis.
- **Chronic paronychia** (Figure 10.25)
  - There are erythema and edema of the proximal nail fold.
  - The cuticle is absent.
  - There is nail dystrophy.
  - Chronic paronychia is seen in individuals with an altered immune status (e.g., diabetic) or in people whose hands are constantly in water (e.g., dishwashers).
  - Culture is positive for *Candida* and/or bacteria.
- *Pseudomonas infection of the nail* (green nail; Figure 10.26). There is onycholysis with secondary bacterial (pseudomonas) colonization.
- **Onycholysis** unrelated to a fungus or psoriasis (Figure 10.27) can be idiopathic or associated with the following:
  - Nail trauma
  - Thyroid disease
  - Use of nail polish and /or nail hardeners
  - Oral tetracyclines (especially demeclocycline) coupled with sun exposure

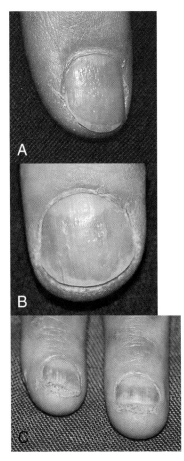

Figure 10.24.
Psoriasis of the nails. (*A*) Pitting; (*B*) oil spots, pits, and distal onycholysis; (*C*) subungual hyperkeratosis and oil spots.

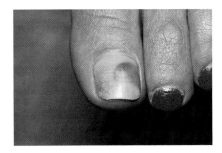
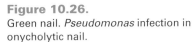

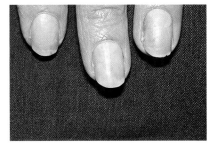

Figure 10.25.
Chronic paronychia. Note loss of cuticle, onycholysis, and nail dystrophy

Figure 10.26.
Green nail. *Pseudomonas* infection in onycholytic nail.

Figure 10.27.
Onycholysis.

MANAGEMENT

- **Surgical ablation** is rarely indicated and is often ineffective.
- **Topical agents** are generally ineffective because of poor nail penetration.
  - They may be used as adjuvant therapy or used to prevent recurrences after clearing with oral agents.
  - They are sometimes useful in cases of SWO.
  - A topical nail lacquer containing the antifungal agent ciclopirox (which is not presently approved for use in the United States) may soon have an important role in the treatment of DSO. It can be used in conjunction with oral antifungal agents or used alone for the prevention of recurrent DSO.
- **Oral agents**
  - **Itraconazole (Sporanox) capsules**
    - Broad-spectrum fungistatic agent
    - Long-term cure reported at greater than 80%
    - Significant drug interactions
    - Minimal side effects
    - **Dosage**
      Pulse dosing with 200 mg twice daily
      Taken with full meals for 7 days of each month; 3 months for fingernails, 4 months for toenails
      Or 200 mg once daily continuously for 12 consecutive weeks
    - Baseline liver function tests; repeated in 6 to 8 weeks
    - Reservoir effect; no need to wait until nail is clinically normal (drug persists in nail for up to 4 to 5 months; thus, there is continued clearing even after cessation of therapy)
  - **Terbinafine (Lamisil) tablets**
    - Fungicidal, especially against dermatophytes
    - Long-term cure reported at greater than 80%
    - **Dosage**
      250 mg per day for 6 weeks for fingernails
      250 mg per day for 12 weeks for toenails

    — Baseline liver function tests; repeated in 6 to 8 weeks
    — Reservoir effect; no need to wait until nail is clinically normal (drug persists in nail for up to 4 to 5 months; thus, there is continued clearing even after cessation of therapy)
- **Fluconazole (Diflucan) tablets**
    — Broad-spectrum fungistatic agent
    — More extensively used in HIV patients
    — **Dosage**
        50 to 100 mg daily for 1 to 4 weeks
        150 mg once per week for 9 to 10 months
    — Many fewer drug interactions
    — Minimal side effects
    — Liver toxicity possible with long-term use

POINTS TO REMEMBER

- Abnormal-appearing nails are not always the result of a fungal infection.
- A diagnosis should not be made based solely on clinical grounds without benefit of either fungal culture or KOH examination.
- Positive results of KOH examination and fungal culture, and even nail plate histopathology, are not necessarily proof of pathogenesis because some organisms, especially yeasts and molds, may be saprophytes or contaminants.
- Onychomycosis is generally asymptomatic, and treatment with the newer systemic antifungal agents is expensive and not always curative.
- Coexistent bacterial infection may be present in onychomycosis.
- Immunosuppressed patients and diabetics appear to have a greater prevalence of onychomycosis than the normal population.
- A complete cure of onychomycosis is probably more difficult in patients with a positive family history of nail or other dermatophyte infections.
- **Important factors to consider before starting oral therapy**
  - Patient motivation and compliance
  - Family history of onychomycosis
  - Patient age and health
  - Drug cost
  - Possible drug interactions and side effects

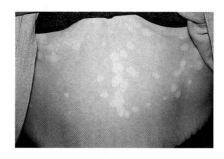

Figure 10.28.
White tinea versicolor (TV).

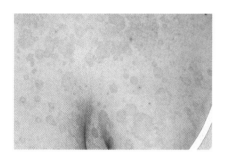

Figure 10.29.
Tan, faun-colored tinea versicolor (TV).

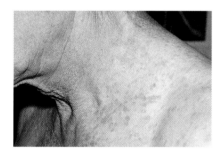

Figure 10.30.
Reddish tinea versicolor (TV).

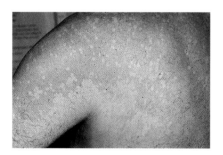

Figure 10.31.
Brown, confluent tinea versicolor (TV).

BASICS

- TV is a common opportunistic superficial yeast infection caused by *Pityrosporum orbiculare*.
- It is seen mostly in young adults, and it is unusual in the very young and elderly. It is also seen more commonly in immunocompromised patients.
- The condition is more common in tropical climates and recurs during the summer months in more temperate zones.
- TV is primarily of cosmetic concern and is generally asymptomatic.
- The term "versicolor" refers to the varied coloration that TV can display. The color of lesions may vary from whitish to pink to tan or brown (Figures 10.28–10.31).

DESCRIPTION OF LESIONS

- The **primary lesions** are well-defined **round** or **oval macules**, with an overlay of fine scales.
- The lesions often coalesce to form larger patches.

DISTRIBUTION OF LESIONS

Lesions are most often distributed on the trunk, upper arms, and neck; however, they may also be seen on the face.

CLINICAL MANIFESTATIONS

- There is occasional mild pruritus.
- Patients usually come for treatment because of blotchy pigmentation.
- TV is minimally, if at all, contagious.

DIAGNOSIS

- If scale is present, **KOH examination** is positive, and the typical "spaghetti and meatball" hyphae are abundant and easily found (see Chapter 26, "KOH Examination and Fungal Culture").
- **Wood's light examination** is used to demonstrate the extent of the infection and may help to confirm the diagnosis, because lesions often fluoresce an orange–mustard color when the Wood's light is held close to lesions in a darkened room.

DIFFERENTIAL DIAGNOSIS

- **Vitiligo** (Figure 10.32).
  - Vitiligo lacks scale.
  - There is complete depigmentation with vitiligo.
- **Seborrheic dermatitis** of the presternal area (Figure 10.33)
  - Seborrheic dermatitis is KOH negative.
  - Usually seborrheic dermatitis tends to occur elsewhere on the body as well.

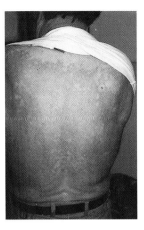

Figure 10.32.
Vitiligo. Note complete depigmentation, no scale.

MANAGEMENT

- **Mild, limited TV**
  - Daily application of topical over-the-counter selenium sulfide should be left on for 15 minutes and rinsed off. Afterwards,
  - Application of a topical antifungal agent such as Micatin or Lamisil Cream or Spray (a spray allows for easy application to the back) should be made once or twice daily.
  - Treatment may be repeated for 3 to 4 weeks. It is also a good idea to repeat this regimen before the next warm season or before a tropical vacation.
  - If this fails, prescription therapy with Nizoral Cream or Shampoo may be tried.
- **Stubborn or widespread disease** may be treated with systemic therapy with itraconazole 200 mg for 5 days.
- **Prophylactic therapy** with selenium sulfide lotion or shampoo or zinc pyrithione bar or shampoo may be used twice monthly.

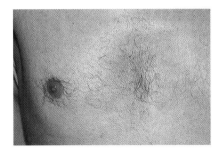

Figure 10.33.
Seborrheic dermatitis localized to the presternal area.

POINTS TO REMEMBER

- Patients should be advised that the uneven coloration of the skin may take several months to disappear after the fungus has been successfully eliminated.
- Recurrences are common, especially in warm weather.
- In physically active individuals, TV may persist year round.
- Systemic therapy should not be given routinely for this essentially cosmetic problem.

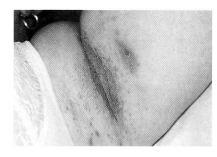

Figure 10.34.
Cutaneous candidiasis (CC) of the axillae. Note satellite pustules.

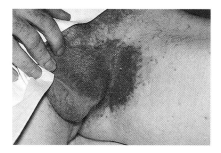

Figure 10.35.
Cutaneous candidiasis (CC) of the groin.

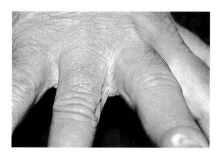

Figure 10.36.
"Erosio interdigitalis blastomycetes."
Cutaneous candidiasis (CC) of the web spaces of the fingers.

BASICS

- Cutaneous candidiasis (CC) is a superficial fungal infection of the skin and mucous membranes caused by *C. albicans,* and, uncommonly, other *Candida* species. The organism thrives on moist occluded sites, particularly as a secondary invader.
- **It occurs in:**
  - People who continually expose their hands to water (e.g., dishwashers, health care workers)
  - Obese individuals (in skin folds)
  - Infants (in the diaper area, mouth)
- It is also found on hosts with an **altered immune status,** such as:
  - Diabetics
  - Patients on long-term systemic steroids
  - Patients with AIDS
  - Patients with polyendocrinopathies

DESCRIPTION AND DISTRIBUTION OF LESIONS

The lesions vary according to location.
- **Intertriginous (occluded) areas**
  - Initially pustules appear, followed by well-demarcated erythematous plaques with small papular and pustular lesions at the periphery ("satellite pustules").
  - Erythematous areas later become eroded and beefy red. Lesions are seen under the breasts, in the axillae, and in the groin, including the intergluteal area and the scrotum (Figures 10.34 and 10.35). They may also be seen in the corners of the mouth (perlèche).
  - The mucous membranes of the oral cavity, vagina, and glans penis may be affected.
  - Lesions are not annular (they have no central clearing), as seen in tinea infection.
- **Other variants of CC**
  - **"Erosio interdigitalis blastomycetica."** Superficial interdigital scaly, erythematous erosions or fissures occur in the web spaces of the fingers (Figure 10.36).
  - **Candidal folliculitis** is characterized by follicular pustules.

- **Candidal balanitis** is seen in men with diabetes. Erythema, edema, and moist curdlike accumulations occur on the glans penis, with possible fissuring and ulceration of the foreskin.
- **Candidal paronychia** (see Chapter 13, "Diseases and Abnormalities of Nails") occurs with edema, erythema, and purulence of the proximal nail fold with secondary nail dystrophy.
- **Oral candidiasis ("thrush")** is characterized by white, creamy exudate or plaques, which, when removed, appear eroded and beefy red.

CLINICAL MANIFESTATIONS

CC is characterized by itching and burning.

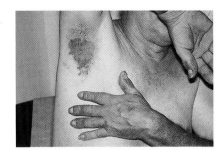

Figure 10.37.
Inverse psoriasis. Note typical psoriatic lesions on the hands.

DIAGNOSIS

- CC is **KOH positive** for **pseudohyphae, budding yeast,** or **mycelia** (see Chapter 26, "KOH Examination and Fungal Culture").
- **Fungal culture** on **Sabouraud's media** reveals creamy dull-white colonies.

DIFFERENTIAL DIAGNOSIS

The differential diagnosis varies with the location of the lesions.
- **Inverse psoriasis, irritant intertrigo,** and **seborrheic dermatitis** (Figure 10.37) are all KOH negative.
- **Lichen simplex chronicus (eczematous dermatitis;** Figure 10.38)
  - Lichen simplex chronicus is KOH negative.
  - There is lichenification of the scrotum or vulva.
- **Tinea infections**
  - There are well-defined, KOH-positive borders.
  - The scrotum is not involved in tinea cruris.
- **Oral candidiasis** and **candidal balanitis** appear in the clinical settings of immunosuppression and diabetes.

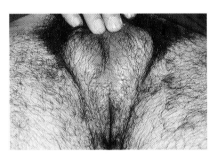

Figure 10.38.
Lichen simplex chronicus (eczematous dermatitis). Lichenification of the scrotum.

MANAGEMENT

- **CC**
  - Burow's solution in cool wet soaks can be applied if there is maceration two to three times daily.
  - The intertriginous area should be kept dry with powders (e.g., Zeasorb-AF Powder) and by drying with a hair dryer after bathing.
  - Topical broad-spectrum antifungal creams, such as prescription Nizoral Cream or the over-the-counter preparations Lotrimin and Micatin, can be applied.
  - Systemic antifungal agents, such as itraconazole or fluconazole, are used for widespread involvement or recalcitrant infections.
- **Oral candidiasis**
  - Oral nystatin for 10 to 14 days
    - Infants: 1 ml in each side of the mouth three times daily
    - Adults: 2 to 3 ml in each side of the mouth three times daily
  - **Or**
  - One Clotrimazole troche orally five times daily for 2 weeks
  - **Or**
  - Fluconazole
    - Children: 6 mg/kg day 1; 3 mg/kg days 2 to 14
    - Adults: 200 mg day 1; 100 mg days 2 to 14
  - **Or**
  - Itraconazole (approved for adults only) 100 to 200 mg/day for 1 to 3 weeks

POINTS TO REMEMBER

- **CC** is much less common than tinea infections; however, it is one of the more over-diagnosed cutaneous conditions. It is also often confused with inverse psoriasis and irritant intertrigo.
- Griseofulvin is ineffective against *Candida* species.

FORMULARY: ANTIFUNGAL AGENTS

TOPICAL AGENTS: *OVER-THE-COUNTER*

AGENT	APPLICATION	FORMS	COMMENTS
Lotrimin *clotrimazole*	Twice daily	Cream, lotion, solution	Tinea, *Candida*, tinea versicolor
Micatin *miconazole*	Twice daily	Cream, lotion, spray	Tinea, *Candida*, tinea versicolor
Tinactin *tolnaftate*	Twice daily	Cream	Tinea (**not indicated for** tinea versicolor)
Selsun Blue *selenium sulfide 1%*	As directed	Shampoo	Tinea versicolor (TV)
Zeaborb A-F Powder *miconazole*	As needed	Powder	Tinea, *Candida*, tinea versicolor; antifriction/drying agent
Desenex AF *clotrimazole*	As needed	Powder	Tinea, *Candida*, tinea versicolor; antifriction/drying agent

TOPICAL AGENTS: *PRESCRIPTION*

AGENT	APPLICATION	FORMS	COMMENTS
Lamisil *terbinafine*	1 to 4 weeks, twice daily	Cream, spray	Tinea (**not indicated for** *Candida*)
Nizoral *ketoconazole*	6 weeks, once daily	Cream	Tinea, *Candida*, tinea versicolor
Spectazole *econazole*	4 weeks, once daily	Cream	Tinea, *Candida*, tinea versicolor, gram-positive bacteria
Loprox *ciclopirox*	4 weeks, as needed	Cream, lotion	Lotion preferred for nail penetration
Naftin *naftifine*	4 weeks, once daily	Cream, gel	Gel preferred for nail penetration
Exelderm *sulconazole*	4 weeks, twice daily	Cream, solution	Tinea, *Candida*, tinea versicolor
Monistat-Derm *miconazole*	4 weeks, twice daily	Cream	Tinea, *Candida*, tinea versicolor (TV)
Oxistat *oxiconazole*	4 weeks, once to twice daily	Cream, lotion	Tinea, *Candida*, tinea versicolor
Selsun 2.5% *Selenium sulfide 2.5%*	As directed	Shampoo	Tinea versicolor (TV); may be irritating

FORMULARY: TINEA VERSICOLOR (TV)

TOPICAL THERAPY

Over-the-Counter
Selsun Blue (selenium sulfide 1%) Shampoo
Head & Shoulders (zinc pyrithione 1%) Shampoo
Zinc pyrithione bar or shampoo
Micatin Cream or Spray
Lotrimin Cream or Solution

Prescription
Nizoral Cream or Shampoo (ketoconazole)
Lamisil Spray

SYSTEMATIC THERAPY

Sporanox (itraconazole); supplied as 100-mg capsules
Diflucan (fluconazole); supplied as 150-mg tablets

Oral Antifungal Agents

Griseofulvin: *Fulvicin, Grisactin, Gris-Peg*
- Effective only against dermatophytes
  - Fungistatic
  - Taken with fatty meals
- Avoid alcohol
- Side effects
  - Occasional headache
  - Gastrointestinal upset
  - Elevation of liver function test (LFT) results
  - Photosensitivity
- Contraindicated in pregnancy
- Significant drug interactions (phenobarbital, warfarin, other drugs metabolized in liver)
- For long-term use, monitor LFTs and complete blood count (CBC) every 3 to 4 months
- Well-tolerated in young children
  - Monitoring of LFTs and CBC is unnecessary with short-term use
- Adult dosage:
- Supplied as microsized: 250-mg, 500-mg tablets
  - Supplied as utramicrosized: 125-mg, 250-mg, 333-mg tablets
- Pediatric dosage: supplied as microsized: 125 mg/tsp pediatric suspension

Terbinafine: *Lamisil*
- Fungicidal, especially against dermatophytes
- Baseline LFTs; repeat in 6 to 8 weeks if therapy is chronic
- Many fewer drug interactions than with itraconazole (terbinafine clearance is decreased by cimetidine and terfenadine; it is increased by rifampin)
- Side effects minimal: reversible taste loss, rare hepatotoxicity
- Supplied as: 250-mg tablets

Itraconazole: *Sporanox*
- Broad-spectrum fungistatic
- **Significant drug interactions and contraindications**: drugs **not** to be taken with itraconazole include: astemizole, cisapride, terfenadine, triazolam, midazolam, lovastatin, and simvastatin
- Side effects minimal: rare hepatotoxicity
- Baseline and follow-up LFTs with long-term use
- Supplied as: 100-mg tablets

Fluconazole: *Diflucan*
- Broad-spectrum fungistatic
- Monitor LFTs with long-term use
- More extensively used in HIV patients
- Supplied as: 50-mg, 100-mg, 150-mg, 200-mg tablets

CHAPTER 11

HAIR AND SCALP DISORDERS RESULTING IN HAIR LOSS

OVERVIEW

Although hair has no vital function in humans, its powerful role in a person's psychosexual identity is attested to by the number of hair care products and hair replacement and hair retention methods that are currently available.

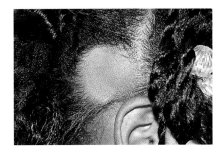

Figure 11.1.
Alopecia areata (AA). Round patch of alopecia. Compare with Figure 11.8.

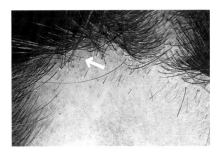

Figure 11.2.
Alopecia areata (AA). "Exclamation mark" hairs at margin of alopecia (*arrow*).

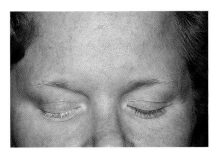

Figure 11.3.
Alopecia areata (AA). White hairs have regrown in eyebrows and eyelashes.

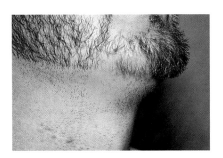

Figure 11.4.
Alopecia areata (AA) of the beard.

BASICS

- Alopecia areata (AA) is an idiopathic disorder characterized by well-circumscribed round or oval areas of **nonscarring** hair loss.
  - **Alopecia totalis** is a loss of all scalp hair and eyebrows.
  - **Alopecia universalis** refers to a loss of all body hair.
- AA most commonly affects young adults and children. A family history of AA is occasionally obtained; often, recent stress or major life crises are attributed to its onset.

Pathogenesis

of AA is generally considered to be **autoimmune**.

This is suggested by biopsy findings demonstrating T-cell infiltrates surrounding hair follicles and the association of AA with putative autoimmune disorders, such as vitiligo, thyroid disease (Hashimoto's disease), and pernicious anemia.

DESCRIPTION OF LESIONS (Figure 11.1)

- Alopecic patches are most often **oval, round,** or **geometric** in shape.
- "Exclamation mark" hairs at the periphery of lesions may sometimes be seen with a hand lens (Figure 11.2).
- A characteristic increased friction (not the expected smoothness) is felt upon gentle stroking of lesional skin. This results from the loss of fine vellus as well as terminal hairs in AA.
- Erythema in lesional skin is unusual.

DISTRIBUTION OF LESIONS

- Alopecia most often involves the **scalp, eyebrows, eyelashes,** and **beard** (Figures 11.3 and 11.4).
- **Alopecia totalis** involves the **entire scalp** (Figure 11.5).
- **Alopecia universalis** involves the **entire body**, including pubic, axillary, and nasal hair.
- **Nails** may demonstrate characteristic **pitting**, or "railroad tracks" (Figure 11.6).

CLINICAL MANIFESTATIONS

- Asymptomatic shedding of hair often is discovered by the patient's barber, hairdresser, or family member.
- Hair frequently regrows spontaneously; however, alopecia recurs in 30% of patients.
- **Poorer prognosis** is suggested by **extensive alopecia**, an **atopic history**, and **chronicity**.
- Initially, regrowing hair is often white (vitiliginous) and thin (Figure 11.7).
- Alopecia universalis is generally a lifelong condition that is refractory to therapy; spontaneous regrowth is rare.

DIAGNOSIS

Diagnosis is made by **clinical appearance** and **scalp biopsy**, if necessary.

DIFFERENTIAL DIAGNOSIS

- **Tinea capitis** (see Chapter 10, "Superficial Fungal Infections.")
  - Most often scaly, inflamed
  - Lymphadenopathy often present
  - Potassium hydroxide (KOH) or culture positive
- **Androgenetic alopecia**. Hair loss is gradual and patterned (in a male or female pattern).
- **Telogen effluvium** (see below)
  - History of antecedent illness, childbirth, or trauma
  - Rapid, diffuse hair loss
- **Traction alopecia** (see below) is characterized by hair loss in areas subject to chronic pulling.
- **Trichotillomania** (Figure 11.8)
  - Hairs broken at different lengths
  - Irregular shape to area of alopecia
  - Asymmetrical loss of scalp hair (more on side of dominant hand)
- **Secondary syphilis**
  - "Moth-eaten" alopecia
  - Reactive VDRL (Venereal Disease Research Laboratories) test

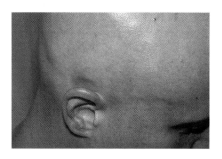
Figure 11.5.
Alopecia areata (AA). Alopecia totalis.

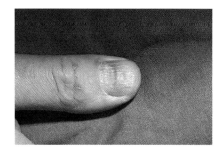
Figure 11.6.
Alopecia areata (AA). Nails with characteristic pitting ("railroad tracks").

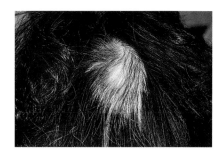
Figure 11.7.
Alopecia areata (AA). White regrowing hair.

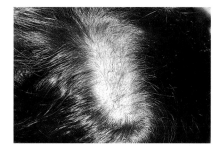
Figure 11.8.
The effects of trichotillomania. Compare with Figure 11.1.

MANAGEMENT

- Mild cases of AA often show spontaneous regrowth, and therapy is often unnecessary.
- **Potent and superpotent topical steroids** may be applied and used under shower cap occlusion, with supervision.
- Intralesional **steroid injections** may be given every 6 to 8 weeks. (This painful approach is difficult to utilize in children.)
- The following have been used to treat severe or recalcitrant AA: topical **minoxidil**, **psoralen plus ultraviolet A (PUVA)**, **irritant therapy** using topical anthralin preparations, **immunotherapy** using topical cyclosporine, and the induction of contact dermatitis with various chemical compounds (e.g., topical diphencyprone). Results with all of these treatments have varied from partial hair regrowth to no regrowth at all.
- **Emotional support** is essential because extreme hair loss evokes loss of self-esteem and personal identity in many people.

POINTS TO REMEMBER

- Alopecia totalis and universalis, the most severe forms of AA, generally raise emotional problems in patients and their families.
- Workup for other diseases (e.g., thyroid disease) should be considered if suggested by a positive history or physical findings.

BASICS

- Androgenetic alopecia (male- and female-pattern **common baldness**) is not a disease but a normal consequence of aging. In the scalp, a significant loss of hair follicles occurs with advancing age.
- Androgenetic alopecia is seen more commonly in men; it tends to be less obvious in women because hair loss in women is generally incomplete and begins at a later age.
- Androgenetic alopecia is **genetically influenced**. It is caused by the action of androgen on hair follicles that results in a shortening of the hair growth, or **anagen** cycle, producing thinner, shorter hairs (miniaturization).
- Androgenetic alopecia is more common in whites than in Asians or African Americans.

DESCRIPTION OF LESIONS

Androgenetic alopecia occurs as **patterned, nonscarring loss of hair**.

DISTRIBUTION OF LESIONS

- **M-shaped frontal** and **vertex pattern** in men (male-pattern baldness; Figure 11.9)
- **Diffuse midparietal pattern** in women (female-pattern baldness; Figure 11.10)

CLINICAL MANIFESTATIONS

- **In men,** balding usually begins in **late adolescence**. It is sometimes associated with seborrheic dermatitis or an increase in dandruff.
- **In women,** balding begins later, most often **after menopause**. Hair loss is more diffuse.

DIAGNOSIS

Diagnosis is made by **clinical appearance** of patterned alopecia and absence of clues to a specific disease to account for hair loss.

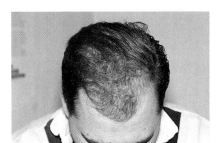

Figure 11.9.
Male-pattern androgenetic alopecia with M-shaped frontal and vertex pattern.

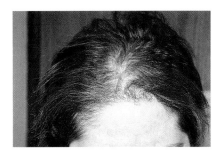

Figure 11.10.
Female-pattern androgenetic alopecia.

DIFFERENTIAL DIAGNOSIS

- **Androgen excess in women**
  - Hirsutism on other areas in a male pattern (beard, chest, groin)
  - Menstrual irregularities, infertility, sudden onset of acne
  - Androgen-secreting tumor
- **Telogen effluvium** (see below). There is a history of an acute event such as illness, childbirth, or trauma 3 to 4 months before the rapid alopecia.
- **Thyroid disease**
  - There is diffuse loss of hair.
  - Hypothyroidism is associated with dull, coarse, brittle hair. Hair loss begins with scalp hair; later, body hair is lost (e.g., sparsity of the eyebrows).
  - Hyperthyroidism is associated with fine, soft hair. Hair loss is rarely severe.
- **Diffuse alopecia areata**, which is rare

MANAGEMENT

- **Minoxidil 2%** solution applied twice daily may reduce shedding and possibly contribute to some regrowth. (**Minoxidil 5%** may be more effective.)
- **Low-dose finasteride** (used for benign prostatic hypertrophy) has recently been approved for use in androgenetic alopecia in men only.
- Hair transplantation or scalp reduction techniques may be helpful.
- Often, patients need emotional support.

POINTS TO REMEMBER

- An evaluation of women with androgenetic alopecia may include a complete blood count and measurement of thyroid stimulating hormone (TSH) and serum iron levels.
- After obtaining a careful history, clinicians should consider an androgen excess syndrome in women with symptoms or signs of virilization. These patients require more extensive hormonal studies.

BASICS

- Hair follicles show intermittent activity. Each hair grows to a maximum length, is retained for a time period without further growth, and is eventually shed and replaced.
- Telogen effluvium is a **temporary shedding** of scalp hairs from resting telogen follicles.
- **Pathogenetic factors** include **major illness, trauma, surgery, crash dieting,** and emotional stress.
- **In women,** telogen effluvium may be associated with **giving birth, aborted pregnancy,** or **discontinuation of oral contraceptives.**
- The precipitating event usually precedes hair loss by **6 to 16 weeks,** which is the time period required for **catagen hair** to become **telogen hair.**

DESCRIPTION OF LESIONS

The condition is seen as **diffuse alopecia**, which is **often not obvious to a casual observer** because only 10% of hairs are in a telogen stage at a given moment.

DISTRIBUTION OF LESIONS

Diffuse, nonpatterned alopecia

CLINICAL MANIFESTATIONS

- There is **noninflammatory, asymptomatic, rapid shedding** of hair.
- Hair is seen on pillows, combs and brushes, and in the bathtub.
- **Regrowth occurs within 1 year,** but hair may not grow back completely.

DIAGNOSIS

- Diagnosis is **made by history** because the diffuse loss associated with telogen effluvium may be subtle.
- A **positive hair-pull** test demonstrates a loss of 400 or more hairs per day (normal shedding is from 40 to 100 hairs per day).

DIFFERENTIAL DIAGNOSIS

- **Androgenetic alopecia** has a **characteristic pattern**.
- **Anagen effluvium**, secondary to drug therapy (e.g., cancer chemotherapeutic and immunotherapeutic drugs), is more extensive and occurs more rapidly than telogen effluvium.

MANAGEMENT

- **Treatment of underlying cause**, if possible
- **Reassurance** that hair tends to grow back normally

POINTS TO REMEMBER

- A careful history should be obtained, looking for antecedent illness, recent child-birth, ingestion of drugs, and recent trauma.
- When the cause of telogen effluvium is not apparent, a complete blood count as well as TSH, VDRL, and antinuclear antibody tests should be obtained.
- Other agents or drugs that may cause a telogen **or** an anagen effluvium include **anticoagulants**, thyroid medication, β-blockers, angiotensin-converting enzyme (ACE) inhibitors, heavy metals, oral contraceptives, lithium, and oral retinoids.

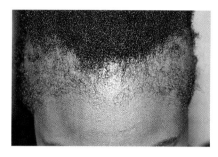

Figure 11.11.
Traction alopecia. Symmetrical loss of hair in frontotemporal distribution.

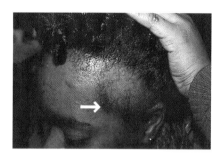

Figure 11.12.
Traction alopecia. Note fringe of residual hairs at the distal margin of alopecia (*arrow*).

BASICS

- A common form of alopecia among African American and African Caribbean women may result from the use of hair reshaping products such as relaxers, straighteners, and permanent wave products.
- **Traction alopecia, chemically-induced alopecia,** and **"hot comb" alopecia** (also known as follicular degeneration syndrome) are common consequences of the following hair grooming methods:
  - Frequent use of hot combs, tight rollers, corn-rowing, and hair extenders may cause hair damage and loss, ultimately resulting in permanent alopecia. It is the persistent prolonged physical stress of **traction** caused by tight rollers and tight braiding or pulling hair back in pony tails that causes hair loss.
  - **Chemicals** such as thioglycolates are found in commercial products used to create curls by destroying disulfide bonds of keratin. These chemicals may also have **irritant effects** on the scalp that can result in inflammation and permanent loss of hair follicles. **Hot comb alopecia** results from the excessive use of pomades with the hot comb or iron. (Hot combing or pomades alone do not cause permanent alopecia.) Upon contact with the hot comb or hot iron (marcelling iron), the pomade liquefies and drips down the hair shaft into the follicle, resulting in a chronic inflammatory folliculitis, which, in time, can lead to scarring alopecia and permanent hair loss.

DESCRIPTION OF LESIONS

- **Traction alopecia** (Figure 11.11) is characterized by the following:
  - **Symmetrical pattern** of alopecia, which is associated with the use of tight curlers, or a more irregular pattern, which is associated with cornrows
  - **Broken-off hairs**
  - Characteristic **fringe of residual hairs** at the distal margin of the alopecia (Figure 11.12)
  - Possibly, scarring alopecia
- **Chemically and hot comb–induced alopecia** is characterized by **scaling, pustules,** and **itching,** which result in temporary or permanent alopecia.

DISTRIBUTION OF LESIONS

- **Traction pattern** most often involves the temples and frontal hairline (marginal alopecia), later involving the vertex and occipital areas.
- **Chemically and hot comb–induced pattern** has a more irregular (less symmetrical) distribution, depending on sites of application.
- **Combination** of both **patterns** exists if traction, hot combs, and chemicals are used.

CLINICAL MANIFESTATIONS

- Asymptomatic **gradual loss** of hair
- Partial, possibly complete, **regrowth** if managed early in the course
- Later, possible **scaling, pustules,** and **itching**
- **Scarring alopecia**

DIAGNOSIS

Diagnois made by **history** of use of hair reshaping techniques and scalp biopsy, if necessary, to rule out other causes, such as cutaneous sarcoidosis.

DIFFERENTIAL DIAGNOSIS

- **Alopecia areata (AA),** with round or oval patches of alopecia
- **Systemic lupus erythematosus (SLE)**
  - Diffuse, sudden loss of hair
  - Positive antinuclear antibody test and other signs and symptoms of SLE
- **Discoid lupus erythematosus**, with focal areas of scarring alopecia
- **Sarcoidosis**
  - May cause a scarring alopecia that closely resembles traction alopecia
  - Signs and symptoms of sarcoidosis

MANAGEMENT

- **Discontinuation of potentially damaging hair styling practices** may result in an abatement of hair loss and partial hair regrowth, depending on how long the insult on the roots has occurred.
- If styling practices are to be continued, the patient should be advised as follows:
  - **Chemicals** should be used **only on hair** and not directly on the scalp.
  - **Looser wrapping of hair** produces less tension on hair roots.
  - Braids should be larger and looser, and they should be undone every 2 weeks.

POINTS TO REMEMBER

- Traumatic alopecia in African American and African Caribbean women is common.
- Traumatic alopecia is sometimes **misdiagnosed as AA** by health care providers who are not familiar with these styling practices.
- Other conditions such as **cutaneous lupus** and **sarcoidosis** may closely resemble or occur concomitantly with traumatic alopecia.
- Patients with alopecia should be routinely asked how they style and manage their hair.

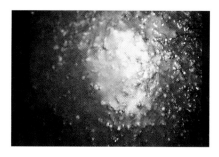

Figure 11.13.
Folliculitis and folliculitis decalvans. Flesh-colored atrophic or hypertrophic plaques are devoid of hairs.

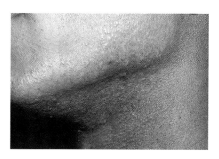

Figure 11.14.
Pseudofolliculitis barbae. Hypertrophic scars from hairs that have penetrated the skin.

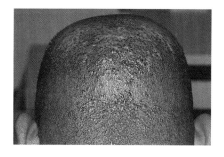

Figure 11.15.
Acne keloidalis. Note papules and hypertrophic scars in occipital area and adjacent scalp.

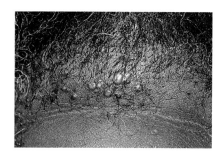

Figure 11.16.
Acne keloidalis. Keloid formation.

BASICS

- **Folliculitis** (see Chapter 9, "Superficial Bacterial Infections"), or hair follicle problems, are common in African Americans. Postadolescent black men, in particular, experience "shaving bumps" (**pseudofolliculitis barbae**) and a characteristic acnelike scarring condition on the occiput (**acne keloidalis**).
- These follicular disorders are thought to be the result of a delayed hypersensitivity reaction targeting the hair follicle. The inflammatory process often results in scarring alopecia (**cicatricial alopecia**).

DESCRIPTION OF LESIONS

Folliculitis and folliculitis decalvans
(Figure 11.13)
- **Focal pustules** often result in scarring.
- Flesh-colored atrophic or hypertrophic **plaques are devoid of hairs**.

Pseudofolliculitis barbae
(Figure 11.14)
- Tight **curly hairs** that have been sharpened by shaving **penetrate the skin**, causing a reaction similar to that caused by a foreign body.
- Inflammatory papules and pustules develop that often result in hypertrophic scars, which appear as flesh-colored papules.

Acne keloidalis
(Figure 11.15)
- A reentry phenomenon similar to that seen in pseudofolliculitis barbae, but that occurs in the occipital area of the scalp, results in inflammatory papules and pustules.
- Ultimately, hypertrophic scarring results, characterized by flesh-colored papules and possibly keloid formation.

DISTRIBUTION OF LESIONS

- **Folliculitis** involves the **scalp, beard,** and other **hairy areas** of the body.
- **Pseudofolliculitis barbae** involves the **beard**, particularly on the neck and submental area.
- **Acne keloidalis** involves the **occipital area** and may extend to the adjacent or entire scalp.

CLINICAL MANIFESTATIONS

- **Gradual evolution** of erythematous papules
- **Itching, tenderness**
- **Pustules,** possibly indicating secondary *Staphylococcus aureus* infection
- Papular, nodular scars become hypertrophic and confluent and may become **keloids** (Figure 11.16)

DIAGNOSIS AND DIFFERENTIAL DIAGNOSIS

In black men and women, the diagnosis of these conditions is readily made on the basis of **clinical appearance**.

Tinea capitis
- This is seen primarily in children.
- Scarring is unlikely; however, severe inflammatory tinea capitis may result in permanent alopecia.

Infectious folliculitis in the immunocompromised setting
This is generally indistinguishable from other types of folliculitis.

It may be the result of other colonizers of the hair follicle, such as *Pseudomonas, Candida,* and *Pityrosporum ovale.*

Tinea faciale and scarring acne should be ruled out.

MANAGEMENT

Folliculitis and folliculitis decalvans
- **Mild**
  - **Topical antibiotics,** such as those used for acne, used for their antiinflammatory effects
  - **Antibacterial shampoo,** such as Betadine
- **Moderate**
  - **Systemic antibiotics,** such as minocycline (dicloxacillin or a cephalosporin to cover *S. aureus* superinfection)
  - Intralesional steroids
- **Severe**
  - Short courses of **systemic steroids**
  - Course of **isotretinoin** (Accutane), similar to that given for cystic acne, may be helpful

Pseudofolliculitis barbae
- **Discontinuation of shaving**
- **Avoidance of close shaving** by using guarded razor (e.g, PFB Bump Fighter)
- **Elevation of penetrating hairs** with a fine needle before they penetrate skin
- **Avoidance of removing hairs with tweezers** because new hairs will grow in the same inflamed sites
- **Topical steroids** to alleviate inflammation and itching
- **Topical antibiotics** such as erythromycin (Akne-Mycin) ointment
- **Systemic antibiotics** such as minocycline
- **Depilatories** such as Magic Shave

Acne keloidalis
- **Topical steroids**
- **Intralesional steroids**
- **Topical antibiotics**
- **Systemic antibiotics** such as minocycline
- **Excisional surgery,** which is reserved for extreme cases and may result in worse scarring

POINTS TO REMEMBER
- Bacteria, when present, is usually a secondary, not a primary pathogen.
- Tinea capitis is unusual in adults.

CHAPTER 12

DISORDERS OF THE MOUTH, LIPS, AND TONGUE

Overview

- Mucous membrane lesions can be **clues to systemic illnesses**, such as AIDS and systemic lupus erythematosus. They may also be helpful in making a diagnosis of dermatologic conditions such as lichen planus.
- Other lesions, such as "canker sores," are most often seen as **isolated phenomena** or, as in Behçet's disease and ulcerative colitis, as an accompaniment or a precursor to the symptom complex.
- It is frequently difficult to make a clinical diagnosis involving the oral cavity because mucous membrane lesions tend to look alike, presenting either as **erythematous erosions** and **ulcers**, or **whitish plaques**. **Pigmentary changes, neoplasms, cystic lesions,** and **normal variants** are also seen on mucous membranes. Examples of each are given below.

APHTHOUS STOMATITIS

BASICS

- Aphthous stomatitis (aphthous ulcers), or **"canker sores,"** consist of shallow erosions of the mucous membranes; they are a common recurrent problem.
- Aphthous stomatitis is seen in children and adults.
- There is **no known cause** for aphthous stomatitis, and most cases heal spontaneously only to recur unexpectedly. Patients often ascribe recurrences to psychological stress or local trauma.
- Oral ulcerations indistinguishable from aphthous stomatitis are sometimes seen in association with Behçet's disease and ulcerative colitis.

DESCRIPTION AND DISTRIBUTION OF LESIONS

- Lesions are small (2 mm to 5 mm), well-demarcated, punched-out erosions occurring on the buccal, labial, and gingival mucosa as well as the tongue.
- There is a ring of erythema, with a yellowish center (Figure 12.1).

CLINICAL MANIFESTATIONS

- The lesions are usually painful.
- They generally heal in 4 to 14 days.
- Lesions may be larger, more extensive, persistent, and painful in patients with HIV and Behçet's disease (Figure 12.2).

DIAGNOSIS

- The diagnosis is made clinically.
- The Tzanck test or herpes simplex virus (HSV) culture is negative.

DIFFERENTIAL DIAGNOSIS

- **Primary HSV infection** (see Chapter 7, "Superficial Viral Infections")
  - Primary HSV infection occurs as a gingivostomatitis.
  - It is seen most often in infants and young children.
  - It is accompanied by pain, fever, a sore throat, and swollen glands.
- **Recurrent HSV infections** and aphthous stomatitis, which it resembles, are often confused by patient and physician alike, as being the same entity. In fact, with the exception of primary HSV and HSV in immune compromised individuals, HSV infection **rarely occurs inside the mouth**

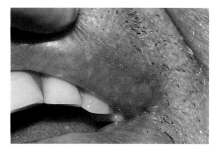

Figure 12.1.
Aphthous stomatitis. Small, punched-out erosions with erythema surrounding a yellowish center.

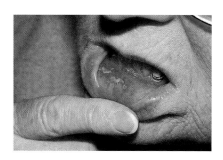

Figure 12.2.
Larger, more persistent aphthous stomatitis lesions in a patient with Behçet's disease.

- **Hand, foot, and mouth disease** (coxsackievirus A16; see Chapter 8, "Exanthems")
  - Lesions are characteristically oval, erythematous erosions.
  - Lesions are asymptomatic because they are shallower than the lesions of aphthous stomatitis.
  - Lesions are located on the pharynx and are associated with similar lesions on the palms and soles.
  - There is a low-grade fever and occasional cervical adenopathy.

MANAGEMENT

- Application of **silver nitrate** directly on the lesions sometimes promotes healing.
- Symptomatic therapy uses the topical anesthetic viscous **lidocaine**.
- **Vanceril** can be sprayed directly on the lesions.
- Superpotent **topical steroids** may be applied directly and held for 10 to 20 minutes to lesions by pressure with a finger.
- **Tetracycline suspension** (250 mg/tsp) is administered in a "swish and swallow" manner.
- **Diphenhydramine suspension** is administered in a "gargle and spit" manner.
- **Intralesional steroid injections** and **systemic steroids** are reserved for recalcitrant ulcers.
- There are reports in the dental literature that the use of sodium lauryl sulfate-free toothpaste may decrease the recurrence rate of aphthae.
- Aphthasol (amlexanox 5%) oral paste, which is available only by prescription, is reported to accelerate ulcer healing.
- Recently, **thalidomide** has been used with some success in healing large, painful, persistent aphthae in persons with HIV disease. (Even a single dose has been known to cause **fetal malformation**; consequently, use in women with childbearing potential requires effective counseling and birth-control measures.)

POINTS TO REMEMBER

- A single, nonhealing ulcer (lasting longer than 2 months) should be biopsied to rule out squamous cell carcinoma.
- Persistent erosions should alert one to the possibility of Behçet's disease, ulcerative colitis, erosive lichen planus, systemic lupus erythematosus, or a primary blistering disease such as pemphigus vulgaris or bullous pemphigoid.

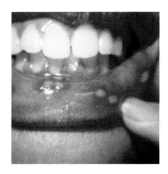

Figure 12.3.
Primary herpes gingivostomatitis. Note erosions of mucosa and swollen gums.

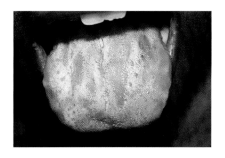

Figure 12.4.
Mucous patches of secondary syphilis. The patches are caused by eroded epithelium of the tongue.

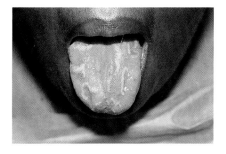

Figure 12.5.
Geographic tongue. Shiny, red patches devoid of papillae, which resemble mucous patches.

PRIMARY HSV

See Chapter 7, "Superficial Viral Infections" (Figure 12.3)
- Lesions are seen frequently in the oral cavity.
- Lesions are often accompanied by fever and swollen glands.

MUCOUS PATCHES OF SECONDARY SYPHILIS

- The lesions of secondary syphilis on the tongue (Figure 12.4) are known as "mucous patches."
- They are characterized by asymptomatic round or oval eroded lesions or papules, which are devoid of epithelium.
- The lesions teem with spirochetes.
- The VDRL is reactive.

GEOGRAPHIC TONGUE

- Geographic tongue (Figure 12.5), or benign migratory glossitis, is a common idiopathic finding.
  - The lesions of geographic tongue are areas that are shiny, red, and devoid of papillae.
  - They resemble mucous patches; however, these lesions move around on the surface of the tongue, changing configuration from one day to the next, accounting for the bizarre varying patterns.
- There have been reports suggesting an association of geographic tongue with psoriasis; however its 2% incidence in patients with psoriasis is no greater than would be expected in the normal population.
- No treatment is necessary.

ERYTHEMA MULTIFORME

- **Erythema multiforme major** (Figure 12.6; see Chapter 18, "Diseases of Vasculature")
  - This condition is also known as Stevens-Johnson syndrome.
  - Hemorrhagic crusts that occur on the lips are seen, in addition to extensive targetoid lesions elsewhere.
- Some cases of **erythema multiforme minor** may exhibit the crusted lesion of recurrent HSV on the vermillion border of the lip (see Figure 7.5).

SYSTEMIC LUPUS ERYTHEMATOSUS

Systemic lupus erythematosus (Figure 12.7) exhibits erosions or ulcerations on the hard palate.

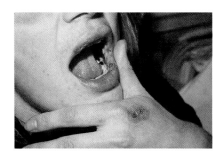

Figure 12.6.
Erythema multiforme major (Stevens-Johnson syndrome). Note the bullae and crusts on the lips.

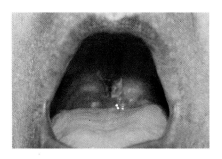

Figure 12.7.
Systemic lupus erythematosus. Note the ulceration on the hard palate.

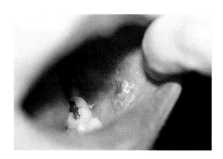

Figure 12.8.
Lichen planus. A white, lacy network of lesions is found on the buccal mucosa and tongue.

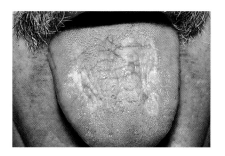

Figure 12.9.
Lichen planus. A white, lacy network of lesions is found on the buccal mucosa and tongue.

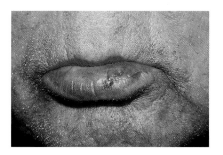

Figure 12.10.
Squamous cell carcinoma of the mucous membranes. Note an ulcer on the lower lip.

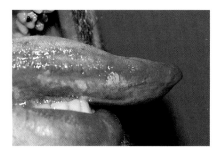

Figure 12.11.
Oral hairy leukoplakia. Note papules on sides of the tongue that resemble white hairs.

LICHEN PLANUS

See Chapter 5, "Eruptions of Unknown Cause."
- There is a white, lacy network of lesions on the buccal mucosa, tongue, and gums (Figures 12.8 and 12.9).
- Lesions may be erosive, ulcerative, and painful.
- Lesions of lichen planus can be found elsewhere on the body.

ORAL LEUKOPLAKIA

- Oral leukoplakia is a white macular or plaquelike lesion, which is considered a precursor to squamous cell carcinoma of the mucous membranes (fewer than 5% of the lesions become squamous cell carcinoma).
- It is characterized by white adherent plaques.
- Lesions occur on the tongue, buccal mucosa, hard palate, and gums.
- Oral leukoplakia may resemble oral lichen planus and oral hairy leukoplakia, or it may resemble the white plaques caused by trauma.
- Smoking, chewing tobacco, and alcohol abuse are all contributing factors.
- Leukoplakia is not a specific diagnosis; rather, it is a lesion that represents a reaction to trauma.

SQUAMOUS CELL CARCINOMA OF MUCOUS MEMBRANES

- Squamous cell carcinoma of the mucous membranes (Figure 12.10) is generally a slow-growing firm papule or ulcer.
- It may be a white plaque or early erosion (i.e., evolving de novo or from leukoplakia).
- Most lesions are found on the lower lip.

ORAL HAIRY LEUKOPLAKIA

See Chapter 24, "The Cutaneous Manifestations of HIV Infection."
- Oral hairy leukoplakia is caused by the Epstein-Barr virus (Figure 12.11).
- It occurs in HIV-positive patients. (There have been some case reports of oral hairy leukoplakia in immunocompromised HIV-negative patients.)
- Filiform papules on sides of the tongue resemble white hairs.
- Usually the lesions are asymptomatic.

CANDIDIASIS ("THRUSH")

See Chapter 24, "The Cutaneous Manifestations of HIV Infection."
- Candidiasis is seen in immunocompromised patients and in neonates.
- Curdlike or erosive lesions are easily removed with gauze.
- It may involve the tongue, oropharynx, and angles of mouth (perlèche).
- The lesion is KOH positive.

BLACK HAIRY TONGUE

- Black hairy tongue (Figure 12.12) represents more than just a pigmentary change. It is actually a benign, asymptomatic hyperplasia (an accumulation of keratin) of the filiform papillae of the tongue.
- It is characterized by a velvety, hairlike thickening of the tongue's surface.
- The pigmentation results from the normal pigment-producing bacterial flora that colonize the keratin. The color can range from a yellowish-brown or green to jet black. A toothbrush can be used to scrape off the excess keratin.
- It has been debatably associated with smoking, excessive coffee or tea drinking, and the prolonged use of oral antibiotics and psychotropic agents. It is considered by some clinicians as a possible marker for AIDS.

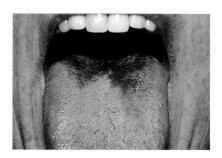

Figure 12.12.
Black hairy tongue.

ANTIMALARIAL THERAPY

The pigmentation that is sometimes seen while a patient is on antimalarial therapy is distinguished by a bluish-gray or purple color (Figure 12.13).

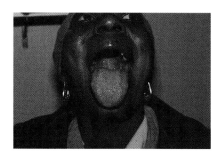

Figure 12.13.
Hyperpigmentation on the tongue is secondary to antimalarial therapy with hydroxychloroquine.

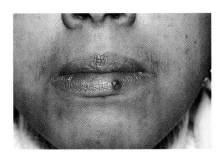

Figure 12.14.
Pyogenic granuloma seen on the lip of a pregnant woman.

PYOGENIC GRANULOMA

Pyogenic granuloma (Figure 12.14; see Chapter 21, "Benign Skin Neoplasms") is seen on the lips and gums, particularly in pregnant women.

MUCOCELE

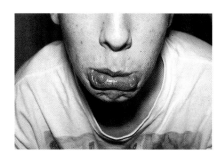

- Mucocele (Figure 12.15) is a common mucous-filled blisterlike lesion. It is not a true cyst and is considered to be the result of trauma to the openings of the salivary glands. It is seen most commonly in infants and young children.
- The lesion is a bluish or clear papule that contains a mucoid material; it can be easily ruptured.
- It occurs on the lip and floor of the mouth.
- The lesion is sometimes recurrent. It may spontaneously disappear, particularly in infants.
- It can be treated with incision and drainage or excision, if necessary.

Figure 12.15.
Mucocele. A cystic lesion is on the lower lip.

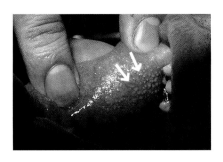

Figure 12.16.
Fordyce spots are yellow papules on the buccal mucosa (*arrows*).

FORDYCE SPOTS

- Fordyce spots (Figure 12.16) are normal findings that represent ectopic mucous glands.
- Yellow papules occur on the lips or buccal mucosa and are more obvious when the skin is stretched.
- They are brought to medical attention when noted by the patient and are an incidental finding that requires no treatment.

CHAPTER 13

DISEASES AND ABNORMALITIES OF NAILS

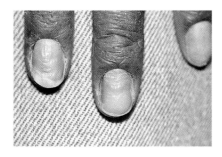

Figure 13.1.
Nail dystrophy secondary to eczematous dermatitis. The characteristic lichenification (exaggeration of normal skin markings) seen in atopic dermatitis (chronic eczematous dermatitis) suggests the cause of the misshapen nails.

BASICS

- Injuries to the matrix of the nail may be caused by microbes, such as fungi, or inflammatory conditions, such as lichen planus. These disorders may result in characteristic deformities, such as nail pitting, "oil spots," and onycholysis as seen in psoriasis. Alternatively, they may result in nonspecific deformities as seen in eczema of the proximal nail fold.
- Nail dystrophy secondary to eczematous dermatitis (Figure 13.1) is a problem that is often overlooked in patients with severe atopic dermatitis. It results when an eczematous dermatitis involves the distal extensor surface of the fingers, the inflammation of which also involves the matrix, or "root," of the nail. The matrix, which underlies the proximal nail fold, consequently gives rise to a dystrophic nail plate. (The resultant nail deformity is analogous to an injury to the root of a tree that causes a deformity to the growing tree trunk.)

MANAGEMENT

The fingernail plate generally grows out normally over a period of time (usually in 4 to 6 months):
- Following control of inflammation with the use of topical steroids, or
- After spontaneous remission of the dermatitis

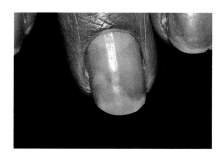

Figure 13.2.
Onycholysis. The separated portion of the nail is white and opaque; the attached portion is pink and translucent.

BASICS

- Onycholysis (Figure 13.2) is a separation of the nail plate from the underlying pink nail bed. The separated portion is white and opaque, in contrast to the pink translucence of the attached portion.
- Physiologic onycholysis is seen at the distal free margin of normal nails as they grow.
- When there is more proximal separation, as can be seen in such conditions as psoriasis, thyroid disease, and onychomycosis, the onycholysis can become more obvious and display a yellow or green tinge (see **green nail** below).
- Onycholysis is most often seen in adult women, particularly those with long fingernails. It may become painful and interfere with a routine function of the nails, for example, picking up small objects such as coins and paper clips.

CAUSES

The causes and associations of onycholysis can be divided into two main groups:
- **External causes**
  - **Irritants** such as nail polish, nail wraps, nail hardeners, and the use of artificial nails may cause onycholysis. It is also seen in individuals who frequently come into contact with water, such as bartenders, hair dressers, manicurists, citrus fruit handlers, and domestic workers.
  - **Physical trauma**, especially injuries to the toes as seen in athletes, may be the result of wearing tight shoes. Fingernail onycholysis may be the result of habitual finger sucking or the use of the fingernails as a tool.
  - **Fungal infections**, as seen in chronic paronychia, yeast infections, and in onychomycosis, may cause onycholysis
  - **Drugs** such as tetracycline, doxycycline, and demeclocycline act as phototoxic agents that may induce onycholysis. Psoralen, the photoactivating drug used in psoralen plus ultraviolet A (PUVA) therapy, and ultraviolet A light are also photoonycholytic agents. Onycholysis has also been associated with thiazide diuretics, sulfa drugs, bleomycin, 5-fluorouracil, doxorubicin, and systemic retinoids.

- **Internal causes**
  - **Psoriasis** is the most common internal cause of onycholysis. Generally, there is evidence of psoriasis elsewhere on the body, or there are other psoriatic nail findings, such as pitting.
  - **Eczematous dermatitis, lichen planus,** and other inflammatory skin diseases may induce onycholysis.
  - **Neoplasms** and **subungual warts** may cause onycholysis; however, this is more likely if only one nail is involved.
  - **Thyroid disease**, **pregnancy**, and **anemia** are also possible internal associations.

MANAGEMENT AND PREVENTION

- Nails should be kept dry.
- Avoid unnecessary manipulation of nails.
- If known, the underlying cause of the onycholysis should be treated or avoided.
- Secondary infection, if present, should be treated because it often accounts for the failure of the nail to reattach itself.
- Nails should be cut closely.
- If the fingernails are kept long, avoid repeated trauma (e.g., typing), which may result in further prying of the nail plate away from the nail bed.

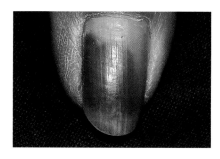

Figure 13.3.
Green nail syndrome. The "dead space" underneath the nail often harbors *Pseudomonas* species.

BASICS

- Green nail syndrome (Figure 13.3) is a consequence of onycholysis. It is a painless discoloration under the nail, not to be confused with a subungual hematoma.
- The "dead space" underneath the onycholytic nail serves as an excellent breeding ground for microbes such as *Pseudomonas* species, which account for the green or green–black nail, and, less frequently, *Candida* species, which can impart a yellow–green or brown color to the nail.

MANAGEMENT AND PREVENTION

- The discoloration can generally be eliminated by soaking the affected nail two times daily in one part chlorine bleach and four parts water, or, similarly, equal parts acetic acid (vinegar) and water.
- The underlying cause (i.e., the factors that lead to onycholysis) should be minimized.

BASICS

- Layered splitting **(onychoschizia;** Figure 13.4) and brittle nails are common findings in adults.
- In some people, nails become fragile and easily break off at the free edge.

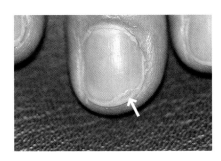

Figure 13.4.
Split nails (onychoschizia). Note distal nail splitting into layers parallel to the nail's surface (*arrow*).

MANAGEMENT

- Brittle nails and distal nail splitting are comparable to scaly, dry skin elsewhere. Thus, many treatment recommendations are similar to those for dry skin:
  - Avoidance of excessive contact with water
  - Wearing gloves in cold winter weather
- As with onycholysis, the nails should be kept short.
- Lactic acid creams in 5 to 12% concentration or other moisturizing creams or ointments may be applied at bedtime.
- Some clinicians claim to have some success in increasing nail integrity and thickness with biotin, 2.5 mg/day.

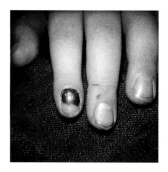

Figure 13.5.
Acute subungual hematoma.
(Slide courtesy of Peter G.
Burk, MD)

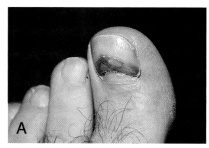

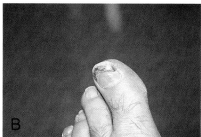

Figure 13.6.
Chronic subungual hematoma. (*A*) Nail
6 months after trauma; (*B*) same nail 10
months after trauma.

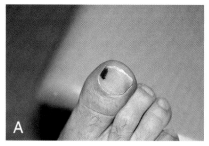

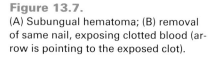

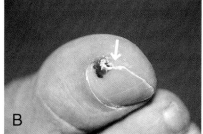

Figure 13.7.
(A) Subungual hematoma; (B) removal
of same nail, exposing clotted blood (arrow is pointing to the exposed clot).

SUBUNGUAL HEMATOMA

Figure 13.5

BASICS

- A subungual hematoma results from trauma to the nail matrix or nail bed, such as repeated minor injuries (e.g., tight shoes, sports injuries) or substantial impact (e.g., from a hammer).
- An acute subungual hematoma that results in a rapid accumulation of blood under the nail plate can be very painful. Small lesions may be painless and go unnoticed for some time.

DIFFERENTIAL DIAGNOSIS

- A chronic, painless subungual hematoma that is not clearly the result of trauma (this is common) may sometimes be confused with a neoplasm such as an **acral lentiginous melanoma,** which is rare.
  If there is a strong suspicion of melanoma, the nail bed should be biopsied.

MANAGEMENT

- An acute, painful, swollen subungual hematoma may be incised and drained by twirling a 27-guage needle on the area that is elevated by the hematoma, thereby creating a small hole through which the blood drains and the pain is quickly relieved.
- Diagnosis may be in doubt because the residue of coagulated blood remains (from 6 to 12 months) until the nail grows out (Figure 13.6).
- A fast method to substantiate the presence of a hematoma is to cut back, gently pare (with a # 15 scalpel), or file down the nail plate until the coagulated blood can be visualized (Figure 13.7).

MEDIAN NAIL DYSTROPHY

- Median nail dystrophy (habit tic deformity of the nail) is caused by repeated trauma to the proximal nail fold of one or both thumbs. It is usually the result of compulsive rubbing by the nail of the adjacent index finger on the thumbs (Figure 13.8). The injured matrix, which underlies the proximal nail fold, consequently gives rise to a dystrophic nail plate.

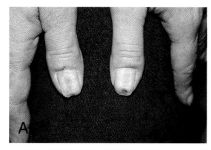

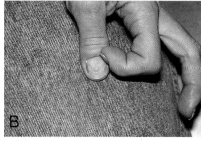

Figure 13.8.
Median nail dystrophy (habit tic deformity of the nail). (*A*) Note the vertical ridging in the nails; (*B*) Note the action of the adjacent index finger that produces the nail deformity.

MANAGEMENT

Treatment of any habit tic deformity is very difficult; the habit tic and resultant nail deformity are usually chronic when medical attention is sought. Because suggestions to willfully "break the habit" usually go unheeded, an alternative activity such as knitting or needlepoint may be suggested as a substitute activity.

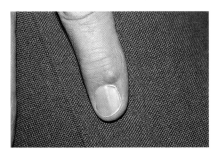

Figure 13.9.
Digital mucous cyst (digital myxoid cyst). Note longitudinal groove in the nail plate.

BASICS

- A **digital mucous cyst** is not a true cyst because it lacks an epidermal lining. It is actually a focal collection of clear, gelatinous, viscous mucin (focal mucinosis), which occurs over the distal interphalangeal joint or, more commonly, at the base of the nail. Myxoid cysts are believed to be a consequence of osteoarthritis and not the result of trauma.
- Pressure from the lesion on the nail matrix results in a characteristic **longitudinal groove** in the nail plate (Figure 13.9).

DESCRIPTION OF LESION

The lesion is dome-shaped and rubbery and occurs exclusively in adults.

MANAGEMENT

- This benign lesion may be ignored.
- Or:
  - Lesions have reportedly resolved after several weeks of daily firm compression.
- Incision and drainage (Figure 13.10), cryosurgery with LN$_2$, and intralesional triamcinolone injections have been tried with varying results.
- Surgical excision is reserved for the occasional painful, or otherwise troublesome, lesions.

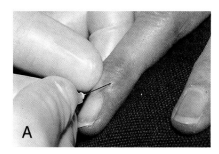

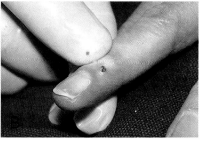

Figure 13.10.
(*A*) Incision of digital mucous cyst; (*B*) incision with a #30 needle reveals blood-tinged, jellylike mucoid material.

PARONYCHIA

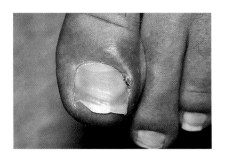

Figure 13.11.
Acute paronychia. Note erythema and edema at lateral nail fold.

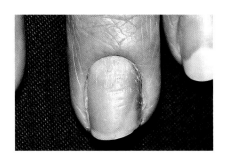

Figure 13.12.
Chronic paronychia. Note onycholysis, greenish discoloration, transverse ridging, and the absence of a cuticle.

Paronychia refers to inflammation of the nail folds surrounding the nail plate.

ACUTE PARONYCHIA

BASICS

- Acute paronychia usually results from an infection with *Staphylococcus aureus*; it is less commonly the result of streptococci and *Pseudomonas* (Figure 13.11).
- Generally, only one nail is involved. An acute paronychia may occur spontaneously, or it may follow trauma or manipulation such as nail biting, a manicure, or removal of a hang nail.
- A rapid onset of a throbbing, intensely painful, tender, bright-red swelling of the proximal or lateral nail fold behind the cuticle heralds an acute paronychia.

MANAGEMENT

- Mild cases may require only warm saline or aluminum acetate (Domeboro 1:40) soaks for 10 to 15 minutes, two to four times daily.
- In more severe cases, simple incision and drainage with a #11 surgical blade usually affords a rapid relief of pain.
- Occasionally, systemic therapy with antistaphylococcal antibiotics such as dicloxacillin, cephalosporin, or erythromycin may be used.

DIAGNOSIS/DIFFERENTIAL DIAGNOSIS

Acute bacterial paronychia can be confused with a herpetic whitlow; thus, a Tzanck preparation and/or bacterial culture may be performed when the diagnosis is in doubt.

CHRONIC PARONYCHIA

BASICS

- Chronic paronychia (Figure 13.12) results primarily from chronic moisture, irritation, and trauma to the nails.
- A secondary problem may result from a low-grade infection caused by *Candida albicans*. Various pathogens and contaminants, including other *Candida* species and/or gram-positive and gram-negative organisms, may be cultured from the pus obtained from under the proximal nail fold.

- Chronic paronychia usually develops slowly and asymptomatically.
- It is much more common in women than men and is seen particularly in people whose hands are chronically exposed to a wet environment, such as housewives, domestic workers, bartenders, janitors, bakers, dishwashers, dentists, dental hygienists, and children who habitually suck their thumbs.
- It is also seen more often in diabetics and in individuals who manicure their cuticles. The predisposing factor is usually trauma or maceration that produces a break in the barrier (cuticle) between the nail fold and the nail plate. This produces a portal of entry, which allows the accumulation of moisture and resultant microbial colonization. Secondary nail plate changes often occur, such as onycholysis, a greenish or brown discoloration along the lateral borders, and transverse ridging.
- Often, one or more fingers are involved.

DIAGNOSIS/DIFFERENTIAL DIAGNOSIS

- Diagnosis is generally made based upon typical clinical appearance and history. On occasion, there may be tenderness and a purulent discharge upon compression of the proximal nail fold.
- Candidal etiology can be confirmed with a KOH preparation or fungal culture, if necessary. The bacterial culture often grows a mixed flora.

MANAGEMENT

- Avoidance of prolonged exposure to moisture and trauma
- Wearing gloves, particularly cotton-under-vinyl gloves
- Avoidance of frequent washing and manicures
- Topical therapy
  - Topical broad-spectrum antifungal agents, such as clotrimazole, ketoconazole, econazole, and miconazole, which are sometimes combined with a potent topical corticosteroid
  - One to two drops daily of 3% thymol in 70% ethanol (compounded by a pharmacist), placed under the proximal nail fold
- Systemic broad-spectrum antifungal therapy
- Systemic antibiotics, pending culture results
- Surgery, which is rarely a treatment option

POINTS TO REMEMBER

- Chronic paronychia is frequently misdiagnosed as an acute staphylococcal paronychia.
- Chronic paronychia is distinct from onychomycosis (tinea unguium), which refers to a fungal infection of the **nail plate**

See Chapters 4 and 10.

CHAPTER 14

PIGMENTARY DISORDERS

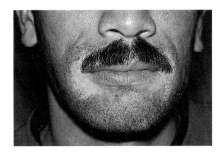

Figure 14.1.
Hypopigmented, perioral chalk-white macules.

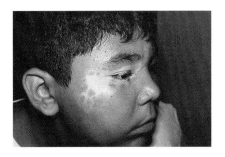

Figure 14.2.
Various shades of hypopigmentation around the eyes. Note the white eyelashes.

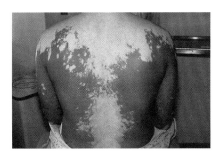

Figure 14.3.
Extensive depigmentation.

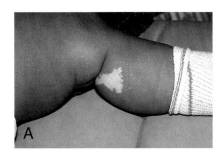

Figure 14.4. (A)
Vitiligo;

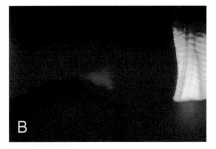

Figure 14.4. (B)
Wood's light examination reveals a "milk-white" fluorescence of lesion.

BASICS

- Vitiligo is an acquired disorder of depigmentation of the skin, which is believed to be caused by an autoimmune process that results in the loss of melanocytes. Another theory holds that vitiligo is caused by an abnormality of nerve endings adjacent to skin pigment cells.
- In support of an immune mechanism in the pathogenesis of vitiligo is its association with other diseases that presumably have an autoimmune basis, such as hyperthyroidism, Addison's disease, alopecia areata, diabetes mellitus, and pernicious anemia.
- The physical appearance of vitiligo can be emotionally devastating, particularly in dark-skinned people. It affects 1 to 2% of the world's population, and 50% of patients report a family history of vitiligo.

DESCRIPTION OF LESIONS

- Hypopigmented, chalk-white macules are more obvious in dark-skinned people (Figure 14.1).
- Occasionally, individual lesions have various shades of color (Figure 14.2).

DISTRIBUTION OF LESIONS

- Vitiligo is bilateral and symmetrical in distribution.
- It appears characteristically around orifices: the mouth, eyes, nose, anus.
- Vitiligo also has predilection for acral areas, such as the hands and feet, body folds, bony prominences, and external genitalia.
- Vitiligo may be even more widespread (Figure 14.3) or total (vitiligo universalis).

CLINICAL MANIFESTATIONS

- The condition is often cyclical, with an early rapid loss of pigment, followed by a stable period, then recurrence.
- Some patients experience spontaneous partial repigmentation; total repigmentation is rare.
- Social stigmatization, embarrassment, and low self-esteem are common.

DIAGNOSIS

- Diagnosis is made by clinical appearance.
- Wood's light examination reveals a "milk-white" fluorescence (Figure 14.4).
- In dark-skinned people, pigmentary loss may be observed at any time of year. In light-skinned people, the tanning effects of the summer sun accentuate the contrast between the light and dark skin.

DIFFERENTIAL DIAGNOSIS

- **Postinflammatory hypopigmentation**
  - Postinflammatory hypopigmentation is off-white in color (the skin is not totally depigmented).
  - The patient may possibly have a history of preexisting inflammatory dermatitis, such as eczema (see Figure 14.11).
- **Tinea versicolor** (Figure 14.5)
  - Scale is associated with tinea versicolor.
  - The lesion is KOH positive.
  - Wood's light may show a yellow–orange fluorescence.
- **Chemically-induced vitiligo** (leukoderma; Figure 14.6) occurs on the hands of people who work with germicidal detergents or with certain rubber-containing compounds that destroy melanocytes. (See Chapter 3, "Occupational Dermatoses.")
- **Tuberculous leprosy**
  - Leprosy is seen in endemic areas.
  - Hypopigmented macules and plaques of tuberculous leprosy are often anesthetic due to sensory nerve destruction.

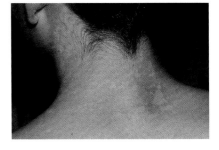

Figure 14.5.
Tinea versicolor. Postinflammatory hypopigmentation.

MANAGEMENT

- **Repigmentation therapy**
  - Potent and superpotent topical steroids used early for limited disease are occasionally helpful.
  - Psoralen plus ultraviolet A (PUVA) photochemotherapy using natural sunlight or artificial PUVA in a phototherapy lightbox (see Chapter 27, "Highly Specialized Procedures") is time-consuming and often ineffective; it is generally not used in children younger than 9 years.
  - **Minigrafting** of normal skin to areas of vitiligo may be useful for certain patients but does not result in total return of normal pigment.
  - There are several clinical reports that aspirin and vitamins B_6, B_{12}, C, E, and folic acid are of some value in treating vitiligo; however, this has not been established.
  - Special cosmetics, such as Dermablend and Covermark, can be used.
  - Self-tanning compounds that contain dihydroxyacetone may be helpful by disguising the lesions.
- **Depigmentation therapy.** Some patients who have greater than 50% loss of pigment may elect to have the remaining pigment "bleached" with the depigmenting agent, Benoquin (the monobenzyl ether of hydroquinone). The results are permanent.

POINTS TO REMEMBER

- People from the Indian subcontinent who have vitiligo have an additional potential stigma because vitiligo often resembles leprosy.
- Health-care providers should resist the tendency that exists among medical professionals to trivialize vitiligo as being only a cosmetic disorder.
- Sunscreens (see Appendix 2) are used to control tanning, which lessens the contrast between lesional and normal skin (they also protect sun-sensitive vitiliginous skin).
- If indicated by positive findings in the patient's history or on physical examination, screening for autoimmune diseases should be undertaken.
- Response to therapy is often disappointing.

Figure 14.6.
Chemically-induced vitiligo due to phenol contained in a cleaning product.

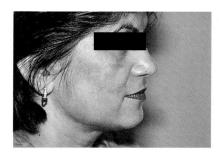

Figure 14.7.
Melasma of the cheeks.

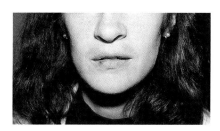

Figure 14.8.
Melasma of the moustache area.

BASICS

- Melasma, formerly known as chloasma, or the "mask of pregnancy" is an acquired hyperpigmentation, which is seen most commonly on the face. It may result from long-term exposure to sunlight, pregnancy, and oral contraceptives, or it may be idiopathic.
- Melasma is seen primarily in young women during their child-bearing years, particularly those who have darker complexions and live in sunny climates.
- It is seen in Asia, the Middle East, South America, Africa, and the Indian subcontinent. In North America, it is a problem seen most often in Hispanics, African Americans, and numerous recent immigrants from the aforementioned regions.

DESCRIPTION OF LESIONS

- Macular tan to brown hyperpigmentation
- Well-demarcated

DISTRIBUTION OF LESIONS

The face is affected, with symmetrical hyperpigmentation primarily on the cheeks, forehead, upper lip, nose, and chin (Figures 14.7 and 14.8).

CLINICAL MANIFESTATIONS

- Asymptomatic darkening of skin, usually after sun exposure.
- Although melasma is a cosmetic problem, it is sometimes as troubling as vitiligo.
- It may disappear after termination of pregnancy or discontinuance of oral contraceptives.

DIAGNOSIS

Diagnosis is based upon clinical appearance.

DIFFERENTIAL DIAGNOSIS

- **Postinflammatory hyperpigmentation**
  - There may be a history of preceding inflammatory eruption or injury.
  - Lesions roughly correspond to the location of the inflammation or injury.
  - The lesions usually have less well-defined margins than those of melasma.

MANAGEMENT

- Sun avoidance or opaque sun blocks
- "Bleaching creams"
  - A 3 to 4% hydroquinone, such as Melanex or Eldoquin Forte (Eldopaque Forte has a sun block), is applied twice daily.
- Forty-eight hours before application, the preparation should be tried out on a limited area (e.g., the flexor forearm) to avoid the chances of contact dermatitis.
- Chemical peels and laser treatment may be used in recalcitrant cases.

POINTS TO REMEMBER

- As with vitiligo, melasma should not be considered a frivolous concern.
- Treatment often requires many months of application of hydroquinone; however, it will not work well without concomitant sun protection.

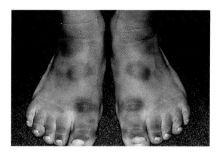

Figure 14.9.
Postinflammatory hyperpigmentation caused by contact dermatitis from sandals.

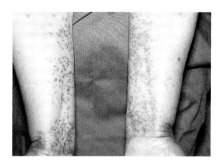

Figure 14.10.
Postinflammatory hyperpigmentation from resolved lichen planus.

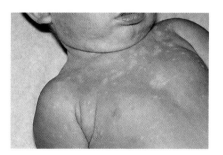

Figure 14.11.
Postinflammatory hypopigmented macules in an infant with atopic dermatitis.

- **Postinflammatory hyperpigmentation**
  - Darkening of the skin may follow nearly any inflammatory eruption, such as eczema and lichen planus (Figures 14.9 and 14.10) or injury, such as a burn.
  - Lesions roughly correspond to the location and the shape of the eruption or burn, although the margins are less well defined.
- **Postinflammatory hypopigmentation**
  - Lightening of the skin may follow nearly any inflammatory eruption (Figure 4.11). It may be noted after an injury such as a burn, or be associated with a surgical scar or following liquid nitrogen (LN_2) therapy; or the hypopigmentation may be idiopathic.
  - Hypopigmented areas roughly correspond to location and the shape of the eruption.

POINTS TO REMEMBER

- Postinflammatory hypopigmentation and hyperpigmentary alterations are the result of inflammation and/or injury to the skin. Recovery to normal pigmentation depends on the degree and type of injury.
- Treatment is generally unrewarding in long-standing cases.

CHAPTER 15

PRURITUS, THE "ITCHY" PATIENT

BASICS

- Pruritus is an unpleasant sensation that elicits the **urge to scratch**.
- The source of pruritus may be one of the following:
  - **Primary skin disorders,** such as eczema, xerosis (dry skin), and dermatitis herpetiformis
  - **Exogenous causes,** such as drugs, scabies, lice, fabric softeners, and fiberglass, and even water (aquagenic pruritus)
  - **Internal disorders,** such as chronic renal disease, AIDS, polycythemia vera, cholestasis, pregnancy-related disorders, primary biliary cirrhosis, diabetes mellitus, thyroid disease, and carcinoid syndrome
  - **Psychogenic** causes, such as delusions of parasitosis, neurotic excoriations, and obsessive–compulsive disorder
  - **Associated malignancies,** such as Hodgkin's disease, leukemia, and multiple myeloma
  - **Pruritus of unknown origin (PUO),** or itching lasting more than 2 to 6 weeks with no determined cause

DESCRIPTION OF LESIONS

- Linear excoriations, crusts, lichenified plaques, and wheals
- Commonly, simply pruritus, without lesions

DISTRIBUTION OF LESIONS

- Local
- Generalized

CLINICAL MANIFESTATIONS

- Associated with a primary skin disease
- Associated with underlying systemic disease
- Associated with underlying malignancy
- A symptom with no objective skin findings

DIAGNOSIS

- Diagnosis is made by **history** and **physical evidence** (i.e., linear excoriations, crusts).
- **Workup for PUO** includes the following:
  - Careful history
  - Physical examination, including rectal and pelvic examinations, if indicated
  - Complete blood count
  - Study of stool for parasites and occult blood
  - Chest radiograph
  - Thyroid and renal tests and liver function tests
  - Patient follow-up

MANAGEMENT

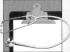

- **General principles**
  - **Treatment of the underlying systemic disease** often relieves the pruritus.
  - **Antihistamines** are of more benefit in the treatment of allergic conditions, urticaria, and drug reactions than they are for the treatment of itching and may be no more effective than a placebo. Even so, the powerful effect of antihistamines as placebos should not be overlooked.
- **Pruritus of chronic renal disease**
  - Ultraviolet B therapy
  - Oral ingestion of activated charcoal or cholestyramine
- **Pruritus of liver disease** may respond to cholestyramine.
- **Pruritus of xerosis** (Figure 15.1) may respond to moisturizers and topical steroids (when there are inflamed skin lesions).
- **Topical therapy**
  - Menthol, phenol, camphor, and calamine lotions (e.g., Sarna Anti-Itch, Prax, PrameGel) are soothing and helpful in some patients.
  - Topical steroids are generally not helpful when no lesions are apparent.
  - Topical doxepin (Zonalon) cream four times daily may help, although it may cause contact dermatitis.
  - Cold applications (e.g., with frozen vegetable packages) may give relief.

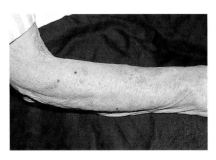

Figure 15.1.
Xerosis. Excoriations, scale, and crusts in an elderly person with pruritus.

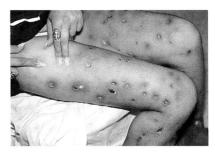

Figure 15.2.
Neurotic excoriations (factitia). Self-induced ulcers in a patient with a severe psychiatric disorder.

POINTS TO REMEMBER

- Antihistamines often exert their antipruritic action by inducing sleep (soporific effect).
- The dosage of antihistamines should be titrated gradually upward using nonsedating agents during the daytime and sedating agents at bedtime.
- Scabies should be considered when more than one family member itches.
- Hodgkin's disease may occur with a pruritus that precedes the diagnosis by as many as 5 years.
- Neurotic excoriations (factitia; Figure 15.2) are self-induced and occur more commonly in women.

CHAPTER 16

XEROSIS, THE "DRY" PATIENT

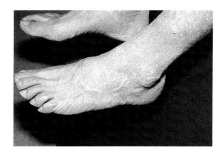

Figure 16.1.
Dry, scaly legs in an elderly person.

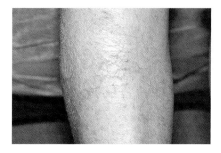

Figure 16.2.
Asteatotic eczema.

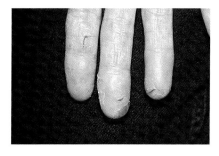

Figure 16.3.
Painful fissures of fingertips in a patient with hand eczema.

BASICS

- Xerosis, or dry skin, is a common observation in northern winter climates, particularly in conditions of cold air, low relative humidity, and indoor heating.
- **Dry, rough,** or **scaly skin** is most frequently seen on the hands and lower legs. (The word "dry" is probably misused because persistent scale is caused by an overadherence, or build-up, of scale, rather than by true dryness, or lack of water.)
- Xerosis becomes particularly evident in **atopic individuals** and in individuals **older than 70 years**.

Xerosis in the elderly

- The reason skin becomes dry, or appears to be dry, is not well-understood. In the elderly, xerosis (Figure 16.1) may be secondary to a **diminished production of sebum (asteatosis)**, as well as to **reduced eccrine sweat gland activity**, but other biochemical factors related to aging skin have also been implicated.
- In most cases of dry skin, such factors as overheated indoor spaces in winter, overbathing, and the use of harsh soaps and hot water tend to exacerbate the problem.

Asteatotic eczema (Figure 16.2)

- Asteatotic eczema **(winter eczema)** is also called erythema craquelé (also see Figure 2.30) and resembles an old cracked porcelain vase.
- It is a common, often pruritic, dermatitis that appears in dry, cold winter months.
- It occurs **exclusively in adults** and is located most commonly on the shins, arms, hands, and trunk.
- A relative loss of water from the skin through evaporation and possibly the decline in production of sebum, the skin's natural lubricant and sealant, result in **lack of normal desquamation**.

Atopic dermatitis

- **Dry, exquisitely sensitive, itchy skin** is a major feature of atopic dermatitis (eczema).
- Individuals with a personal or family **history of allergies, asthma,** or **hay fever** may, in addition to having scaly eczematous plaques, also have painful linear cracks or fissures, particularly on the palms, soles, and fingertips (Figure 16.3).

DESCRIPTION OF LESIONS

- **Scale**, with or without underlying erythema
- **Linear excoriations** and **crusts** after scratching
- **Painful fissures**

DISTRIBUTION OF LESIONS

- Most commonly on the hands, arms, and lower legs
- Often involve the palms, soles, and fingertips
- May be generalized

CLINICAL MANIFESTATIONS

- **Itching** is a primary manifestation.
- **Fissures** can be an isolated, recurrent, or **seasonal** finding in some individuals.
- Fissures are **painful**, often involving the fingertips in winter months, and are slow to heal.

DIAGNOSIS

Diagnosis is based on **clinical observation**.

DIFFERENTIAL DIAGNOSIS

- **Atopic dermatitis or nonspecific eczematous dermatitis**
  - There is often an atopic history.
  - Lichenification may be seen.
- **Scabies** should be considered in the differential, particularly, if the patient is pruritic or if the problem occurs in an institutional setting, such as a nursing home.

MANAGEMENT

- **Moisturizers** do not add water to the skin, but they do help retain, or "lock in", water that is absorbed while bathing. Therefore, **applying a moisturizer when the skin is still damp** helps seal in the absorbed water.
  - There are numerous **over-the-counter preparations** (e.g., Aquaphor, Eucerin, Alpha-Keri, Lubriderm, Vaseline Pure Petroleum Jelly, Vaseline Dermatology Formula, cocoa butter, Crisco shortening). Some are in ointment bases, cream bases, and lotion form, and others contain alpha-hydroxy acids. The product is chosen based on personal preference, ease of application, cost, and effectiveness.
  - Prescription Lac-Hydrin 12% Lotion, an **alpha-hydroxy acid preparation**, may be applied.
- **Topical steroids**, low-to-medium potency, are valuable in treating itch and erythema. In severe cases or if fissuring is present, more potent topical steroids may be applied.
- **Tepid water** should be used for showers and baths, which should be taken less frequently and for a short duration.
- **Mild soaps** (e.g., Dove, Basis) or a soap substitute (e.g., Cetaphil Lotion) may be used. **Excessive use of any soap should be avoided**, especially on affected areas.
- **Adhesive bandages** are effective in promoting healing of fissures.
- Adults may wear lined gloves while washing dishes.
- Skin should be protected from outdoor cold exposure by wearing gloves and other protective clothing.
- The value of room humidifiers is probably overestimated.
- Ingestion of copious amounts of fluid is also of questionable value.
- Vitamins also have not been shown to be of any benefit; in fact, overingestion of vitamin A can produce a dry skin–like condition known as phrynoderma.

 POINT TO REMEMBER

Dry skin and persistent pruritus, particularly when seen in elderly patients, should be investigated for possible systemic disease such as thyroid disease, renal disease, or underlying malignancy.

CHAPTER 17

DRUG ERUPTIONS

BASICS

- An **adverse drug reaction** is any nontherapeutic deleterious effect of a prescribed medication.
- Drug reactions may be **allergic (immunologic)** or **nonallergic (toxic)** in nature.
- Most drug eruptions are **exanthematous** (red rashes) and usually fade in a few days.
- **More serious reactions** include erythema multiforme major (Stevens-Johnson syndrome), toxic epidermal necrolysis, and serum sickness.
- The presence of urticaria, mucosal involvement, extensive or palpable purpura, or blisters almost always requires **discontinuation of the drug**.

Risk factors

- **Age.** Drug eruptions are more commonly seen in the elderly because they often take more drugs than younger people, they often take more than one drug at a time, and they are more likely to have been previously sensitized.
- **A history of previous drug reactions**
- **A family history of drug eruptions**
- **Prolonged use** of the drug

Characteristic skin reactions

Adverse cutaneous drug reactions can mimic many common non–drug-related skin eruptions, and certain drugs are more likely to cause characteristic reactions in the skin:

- **Exanthems:** sulfonamides, penicillins, hydantoins, allopurinol, quinidine
- **Urticarial:** penicillins, salicylates, blood products
- **Acneiform eruptions:** systemic steroids, topical steroids, lithium, oral contraceptives, androgenic hormones
- **Photosensitivity:** tetracyclines, particularly demethylchlortetracycline and doxycycline, griseofulvin, sulfonamide diuretics, sulfonylurea agents used to treat diabetes, nonsteroidal antiinflammatory drugs (NSAIDs), and phenothiazines
- **Erythema nodosum:** iodides, oral contraceptives, penicillin, gold, amiodarone, sulfonamides, opiates
- **Bullous eruptions:** penicillin, sulfonamides, captopril, iodides, gold, furosemide
- **Purpura:** anticoagulants, thiazides
- **Erythema multiforme major (Stevens-Johnson syndrome) and erythema multiforme minor:** sulfonamides, penicillins, tetracyclines, hydantoins, barbiturates

- **Fixed drug eruptions:** tetracyclines, sulfonamides, griseofulvin, barbiturates, phenolphthalein, NSAIDs
- **Contact dermatitis:** neomycin, preservatives in topical medications

DESCRIPTION OF LESIONS

- **Exanthematous drug eruption** (Figure 17.1)
  - Lesions are morbilliform (measleslike, macular and/or papular).
  - There are areas of confluence.
  - Lesions are pink, "drug red," or purple in color.
- **Urticarial drug eruption** (Figure 17.2) often manifests in bizarre, changing shapes.
- **Drug photosensitivity** may be erythematous (an exaggerated sunburn; Figure 17.3), eczematous, or lichenoid (lichen planus–like).
- **Fixed drug eruption** (Figure 17.4) is a reaction of red plaques or blisters that recur at the same cutaneous site each time the drug is ingested. In other words, a rechallenge of the drug results in an identical eruption at the same site or sites.
  - Lesions may be round or oval, single or multiple.
  - Lesions initially are erythematous; later they become violaceous.
  - Lesions often blister and erode.
  - The eruption often heals with postinflammatory hyperpigmentation.
- **Other drug eruptions** are discussed in Chapters 1 (acneiform), 2 (contact dermatitis), 18 (urticarial, purpuric, erythema multiforme), and 25 (erythema nodosum).

DISTRIBUTION OF LESIONS

Drug eruptions tend to be symmetrical and possibly generalized in distribution; however, certain eruptions have specific regional predilections.
- **Exanthems** are noted particularly on the trunk, thighs, upper arms, and face.
- In **contact dermatitis**, the distribution may be focal or random.
- A **fixed drug eruption** may present as a solitary, isolated lesion occurring most often on the extremities, glans penis, or trunk. Multiple lesions may also occur (multiple fixed drug eruptions; Figure 17.5).
- A **photosensitivity drug eruption** occurs on the face, dorsal forearms, and "V" of the neck and upper sternum.
- **Erythema nodosum** occurs characteristically in the pretibial area.
- **Purpura** also tends to occur on the lower extremities.
- **Steroid rosacea** occurs on the face.
- **Steroid atrophy** occurs in body folds (axillae and inguinal creases).
- **Urticaria** can be seen anywhere on the body.
- **Angioedema** occurs in a periorbital, labial, and perioral distribution.
- **Erythema multiforme** and other forms of **primary bullous eruptions** (e.g., pemphigus vulgaris) commonly manifest lesions of the oral mucous membranes and on other areas of the body.

CLINICAL MANIFESTATIONS

- Pruritus is a common complaint.
- Painful mucous membrane lesions (e.g., erosions, ulcers)
- Depending on the drug, serum sickness consisting of fever ("drug fever") and arthralgias

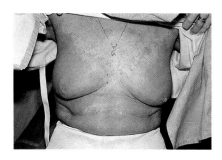

Figure 17.1.
Exanthematous ampicillin reaction. Note the "drug-red" symmetrical eruption, with areas of confluence.

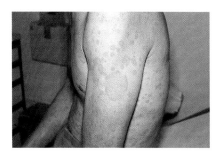

Figure 17.2.
Urticarial drug eruption. Note the bizarre shapes of the urticarial plaques.

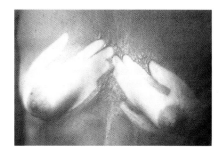

Figure 17.3.
Drug photosensitivity eruption. Erythematous (exaggerated sunburn) reaction in a person who was taking tetracycline and fell asleep on the beach. (Courtesy of the Albert Einstein College of Medicine, Division of Dermatology)

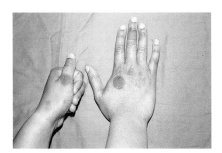

Figure 17.5.
Fixed drug eruption with multiple lesions.

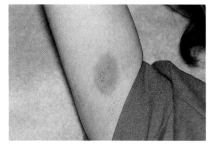

Figure 17.4.
Fixed drug eruption. An oval lesion occurred at the identical site where it had occurred previously. In both episodes, the rash emerged after ingesting a sulfonamide antibiotic. Note eroded blister in the center of the lesion.

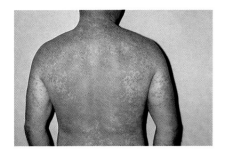

Figure 17.6.
Viral exanthem. (Courtesy of the Albert Einstein College of Medicine, Division of Dermatology)

DIAGNOSIS

- **History** is generally diagnostic.
- There may be a **characteristic rash**.
- There is occasional **eosinophilia**.
- Skin biopsy of an exanthem **showing perivascular lymphocytes** and **eosinophils** may be helpful but is not diagnostic.
- **Characteristic histopathologic changes** may occur in some cases (e.g., leukocytoclastic vasculitis in palpable purpura and a panniculitis in erythema nodosum; however, they are not necessarily diagnostic of a drug etiology).

DIFFERENTIAL DIAGNOSIS

Viral or **bacterial exanthems** occur with fever and other symptoms; however, they are often indistinguishable from a drug eruption (Figure 17.6).

MANAGEMENT

- **Discontinuation of the drug**
- **Oral antihistamines**
- **Systemic steroids**, only if necessary

POINTS TO REMEMBER

- Prompt recognition and withdrawal of an offending drug is important, particularly in instances of severe reactions.
- If a patient is taking multiple medications, it is often impossible to identify the agent responsible for an adverse reaction. In these instances, the drug that is most likely to cause the reaction should be suspected.
- If it is necessary to continue the drug (i.e., there is no alternative medication) and the adverse reaction is mild or tolerable, the difficulty may be minimized by decreasing the dosage or treating the adverse reaction.
- Trimethoprim–sulfamethoxazole (Bactrim or Septra), dapsone, and rifampin commonly cause hypersensitivity reactions in patients with AIDS.
- Drug reactions can occur after years of continuous therapy with the same drug.
- Drug reactions can occur days after the drug has been discontinued.
- A drug eruption may easily be confused as being a feature of the condition that it is intended to treat (e.g., a viral exanthem treated with an antibiotic).

CHAPTER 18

DISEASES OF VASCULATURE

BASICS

- **Urticaria**, commonly known as **hives**, is a reaction of cutaneous blood vessels that produces a transient dermal edema consisting of papules or plaques of different shapes and sizes **(wheals)**.
- **Angioedema** refers to edema that is deeper than urticaria and **involves the dermis and subcutaneous tissue**.
- By definition, an individual **urticarial lesion lasts less than 24 hours**.
- A total of 10 to 20% of the population has at least one episode of urticaria/angioedema at some point in their lifetime.

Causes

- Causes of urticaria/angioedema include:
  - Immunologic (IgE mediated), associated with food, drugs, or parasites
  - Complement mediated, associated with serum sickness or whole blood transfusions
  - An association with physical stimuli, such as cold, sunlight, and pressure
  - Occult infections, such as sinusitis, dental abscesses, and tinea pedis are rarely associated with chronic urticaria.
  - In 85 to 90% of patients with chronic urticaria, the etiology is unknown (chronic idiopathic urticaria [CIU]); however, there is increasing evidence that CIU may be an autoimmune disease because approximately 33% of patients have recently been shown to have histamine-releasing circulating IgG autoantibodies.

CLASSIFICATION

Urticaria may be classified as **acute** or **chronic** urticaria, **physical** urticaria, urticarial **vasculitis,** and **hereditary angioedema** (rare).

Acute and chronic urticaria

- **Acute urticaria** lasts less than 4 to 6 weeks.
  - Outbreaks are often **IgE mediated**.
  - Many patients have an **atopic history**.
  - There may be often an obvious precipitant such as an acute upper respiratory infection or a bee sting.
  - The most common **causal drugs** are antibiotics, aspirin, nonsteroidal antiinflammatory drugs (NSAIDs), narcotics, and radiocontrast dyes.
  - Milk, wheat, eggs, chocolate, shellfish, and nuts are **foods** that may initiate acute or recurrent lesions.
  - Anaphylaxis or an anaphylactoid reaction may occur.
- **Chronic urticaria** by definition lasts longer than 4 to 6 weeks.
  - There is a 2:1 female-to-male ratio of occurrence.
  - The cause is usually unknown; however, chronic urticaria may infrequently be a sign of one of the following systemic diseases: **systemic lupus erythematosus, serum hepatitis, lymphoma, polycythemia, macroglobulinemia,** or **thyroid disease**.

DESCRIPTION OF LESIONS

- Papules and plaques are of varying sizes.
- Wheals are flesh-colored or pale red; a halo may be noted at the periphery of lesions (Figure 18.1).
- Lesions have various shapes; they can be annular, linear, arciform, or polycyclic, and frequently they are multiple with bizarre shapes (Figure 18.2).
- Individual lesions disappear within 24 hours.
- Lesions may be accompanied by angioedema (Figure 18.3).

DISTRIBUTION OF LESIONS

- Angioedema is noted in the periorbital area (see Figure 18.3), lips, and tongue.
- Urticarial lesions may occur anywhere on the body and may be localized or generalized.

CLINICAL MANIFESTATIONS

- Lesions generally itch.
- Arthralgia, fever, malaise, and other symptoms may accompany urticaria when it is caused by those disorders in which circulating immune complexes are present (e.g., serum sickness).
- Scratching and rubbing of lesions generally does not produce crusts similar to those seen in atopic dermatitis.
- Acute urticaria lasts for hours to days (generally less than 30 days).
- Approximately 50% of patients with chronic urticaria are free of lesions in 1 year; in the others, lesions may recur for many years.
- Emotional stress may trigger recurrences.

DIAGNOSIS

- Diagnosis is usually made on **clinical observation** and **history**.
- If a complete review of systems is normal, it is often futile to perform multiple laboratory tests to determine a cause for chronic urticaria.
- A positive symptom-directed search for underlying illness (e.g., systemic lupus erythematosus, thyroid disease lymphoma, necrotizing vasculitis) may warrant evaluations such as:
  - Complete blood count
  - Erythrocyte sedimentation rate (ESR)
  - Fluorescent antinuclear antibody test
  - Throid function studies, including antithyroglobulin and antimicrosomal antibodies
  - Hepatitis-associated antigen test
  - Assessment of the complement system
  - Radioallergosorbent test for IgE antibodies
  - In the presence of eosinophilia, stool examination for ova and parasites

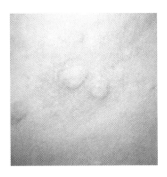

Figure 18.1.
Urticaria. Flesh-colored wheals.

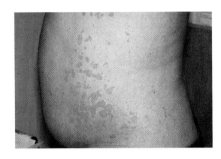

Figure 18.2.
Multiple erythematous lesions with various shapes and sizes.

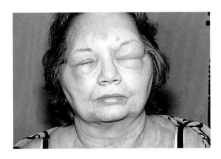

Figure 18.3.
Marked angioedema.

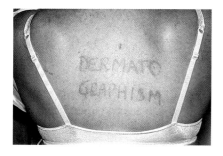

Figure 18.4.
Dermatographism ("skin writing").

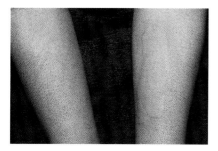

Figure 18.5.
Cold urticaria. Wheal and surrounding erythema 5 minutes after application of an ice cube. The "ice cube test."

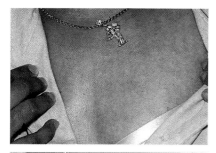
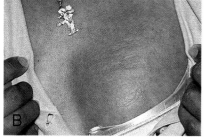

Figure 18.6.
Solar urticaria induced by UVA light. (*A*)Before sun exposure and (*B*) after 15 minutes of sun exposure through a glass window.

DIFFERENTIAL DIAGNOSIS

- **Insect bite reactions** (also known as **papular urticaria**; see Chapter 20, "Infestations, Bites, and Stings")
    - Reactions to insect bites may be indistinguishable from ordinary hives.
    - Bites are generally seen on exposed areas.
    - They may have a central punctum and crust; they also may blister.
    - Individual lesions may last more than 24 hours.
- **Erythema multiforme minor** (see below)
    - Lesions are targetlike.
    - Lesions last more than 24 hours.
    - Lesions are generally nonpruritic.
- **Erythema migrans (acute Lyme disease**; see Chapter 20, "Infestations, Bites, and Stings")
    - Erythema migrans may be indistinguishable from urticaria.
    - The lesion is usually solitary.
    - Lesions last more than 24 hours.
    - Lesions are generally nonpruritic.
- **Urticarial vasculitis**
    - Persistent hivelike lesions last for more than 24 hours.
    - Evidence of vasculitis (e.g., purpura) is occasionally seen in the lesions.
    - Diagnosis is confirmed by skin biopsy.
    - Patients may have hypocomplementemia and an elevated ESR.
    - Urticarial vasculitis may be associated with collagen vascular diseases.

CLINICAL VARIANTS

Physical urticaria

- **Dermatographism** ("skin writing"; Figure 18.4)
    - Dermatographism affects more than 4% of the normal population, in whom it is physiologic and asymptomatic.
    - Hives occur after firmly stroking the skin with the wooden handle of a cotton swab; they fade within 30 minutes.
    - Hives are seen under constrictive garments, such as belts and bras.
    - In some individuals, itching is the primary symptom.
    - Episodes of dermatographism may persist for years.
    - Dermatographism can occur with other forms of hives. When another form of hives is associated with the dermatographism, finding or eliminating the cause of the hives may clear the dermatographism.
- **Cold urticaria** (Figure 18.5)
    - Cold urticaria occurs in young adults and children.
    - Itchy hives occur at sites of cold exposure, such as areas exposed to cold winds or immersion in cold water.
    - In the "ice cube test," a wheal arises on the skin after application of an ice cube.
- **Light-induced solar urticaria** (Figure 18.6) is urticaria resulting from sun-exposure. Itchy, pale or red swelling occurs at the site of exposure to ultraviolet or visible light. Different subtypes of solar urticaria are triggered by different wavelengths of light.
- **Cholinergic urticaria**
    - Exercise to the point of sweating provokes lesions and establishes the diagnosis.
    - Typical lesions are multiple small wheals.
    - Lesions have various shapes—annular, linear, arciform, polycyclic; they are frequently annular or multiple with bizarre shapes.
    - Individual lesions disappear within 24 hours.
- **Other physical urticarias** include those induced by pressure, vibration, and water (aquagenic urticaria).

MANAGEMENT

- If possible, the **cause** of the hives **should be eliminated**, and **tight clothing** and **hot baths** and **showers** should be **avoided**.
- **H₁ blockers** include hydroxyzine, diphenhydramine, and cyproheptadine; **H₁** and **H₂** blockers **may be used in combination** (e.g., cimetidine plus hydroxyzine).
- Newer, **nonsedating antihistamines**, such as loratadine and cetirizine, may be used during the day and a more sedating **tricyclic drug**, such as doxepin, can be given at bedtime at a much lower dosage than when it is used as an antidepressant.
- Oral doxepin alone, at doses ranging from 5 mg twice daily to 50 mg three times daily, have been used to successfully suppress chronic urticaria.
- **Systemic steroids** are sometimes used for short periods to "break the cycle" of chronic urticaria.
- Salicylates, NSAIDs, and narcotics, which are all **histamine-releasing agents**, may aggravate acute and chronic urticaria and **should be avoided**.
- A diary of daily foods eaten may be kept, with subsequent food and food additive elimination tried, if all else fails; however, this is rarely successful.

 POINTS TO REMEMBER

- Except for physical urticaria and urticaria that is obviously associated with drugs and systemic disease, determining the cause of chronic urticaria is generally a fruitless task. Allergy testing is expensive, and often tests are positive for allergies that have nothing to do with urticaria.
- When individual wheals persist for more than 24 hours, the process is unlikely to be urticaria.
- The **mainstay of treatment for chronic urticaria is the use of antihistamines**. Infrequently, short courses of systemic steroids are necessary. Immunotherapy using plasmapheresis, intravenous immunoglobulin, and cyclosporine may be valuable in severe recalcitrant cases.
- Epinephrine, which is often administered through intramuscular or subcutaneous injections for acute urticaria, should not be used for routine cases of hives. It should be reserved for cases of acute anaphylaxis.
- People with documented cold urticaria should be advised not to abruptly immerse themselves in cold water.
- People with severe reactions should consider wearing a MedicAlert bracelet.

BASICS

- Erythema multiforme is a confusing condition for many health care providers. What many diagnose as erythema multiforme is, instead, urticaria and frequently urticaria with lesions of many shapes and sizes. There is the erroneous belief that the term "multiforme" refers to the many shapes of lesions. The classic description of erythema multiforme made by Ferdinand von Hebra in the late nineteenth century was very specific: a **self-limited eruption characterized by symmetrically distributed erythematous papules, which develop into the targetlike lesions consisting of concentric color changes with a dusky central zone that may become bullous.** This classic form of erythema multiforme is currently defined as **erythema multiforme minor**.
- The more serious variant, with mucous membrane involvement, systemic symptoms, and more extensive lesions, is called **erythema multiforme major (Stevens-Johnson syndrome)**.
- Erythema multiforme is a reaction pattern of dermal blood vessels with secondary changes noted in the epidermis, which result clinically in curious targetlike shapes.
- Erythema multiforme is most commonly seen in **late adolescence** and in **young adulthood**. Affected individuals are generally in good health.

Causes.

The list of causes of erythema multiforme is long and is, in many cases, a duplication of the list of causes of urticaria. The following are the most well-documented associations.

- The most common precipitating cause of **erythema multiforme minor** is recurrent labial **herpes simplex virus (HSV)** infection (Figure 18.7); recurrences of herpes progenitalis have also been reported to precede or sometimes occur simultaneously with episodes of recurrent erythema multiforme minor.
- Precipitating factors in **erythema multiforme major** are **drugs** (sulfonamides, penicillin, hydantoins, barbiturates, allopurinol, NSAIDs), *Mycoplasma* infection, **pregnancy,** *Streptococcus* infection, **hepatitis A and B, coccidiomycosis,** and **Epstein-Barr virus infection**.
- Many cases are idiopathic.

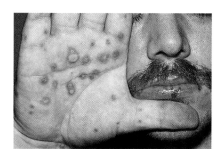

Figure 18.7.
Erythema multiforme minor in patient with recurrent herpes simplex virus (HSV) infection. Note drying crust of HSV "cold sore" on lip.

DESCRIPTION OF LESIONS

- Lesions begin as round erythematous macules.
- Some lesions evolve to form targetoid plaques (iris lesions) with a dark center, which may become vesicobullous.
- Lesions persist (are "fixed") for at least 1 week.
- Erosions and crusts form.

DISTRIBUTION OF LESIONS

- Bilateral and symmetrical
- Palms and soles, dorsa of hands and feet, extensor forearms and legs, face, and genitalia
- Mucous membrane lesions, limited to the mouth in erythema multiforme minor
- Extensive mucous membrane lesions in erythema multiforme major, located in multiple sites including the mouth, pharynx, eyes, and genitalia (Figure 18.8)

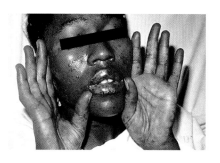

Figure 18.8.
Extensive hemorrhagic crusting on mucous membranes in a patient with erythema multiforme major.

CLINICAL MANIFESTATIONS

- **Erythema multiforme minor**
  - Acute, self-limited, often recurrent eruption
  - Possible evidence of herpes labialis
  - Little or no mucous membrane involvement
- **Erythema multiforme major**
  - Often accompanied by symptoms of fever, malaise, and myalgias
  - Severe, painful mucous membrane involvement
  - Possible complications of keratitis, corneal ulcers, upper airway damage, and pneumonia
  - In extensive involvement of the body surface, a sheetlike loss of epidermis, resulting in **toxic epidermal necrolysis**, which is associated with a significant risk of death from sepsis

DIAGNOSIS

- Typical **target lesions**
- **Skin biopsy**, if necessary

DIFFERENTIAL DIAGNOSIS

- **Urticaria**
  - The center of annular lesions is normal, not dusky.
  - Lesions are transient, not "fixed."
  - Angioedema is possible.
  - Lesions are pruritic.
- **Primary herpes gingivostomatitis and primary bullous diseases of the oral cavity**
  - In the absence of skin lesions, other diseases of the mucous membranes may be clinically indistinguishable from those of erythema multiforme.
  - Mucous membrane biopsy may distinguish oral bullous erythema multiforme from primary bullous disease such as pemphigus vulgaris or bullous pemphigoid.

MANAGEMENT

- If known, the **precipitating cause should be treated**.
- Suspected **etiologic drugs should be discontinued**.
- Empirical treatment with oral acyclovir famciclovir or valacyclovir may prevent or mitigate recurrences.
- Wet dressings and topical steroids may be applied.
- Many recurrences are mild and self-limiting and require no treatment.
- In **life-threatening situations**, such as **erythema multiforme major** or **toxic epidermal necrolysis**, hospitalization is often essential; patients can then be given topical skin care, eye care, fluid restoration, and antibiotics, if necessary.
- The use of systemic steroids is controversial, and their effectiveness has not been established.

POINTS TO REMEMBER

- Erythema multiforme is not a disease but a syndrome with multiple causes and various degrees of severity.
- Even in the clinical absence of HSV infection, recurrent erythema multiforme may be suppressed with oral acyclovir, famciclovir, or valacyclovir.

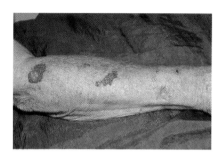

Figure 18.9.
Senile, or actinic, purpura on the dorsal forearms in an elderly person.

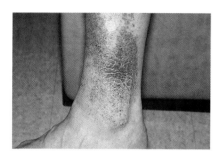

Figure 18.10.
Stasis dermatitis. Purpura and lichenification.

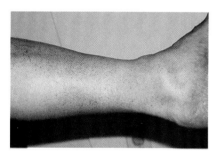

Figure 18.11.
Schamberg's purpura. "Cayenne pepper" petechiae seen on lower extremities.

BASICS

Purpura is **hemorrhage of blood into the skin**. It may be seen after:
- Minor **trauma** to the skin, particularly when an individual is taking drugs such as aspirin or other NSAIDs and warfarin (Coumadin), which decrease clotting time.
- Long-term application of potent topical steroids in the elderly
   or in association with:
- **Blood dyscrasias** and **coagulopathies** such as thrombocytopenia, leukemia, and disseminated intravascular coagulopathy
- **Senile**, or **actinic, purpura,** a prevalent finding on the dorsal forearms in elderly persons (Figure 18.9)
- **Chronic venous insufficiency** of the lower extremities (Figure 18.10)
   or as benign variants such as:
- **The benign pigmented purpuras**, of which there are several varieties, caused by a capillaritis, which allows blood to exit small vessels (extravasation), creating petechiae
  - As their name implies, these benign purpuras are not associated with any systemic disease.
  - **Schamberg's purpura** is the most common benign pigmented purpura, characterized by so-called "cayenne pepper" purpura.

DESCRIPTION OF LESIONS

- Lesions begin as nonblanching, red, pinpoint macules **(petechiae)**, or bruises **(ecchymoses)**, which may coalesce.
- Older lesions become purple, then brown as hemosiderin forms.

DISTRIBUTION OF LESIONS

- Blood dyscrasias and coagulopathies are noted more commonly on dependent areas (i.e., lower legs and ankles; buttocks in bedridden patients).
- Senile, or actinic, purpura is seen on the dorsa of forearms (see Figure 18.9).
- Chronic venous insufficiency (often with secondary stasis dermatitis) is seen on the lower legs (Figure 18.10; see Chapter 2, "Eczematous Rashes").
- Schamberg's purpura and other variants of benign pigmented purpura are most commonly seen on the lower extremities (Figure 18.11).

CLINICAL MANIFESTATIONS

- Lesions are asymptomatic but may be mildly pruritic.
- Pruritus is more severe when stasis dermatitis complicates chronic venous insufficiency.
- Purpuric lesions are of cosmetic concern. Some patients want to be reassured that purpura is not a sign of a serious disease.
- Lesions may persist for months to years.

DIAGNOSIS

- Diagnosis is made on the basis of **clinical presentation.**
- Lesions are **not palpable** and are **nonblanching** on diascopy.
- A coagulopathy or blood dyscrasia should be ruled out if clinically suspected.

DIFFERENTIAL DIAGNOSIS

Biopsy may be necessary at times to distinguish benign purpura from palpable purpura (see below).

MANAGEMENT

- Benign pigmented purpura generally requires **no workup**; however, if a coagulopathy, macroglobulinemia, or cryoglobulinemia is suspected, appropriate laboratory tests should be ordered.
- **Offending drugs should be evaluated** regarding their risk-to-benefit ratio.
- If a blood dyscrasia or coagulopathy is found, appropriate evaluation and treatment are necessary.

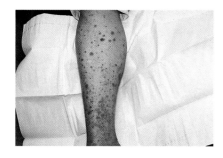

Figure 18.12.
Leukocytoclastic vasculitis. Palpable purpura.

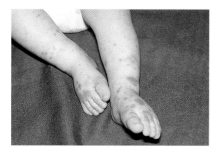

Figure 18.13.
Henoch-Schönlein purpura (HSP). Resolving palpable purpura in an infant.

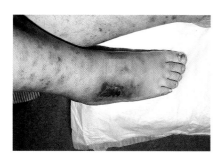

Figure 18.14.
Ulceration in patient with vasculitis.

BASICS

- **Hypersensitivity vasculitis (HV)** refers to a group of vasculitic conditions involving the vessels that lie within the middle to upper dermis.
  - Clinically, HV is manifested in the skin as palpable purpura that is caused by deposition of circulating immune complexes in the postcapillary venules (Figure 18.12).
  - The circulating immune complexes may also deposit in internal organs, causing a vasculitis with resultant gastrointestinal bleeding, hematuria, and arthralgias.
- **Henoch-Schönlein purpura (HSP)** is a type of HV usually caused by group A streptococci that demonstrate an IgA immunofluorescent pattern. "HSP" (Figure 18.13) is a term that should be reserved for disease that follows an upper respiratory infection (generally in children).
- Vasculitis may be associated with a **hypersensitivity to antigens** from drugs, infectious agents, neoplasms, or other underlying diseases such as collagen vascular disease and cryoglobulinemias, or it may be idiopathic in origin. (HV is idiopathic in more than 50% of cases.)
- **Leukocytoclastic vasculitis** is the histopathologic hallmark of HV.

DESCRIPTION OF LESIONS

- Lesions are frequently palpable and do not blanche (palpable purpura).
- Ulceration may develop (Figure 18.14).

DISTRIBUTION OF LESIONS

- Dependent areas of the lower legs and ankles and on the buttocks in bedridden patients
- In severe forms, lesions can be generalized.

CLINICAL MANIFESTATIONS

- Lesions are asymptomatic, slightly painful, or mildly pruritic.
- Lesions sometimes recur.
- There may be associated malaise and possible fever.
- In HSP, abdominal pain, arthralgia, hematuria, and proteinuria may be present.
- In systemic vasculitis, symptoms are referable to the organ involved.

DIAGNOSIS

- **Laboratory investigation** is made for underlying disease: complete blood count, ESR, urinalysis, stool examination for occult blood. Further studies should be symptom directed.
- Biopsy of lesions shows characteristic leukocytoclastic vasculitis ("nuclear dust").
- HSP caused by group A streptococci demonstrates a **perivascular IgA immunofluorescent deposition in the skin and kidneys.**

DIFFERENTIAL DIAGNOSIS

Palpable and nonpalpable purpura may also be seen in **septic vasculitis,** in which lesions are generally acral and tend to be few in number (e.g., gonococcemia; Figure 18.15).

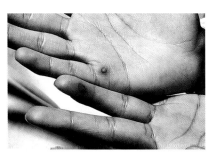

Figure 18.15.
Disseminated gonococcemia; an example of septic vasculitis. Note two palpable purpuric hemorrhagic vesicles.

MANAGEMENT

- If known, the **precipitating cause should be eliminated.**
- In general, **no treatment** is necessary for mild, self-limited episodes.
- **Systemic steroids** and appropriate **antibiotics** are administered, if indicated.
- **Nonsteroidal medications** may include dapsone or colchicine.
- **Immunosuppressants** are sometimes used in conjunction with systemic steroids as steroid-sparing agents.

POINT TO REMEMBER

Palpable purpura may be a sign of systemic vasculitis, sepsis, drug allergy, underlying disease, or an idiopathic reaction pattern.

CHAPTER 19

SEXUALLY TRANSMITTED DISEASES

Mary Ruth Buchness

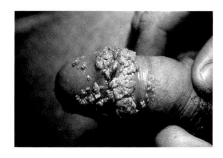

Figure 19.1.
Condyloma acuminata with appearance of small cauliflowers. Compare with Figure 19.7.

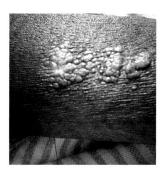

Figure 19.2.
Condyloma acuminata. Smooth, dome-shaped papular lesions. Compare with Figure 19.8.

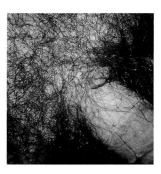

Figure 19.3.
Condyloma acuminata. Verrucous papules or plaques that resemble a common wart.

BASICS

Condyloma acuminata are **sexually transmitted viral warts** caused by infection with specific types of human papillomavirus (HPV).

It is estimated that 1% of the United States population have clinically evident condyloma acuminata and that 15% have latent HPV infection.

The incubation period is variable, ranging from 3 weeks to 8 months, with an average of 2.8 months in one study.

With the aid of the electron microscope, HPV particles have been identified in the skin of infected persons at a distance of up to 1 cm from the actual lesion, which may account for the high recurrence rate.

HPV types 16, 18, 31–35, 39, 42, 48, and 51–54 have been identified in cervical and anogenital cancers.

Lesions tend to be more extensive and recalcitrant to treatment in immunocompromised persons; they also tend to grow larger and more numerous during pregnancy.

DESCRIPTION OF LESIONS

- There are **five morphologic types** of condyloma acuminata:
  - Condyloma acuminata may have the appearance of **small cauliflowers** (Figure 19.1).
  - The lesions may appear as **smooth dome-shaped papules** (Figure 19.2).
  - **Verrucous papules** or **plaques** may resemble a common wart or seborrheic keratosis (Figure 19.3).
  - Occasional **flat papules** may be hyperpigmented.
  - **Lesions of mucous membranes** may appear white from maceration.
- The appearance of a given wart depends on its location (e.g., condyloma acuminata type tends to occur on moist surfaces).
- A patient may manifest more than one morphologic type of condyloma acuminata.

DISTRIBUTION OF LESIONS

Anogenital
- In **men**, these lesions can appear on the penis, the scrotum, and the mons pubis; in the inguinal crease; and in the perianal area (Figure 19.4).
- In **women**, these lesions can appear on the vagina, labia, mons pubis, and uterine cervix; and in the perianal area.
- **Intra-anal warts** occur predominantly in patients who have had anoreceptive intercourse.
- **Periurethral** and **intraurethral warts** can also occur (Figure 19.5).

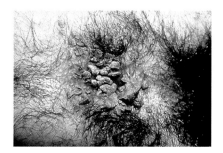

Figure 19.4.
Condyloma acuminata. Perianal lesions. Compare with Figure 19.18.

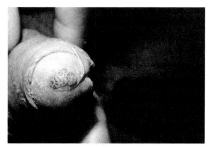

Figure 19.5.
Condyloma acuminata. Periurethral warts.

Outside the genital area

- HPV infection has been associated with **conjunctival, nasal, oral,** and **laryngeal warts**.
- **Oral–anal warts** may be present without a history of anal intercourse.

CLINICAL MANIFESTATIONS

- Usually asymptomatic
- May be pruritic, particularly perianal and inguinal lesions
- May be painful or bleed if traumatized
- May resolve spontaneously, or rarely, progress to invasive squamous cell carcinoma

DIAGNOSIS

- Diagnosis is usually made on **clinical grounds**.
- **Biopsy** is sometimes necessary to rule out anogenital bowenoid papulosis or squamous cell carcinoma in cases of unusual or recalcitrant lesions.
- **Acetowhite test**
  - **Women.** Colposcopy is performed in areas of mucous membranes in women after applying a 3 to 5% solution of acetic acid, which produces an acetowhitening of subclinical lesions on the vaginal and cervical mucosa (Figure 19.6).
  - **Men.** In this test, 5% acetic acid is applied to suspected warts on nonmucous-membrane skin. There is a high rate of false-positive results, and this test is no longer recommended for routine screening.
- **Papanicolaou (Pap) smears** may demonstrate atypia or koilocytosis, representing early changes resulting from HPV infection.

DIFFERENTIAL DIAGNOSIS

Normal anatomic structures

- **In men, pearly penile papules (angiofibromas;** (Figure 19.7) are frequently mistaken for and treated as warts.
  - Lesions are small, shiny flesh-colored or pearly papules.
  - They are most often located around the rim of the corona of the glans penis and on the distal shaft and frenum of the penis.
- **In women, vestibular papillae and sebaceous (Tyson's) glands** are frequently mistaken for and treated as warts.

Molluscum contagiosum (Figure 19.8)

- Papules are shiny and dome-shaped.
- There is often a central white core or umbilication.

Skin tags

- Skin tags are smooth and most often flesh-colored.
- They are seen in skin fold areas affected by friction.

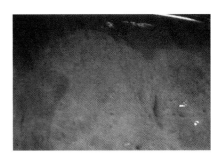

Figure 19.6.
Acetowhitening of subclinical lesions on the cervical mucosa.

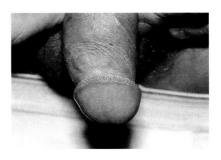

Figure 19.7.
Pearly penile papules. Shiny papules around the corona of the glans penis.

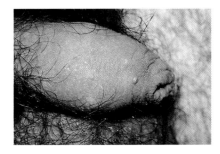

Figure 19.8.
Molluscum contagiosum. Dome-shaped papules with central white core.

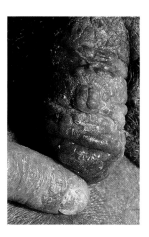

Figure 19.9.
Squamous cell carcinoma.

Bowenoid papulosis

Lesions are associated with HPV types 16, 18, 31, and 33.

They are clinically similar to, and often indistinguishable from, flat or dome-shaped genital warts.

Histologically, Bowenoid papulosis demonstrates squamous cell carcinoma in situ; however, it follows a largely benign clinical course.

Bowenoid papulosis responds to treatment for condylomata (see below).

Squamous cell carcinoma (Figure 19.9)

- Lesions are rapidly growing.
- They may be painful or bleeding.

Condyloma lata of secondary syphilis (see Figure 19.18)

- Lesions are moist and tend to be whitish and flat-topped (see Syphilis, below).
- There is positive syphilis serology.

Hemorrhoids

- Hemorrhoids are bluish in coloration.
- They are smooth and compressible.

MANAGEMENT

Counseling

- Lesions have a long latency period, and the patient may not have developed condyloma from his or her current partner. Thus, sexual partners of patients with condyloma acuminata should be evaluated for genital warts but cannot be assumed to be the source of an HPV infection.
- To avoid sexual transmission, men should use condoms during sexual intercourse for at least 1 year after clinical infection is treated.
- There is a risk of malignant degeneration to cervical intraepithelial neoplasia or squamous cell carcinoma. Affected women should get Pap smears every 6 months.

Surgical treatment

- Liquid nitrogen (LN_2) cryosurgery
- Electrodesiccation and curettage
- CO_2 laser treatment, which is more expensive
- Surgical excision

Topical therapy

- **Physician-applied therapies**
  - Podophyllin 10 to 50% in tincture of benzoin is applied in the physician's office. Podophyllin is an antimitotic agent that causes local tissue destruction. The patient is instructed to wash the area in 4 to 6 hours, and the interval is increased on subsequent treatments. Treatment is most effective on mucosal warts.
  - Trichloroacetic acid 25 to 90% is most effective on small warts and on nonmucosal surfaces, since it causes intense burning of mucosal surfaces. It causes intense burning of mucosal surfaces. It may be followed by application of podophyllin on nonmucosal surfaces.

- ■ Topical or injectable 5-fluorouracil may also be used.
- Patient-applied therapies
  - ■ This course of treatment is best suited for patients who understand the treatment plan and are able to identify the warts.
  - ■ Podofilox, the active ingredient in podophyllin, in a 0.5% solution or gel (condylox) is used twice per day for 3 consecutive days. Treatment is repeated every 3 weeks. Safety for use during pregnancy is unknown.
  - ■ The newer 5% imiquimod (Aldara) cream is applied three times per week until the wart is cleared or for 16 weeks. It is believed to act by enhancing the patient's immunity to HPV by local production of interferon. Efficacy in immunocompromised patients is unknown. Safety for use during pregnancy is unknown.
- Intralesional therapy. Interferon α-2b, 1 to 1.5 units, may be administered three times per week for 3 weeks. This treatment is not recommended by the Centers for Disease Control (CDC) because of high expense and no increased

POINTS TO REMEMBER

- HPV may exist in a latent form in the skin and manifest as condyloma acuminata at any time.
- Anal warts may be present without any history of anal intercourse.
- Condoms are not 100% effective in preventing the spread of HPV.
- Perinatal transmission can occur, and lesions may have an incubation period of up to 2 years.
- The CDC recommends a cesarean section only when the vaginal outlet is obstructed or if vaginal delivery would cause excessive bleeding.
- Immunocompromised patients frequently have recalcitrant, recurrent warts. Warts that begin to respond to treatment indicate improving immunity.
- Malignant degeneration may be indicated by increasing size, pain, or bleeding.
- Patients who have internal anal or rectal warts tend to have continual recurrences of external warts and should be referred to a rectal surgeon.
- Although skin warts are common in the general pediatric population, genital warts are uncommon in children. Diagnosis of genital warts in children should alert the health care provider to the possibility of sexual abuse.

BASICS

- Herpes simplex genitalis is a **genital disease caused most commonly by herpes simplex virus (HSV)-2,** although HSV-1 can also infect genital skin. It is most commonly, but not invariably, sexually transmitted.
- The disease is highly contagious during the prodrome and while the lesions are active and becomes noncontagious when all lesions are crusted over.
  - Risk of neonatal infection is greatest in patients with primary HSV infection at the time of delivery.
  - Recurrent HSV carries less than a 3% risk of neonatal transmission.
- HSV establishes latency in the dorsal root ganglia and reappears following different triggers in individual patients. Triggers include psychological or physiologic stress, physical trauma (e.g., from intercourse), menses, and immunosuppression.
- Affected patients may have recurrences that are infrequent or as frequent as once monthly.
- Patients who have six or more episodes per year are candidates for chronic suppressive therapy.

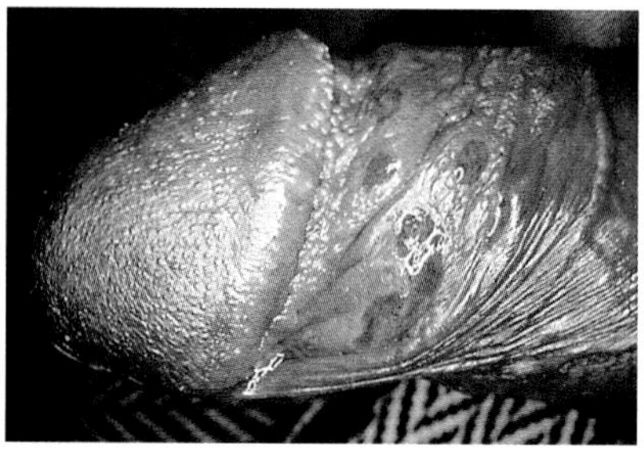

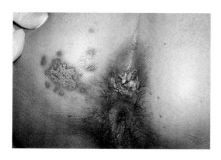

Figure 19.10.
Herpes simplex. Multiple erosions.

DESCRIPTION OF LESIONS

- Grouped vesicles on an erythematous base may become pustular, crusted, and eroded (Figure 19.10).
- Chronic ulcerations, crusted lesions, or verrucous lesions may develop in immunocompromised patients (Figure 19.11).

Figure 19.11.
Chronic ulcerated lesions and scattered intact vesicles in an immunocompromised patient.

DISTRIBUTION OF LESIONS

- In **women**, these lesions may appear on the vulva, perianal area, perineum, inner thighs, upper thighs, buttocks, and sacral area.
- In **men**, these lesions may appear on the penis, scrotum, thigh, sacral area, and buttocks.
- In men and women, anorectal HSV infection may occur resulting from anoreceptive intercourse.

CLINICAL MANIFESTATIONS

Primary HSV infection
- May be more severe than recurrent infections
- Regional adenopathy
- Fever, dysuria, and constipation
- May be asymptomatic so that initial outbreak resembles recurrent HSV infection
- Duration of 10 to 14 days

Recurrent HSV infection
- Prodrome of itching, burning, numbness, tingling, or pain 1 to 2 days before clinical outbreak
- Lesions localized and recurrent at the same site or in close proximity each time
- May have local adenopathy
- Vulvar involvement may cause dysuria
- Duration 3 to 5 days
- Most common cause of recurrent erythema multiforme
- Chronic ulcerative lesions are indicative of immunosuppression

DIAGNOSIS

- Diagnosis is by **clinical appearance, Tzanck preparation** (see Chapter 26 "Basic Procedures"), or **viral culture,** which takes 1 week.
- **Tissue culture** using monoclonal antibodies or polymerase chain reaction is sensitive but expensive.
- Serologic testing is of little value.

DIFFERENTIAL DIAGNOSIS

Herpes zoster (Figure 19.12)

- Herpes zoster is dermatomal; however, herpes simplex may also present in a linear grouping, thus resembling a dermatomal distribution.
- Culture distinguishes the two, but treatment should be initiated before results are obtained.
- History of recurrences indicates HSV infection.

Primary syphilis (chancre)

- Primary syphilis is painless.
- Borders are indurated.
- The chancre is not preceded by vesicles.

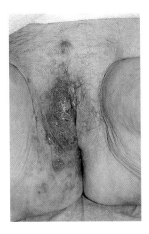

Figure 19.12.
Herpes zoster in a unitlateral dermatomal distribution.

MANAGEMENT

Topical therapy

- Topical antiviral agents have limited effectiveness.
- Symptomatic relief is obtained with cold compresses, viscous Xylocaine, eutectic mixture of lidocaine and prilocaine (EMLA), and oral analgesics.

Systemic therapy

Antiviral agents significantly reduce the duration of symptoms, local pain, dysuria, and viral shedding. They also accelerate the healing of lesions and help to suppress recurrences.

- **Primary HSV infection** is treated as follows:
  - **Acyclovir** 200 mg five times per day or 400 mg three times per day for 10 days
  - **Famciclovir** 250 mg three times per day for 10 days
  - **Valacyclovir** 500 mg twice per day for 10 days
- **Recurrent HSV infection** should be treated at the first sign of the prodrome.
  - **Acyclovir** 200 mg five times per day or 400 mg three times per day for 5 days
  - **Famciclovir** 125 mg twice per day for 5 days
  - **Valacyclovir** 500 mg twice per day for 5 days
- **Recurrent HSV infection** with more than six recurrences per year or **chronic recurrent erythema multiforme** associated with HSV is treated as recurrent HSV infection for 5 days, then therapy is continued as follows:
  - **Acyclovir** 200 mg three times per day or 400 mg twice per day
  - **Famciclovir** 200 mg twice per day
  - **Valacyclovir**, however, **should not** be used in patients who are HIV-positive.
- **Acyclovir-resistant HSV infection** is seen in patients with AIDS and coresistance to famciclovir and valacyclovir.
  - **Foscarnet** 40 mg/kg may be given intravenously two to three times per day.
  - HSV infection after foscarnet administration is often acyclovir-sensitive.
- **HSV infection in pregnant women** should be treated according to the following CDC recommendations:
  - Systemic treatment should be avoided unless the infection is life-threatening.
  - If no symptoms or signs present during labor, vaginal delivery is recommended.
  - If vaginal delivery occurs through an infected birth canal, a viral culture should be taken from the infant within 24 to 48 hours.

POINTS TO REMEMBER

- Episodic antiviral treatment for recurrences of HSV should be initiated during the prodrome.
- Recurrences are generally less severe than initial episodes; recurrence rates tend to decline over time.
- All HSV infections establish latency and are incurable. A current infection may actually be a recurrence of an asymptomatic infection acquired in the past.

BASICS

Syphilis is a **sexually transmitted systemic disease** caused by the spirochetal bacterium *Treponema pallidum*.

Syphilis is divided into **primary, secondary, latent,** and **tertiary stages.**

Latent syphilis is evidenced by positive serologic tests for nontreponemal and treponemal antibodies in the absence of clinical manifestations. It is divided into **early latent syphilis** and **late latent syphilis**.

Early latent syphilis is syphilis documented to be of less than 1 year's duration and is treated with the same regimen as primary and secondary infections.

Late latent syphilis is greater than 1 year's duration or of unknown duration and is treated with the same regimen as tertiary syphilis.

HIV-infected patients with latent syphilis of any duration should have a **cerebrospinal fluid (CSF)** examination to rule out neurosyphilis before treatment.

Tertiary syphilis, which occurs approximately 20 years after the onset of untreated syphilis, is **exceedingly rare** in the modern era, because most infected patients have had exposure to multiple courses of antibiotics during the course of their lives, which probably prevented the infection from progressing.

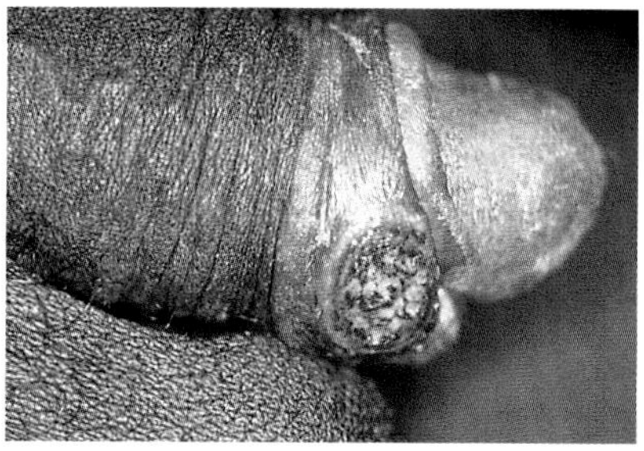

PRIMARY SYPHILIS

DESCRIPTION OF LESIONS

- There is painless ulceration with a rolled, indurated border (chancre; Figure 19.13)
- The lesion is usually single but may be multiple.
- The base of the ulcer is "clean," unless there is superinfection.

DISTRIBUTION OF LESIONS

- Lesions are most common on the **glans penis** in men, less common on the **shaft**. They may occur at the **base of the penis** in condom wearers.
- A visible chancre is less common in women. Lesions may occur on the labia majora or minora, clitoris, or posterior commissure.
- Anal lesions are the most common presentation after receptive anal intercourse (Figure 19.14).
- There may possibly be extragenital chancres.

CLINICAL MANIFESTATIONS

- Usually asymptomatic
- Regional adenopathy
- Healing of untreated chancre within 3 months

DIAGNOSIS

- Diagnosis may be made on **clinical grounds**.
- **Dark-field examination** of ulceration may aid in diagnosis.
- **Skin biopsy** may be performed.
- **Nontreponemal serologic tests** (Venereal Disease Research Laboratory [test] [VDRL], rapid plasma reagin [RPR] test, automated reagin test) are positive at a rate of 25% of patients per week of infection.

DIFFERENTIAL DIAGNOSIS

Herpes simplex

- Painful lesions
- Flat borders, not indurated
- Ulceration preceded by vesicles

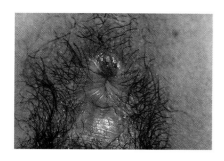

Figure 19.13.
Chancre of primary syphilis. Compare with Figure 19.20.

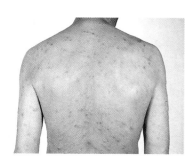

Figure 19.14.
Chancre of primary syphilis on the anus.

Figure 19.15.
Secondary syphilis. Scaly, erythematous oval patches and papules. Compare with Figure 19.19.

Chancroid (See Figure 19.20 below)

- Unusual in the United States
- Often presents as a coinfection in Africa
- Painful lesions

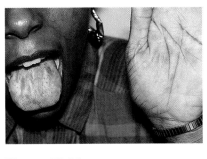

Figure 19.16.
Secondary syphilis. Mucous patches on tongue and characteristic palmar lesions.

MANAGEMENT

- A test for HIV infection should be performed.
- **In non–penicillin-allergic patients,** benzathine penicillin G, 2.4 million units intramuscularly, is administered in a single dose.
- In **penicillin-allergic nonpregnant patients**:
  - **Doxycycline** 100 mg by mouth is administered twice per day for 2 weeks
  - **Tetracycline** 500 mg is administered four times per day for 2 weeks.
- In **penicillin-allergic pregnant patients**:
  - Patients are first **desensitized to penicillin.**
  - Subsequent treatment is given with **benzathine penicillin G**, 2.4 million units intramuscularly with a second dose 1 week later.
- In **HIV-infected patients**:
  - **Benzathine penicillin G**, 2.4 million units intramuscularly, is administered in a single dose.
  - A second treatment with benzathine penicillin G is sometimes recommended.

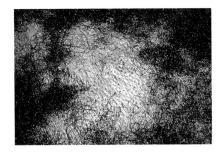

Figure 19.17.
Secondary syphilis. "Moth-eaten" alopecia.

POINTS TO REMEMBER

- In most patients, follow-up at 3 months after treatment of primary or secondary syphilis should demonstrate an RPR that is negative or has decreased fourfold in titer.
- Patients should be reevaluated clinically and with serologic testing at 6 and 12 months or longer after treatment because RPR titers after treatment may remain serofast in 15 to 20% of patients.

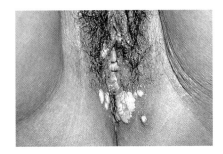

Figure 19.18.
Secondary syphilis. Condyloma lata.

SECONDARY SYPHILIS

DESCRIPTION OF LESIONS

- Scaly, erythematous oval papules (Figure 19.15)
- Mucous patches (Figure 19.16)
- "Moth-eaten" alopecia (Figure 19.17)
- Condyloma lata (Figure 19.18)

DISTRIBUTION OF LESIONS

Distribution of lesions is generalized, including the **palms, soles, scalp,** and **mucous membranes**.

CLINICAL MANIFESTATIONS

- Skin lesions are usually asymptomatic
- Generalized adenopathy
- Mild systemic symptoms

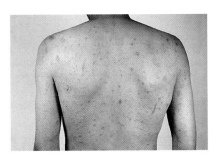

Figure 19.19.
Pityriasis rosea (PR). Note similarity with Figure 19.15.

DIAGNOSIS

- Diagnosis may be made on **clinical appearance**.
- **Dark-field examination** of serum expressed from lesions may aid in the diagnosis.
- Treponemal (fluorescein treponema antibody) and nontreponemal **serologic tests** are positive (in 100% of non–HIV-infected patients and usually at a titer greater than 1:16 for the nontreponemal test).
- **Skin biopsy** is conducted with silver or immunoperoxidase stain.
- Serologic titers in patients who are HIV-infected may possibly be negative.

DIFFERENTIAL DIAGNOSIS

Pityriasis rosea (PR)
(Figure 19.19)
- PR is usually confined to skin above the knees; it generally spares the face, palms, and soles.
- Sometimes it is itchy.
- Serologic testing for syphilis should be performed in patients with PR because it may closely resemble secondary syphilis

Other papulosquamous eruptions
- Psoriasis
- Lichen planus
- Drug eruption

MANAGEMENT

Management is the same as it is for primary syphilis.

TERTIARY SYPHILIS

DESCRIPTION OF LESIONS

- Swelling begins in the subcutis, which spreads to the rest of the skin and ulcerates. The ulcerated tissue degenerates into a slimy, stringy mass, giving rise to the name "**gumma.**"
- **Nodular syphilis** arises as firm, coppery red nodules that form serpiginous plaques.
- **Mucosal lesions** manifest as glossitis and palatal perforations caused by gumma.

DISTRIBUTION OF LESIONS

- **Gumma**: face, scalp, chest, palate, and legs
- **Nodular syphilis**: Extensor aspects of arms, back, and face
- **Mucosal lesions**: tongue and hard and soft palates

CLINICAL MANIFESTATIONS

- Syphilitic glossitis, possibly resulting in malignant degeneration
- Syphilitic aortitis
- Neurosyphilis

DIAGNOSIS

- Clinical appearance
- Serologic testing
- Skin biopsy
- Examination of cerebral spinal fluid (CSF)
- Chest radiograph

DIFFERENTIAL DIAGNOSIS

(of cutaneous manifestations)
- Pyoderma gangrenosum
- Granuloma annulare
- Sarcoid
- Leukoplakia

MANAGEMENT

- In **non–penicillin-allergic patients without evidence of neurosyphilis**, benzathine penicillin G, 2.4 million units per week is administered intramuscularly for 3 weeks.
- In **penicillin-allergic patients**, CSF examination should be performed before treatment.
  - If the CSF examination is negative, the patient should be referred to a specialist in infectious diseases.
  - If the CSF examination is positive, the patient requires desensitization to penicillin and treatment as is given for neurosyphilis.
- In patients with **neurosyphilis**:
  - Aqueous crystalline penicillin G, 12 to 24 million units daily, is administered as 2 to 4 million units intravenously every 4 hours for 10 to 14 days.
  - Procaine penicillin, 12 to 24 million units daily, is administered intramuscularly, plus probenecid, 500 mg by mouth four times per day for 10 to 14 days.
- **Congenital syphilis** can occur in infants born to mothers with:
  - Untreated syphilis
  - Syphilis treated during pregnancy with erythromycin less than 1 month before delivery
  - Syphilis treated with penicillin but without a fourfold decrease in serologic titer
- The CDC recommends testing all pregnant women for syphilis at least once during pregnancy and at the time of delivery in at-risk populations.

POINTS TO REMEMBER

- The only antibiotic used to treat syphilis that achieves therapeutic CSF concentrations in all patients is aqueous crystalline penicillin G.
- In neurosyphilis, the CSF examination should be repeated every 6 months. If results are abnormal 2 years after treatment, retreatment should be considered.

BASICS

- Chancroid is an **ulcerative sexually transmitted disease** that is most common in underdeveloped countries and is rare in the United States and western Europe.
- In the United States, it has been associated with the use of crack cocaine.
- The causative organism, *Haemophilus ducreyi*, a gram-negative rod, is fastidious and requires specific conditions for culture.
- Chancroid occurs as a mixed infection with syphilis or HSV in 10% of cases.
- Clinical infection is more common in men than in women.

DESCRIPTION OF LESIONS

- Earliest manifestation is a papule, which becomes a pustule and ulcerates.
- Fully developed lesions are painful, with undermined borders and peripheral erythema.
- Borders are not indurated.
- There may be satellite ulcers.

DISTRIBUTION OF LESIONS

- Distribution depends on the site of inoculation.
  - In **men**, the lesion may occur on the prepuce, balanopreputial fold, or shaft of the penis (Figure 19.20).
  - In **women,** the lesion may occur on the labia majora, posterior commissure, or perianal area.
- Extragenital lesions may occur.

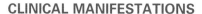

CLINICAL MANIFESTATIONS

Incubation period is 2 to 5 days.
Tenderness and pain
Unilateral or bilateral inguinal adenopathy

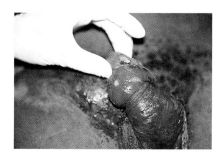

Figure 19.20.
Chancroid. Multiple painful ulcers with sinus tracts and bubo. Compare with Figure 19.13.

DIAGNOSIS

Diagnosis is made with Gram's stain showing characteristic "schools of fish" or "Chinese characters."
Culture is difficult.
Polymerase chain reaction may help in diagnosis.
Negative dark-field examination, syphilis serology, and **HSV culture** all may aid in the diagnosis.

DIFFERENTIAL DIAGNOSIS

Herpes simplex infection
- HSV is preceded by blisters.
- Borders are not undermined.
- Chronic HSV infection in patients with AIDS possibly resembles chancroid.

Primary syphilis
- Borders are indurated, not undermined.
- The lesion is painless.

MANAGEMENT

- All four of the following treatment alternatives are effective in HIV-infected patients
  - **Azithromycin,** 1 g by mouth in a single dose
  - **Ciprofloxacin,** 500 mg twice daily for 3 days
  - **Ceftriaxone,** 250 mg intramuscularly in a single dose
  - **Erythromycin,** 500 mg by mouth four times per day for 7 days (dosage is the same for pregnant women)
- **HIV testing**
- Symptomatic improvement in 3 days, objective improvement in 7 days, and possibly more than 2 weeks for complete healing

POINTS TO REMEMBER

- Chancroid is rare in the United States, but epidemics have been described in crack cocaine users.
- Chancroid predisposes patients to HIV infection because CD4 cells are recruited into the ulcer.
- Patients with chancroid should always be tested for coinfection with HIV, syphilis, and HSV.

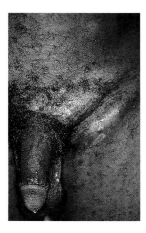

Figure 19.21.
Lymphogranuloma
venereum (LGV). Regional
lymphadenitis ("the
groove sign").

BASICS

- Lymphogranuloma venereum (LGV) is caused by *Chlamydia trachomatis* types L1, L2, and L3, and is most often sexually transmitted.
- LGV is rarely seen in the United States and most commonly occurs in tropical countries.
- An **inconspicuous cutaneous ulceration** occurs at the site of inoculation and often heals without being noticed.

DESCRIPTION OF LESIONS

- Evanescent papulopustule or ulceration
- Regional lymphadenitis (Figure 19.21)
- Development of fluctuance and sinus tracts
- Nodes divided into upper and lower groups by the groin fold ("the groove sign")

DISTRIBUTION OF LESIONS

- **Genital**
- **Perirectal**

CLINICAL MANIFESTATIONS

- Malaise and joint stiffness may be associated.
- Scarring may result in genital lymphedema.
- Erythema nodosum occurs in 10% of women.
- Photosensitivity rashes are common in Caucasian patients.

DIAGNOSIS

- **Serologic testing**
- **Exclusion of other causes** of suppurative adenopathy

DIFFERENTIAL DIAGNOSIS

Cat scratch disease
History of traumatic contact with cats at site proximal to involved nodes

Pyogenic adenitis
Positive Gram's stain and cultures

Tuberculous adenitis
- Positive acid-fast bacillus stain and cultures
- Positive purified protein derivative (PPD)

POINTS TO REMEMBER

- Infection is rare in the United States.
- Cutaneous manifestations are usually inapparent.

MANAGEMENT

- **Doxycycline** 100 mg is administered by mouth twice daily for 21 days.
- An alternative regimen is **sulfisoxazole**, 500 mg by mouth four times per day for 21 days.
- In pregnancy, **erythromycin** is administered, 500 mg by mouth four times per day for 21 days.

GRANULOMA INGUINALE

BASICS

- Granuloma inguinale is a **chronic granulomatous ulcerative disease of the genitalia** caused by the gram-negative bacillus *Calymmatobacterium granulomatis*.
- It is thought to be sexually transmitted, with low infectivity.
- Granuloma inguinale is rare in the United States but is widespread in the tropics and subtropics.
- The frequency of the disease in homosexuals suggests that the causative organism may reside in the gastrointestinal tract.

DESCRIPTION OF LESIONS

- The initial lesion is a papule or a nodule that ulcerates.
- The ulcer is painless and has an undermined border.
- There is no adenitis.

DISTRIBUTION OF LESIONS

- Genital, pubic, perineal, groin, or perianal areas are affected.
- Extragenital lesions occur in 3 to 6% of cases.

CLINICAL MANIFESTATIONS

The clinical manifestations of granuloma inguinale include the presence of pain or adenitis, suggesting superinfection.

DIAGNOSIS

- **Smears** from the edge of the lesion show characteristic Donovan bodies (organisms within macrophages).
- **Biopsy** of edge of lesion will aid in diagnosis.

DIFFERENTIAL DIAGNOSIS

Syphilis
- Syphilis must be excluded by dark-field and serologic examinations.
- Borders are indurated, not undermined.

Chancroid
- Chancroid is associated with adenopathy.
- There is painful ulceration.

MANAGEMENT

- **Tetracycline**, 500 mg four times per day for 10 to 20 days
- For treatment failures, **gentamycin** is administered.

CHAPTER 20

BITES, STINGS, AND INFESTATIONS

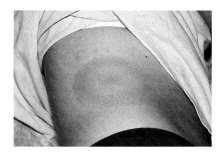

Figure 20.1.
Lyme disease. Solitary annular erythematous plaque of erythema migrans (EM).

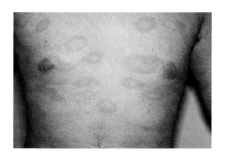

Figure 20.2.
Lyme disease. Multiple lesions of erythema migrans (EM).

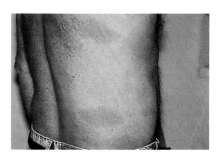

Figure 20.3.
Lyme disease. Morphologically uniform, confluent lesions of erythema migrans (EM).

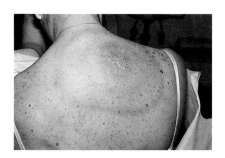

Figure 20.4.
Lyme disease. Erythema migrans (EM). Concentric rings with drying central vesicles.

BASICS

- **Lyme disease, or Lyme borreliosis (LB)**, is an infection caused by the spirochete, *Borrelia burgdorferi*. It is transmitted to humans by the bite of the tiny *Ixodes* tick. *I. dammini* is found in the northeastern and midwestern United States, where most cases are reported. *I. scapularis*, in the southeastern United States, *I. pacificus* on the Pacific coast, and *I. ricinus*, the sheep tick, in Europe are also vectors.
- Reservoir animal hosts include deer, mice, migratory birds, and some domestic animals.
- The ticks cling to vegetation (not trees) in grassland, marshland, and woodland habitats. They transfer to animals and humans that brush against the vegetation.
- LB can occur in any season, although it is most prevalent during the warmer months.
- Successful transmission of the spirochete seems to require 48 to 72 hours, affording the tick (usually the larva or nymph) enough time to embed in the skin.

DESCRIPTION OF LESIONS

- Initially, the LB lesion is a red macule or papule at the site of a tick bite. The bite itself usually goes unnoticed (only 15% of patients report a tick bite). In approximately 2 to 30 days after infection, the rash appears.
- The lesion expands to form an annular erythematous lesion, **erythema migrans (EM)**, which is the classic lesion of Lyme disease (Figure 20.1). The lesion measures from 4 cm to 70 cm in diameter, generally with central clearing. The center of the lesion, which corresponds to the putative site of the tick bite, may become darker, vesicular, hemorrhagic, or necrotic.

DISTRIBUTION OF LESIONS

- Initially, there may be multiple lesions, presumably arising at the sites of multiple tick bites or more likely from bacteremia (Figure 20.2). They may be confluent in morphology (not annular) and, at times, concentric rings may form (Figures 20.3 and 20.4).
- Only 50 to 80% of patients with LB exhibit EM. Multiple lesions occur in approximately 50% of patients.
- Common sites are the thigh, groin, trunk, and axillae.

CLINICAL MANIFESTATIONS

Early Lyme disease

At the early stage of disease, flulike symptoms, such as malaise, arthralgias, headaches, fever, and chills, may occur, as can a stiff neck and muscles, difficulty in concentrating, and fatigue.
- The EM rash is usually asymptomatic.
- Acrodermatitis chronica atrophicans and lymphocytoma are cutaneous findings that are seen in patients in Europe; however, they are rare in the United States, possibly because of the existence of different antigenic strains of the bacterium.

Intermediate and chronic Lyme disease

Some of the signs and symptoms of LB may not appear for weeks, months, or even years after the initial tick bite. These include arthritis in one or more large joints, nervous system problems that may include pain, paresthesias, Bell's palsy, headaches, memory loss, and cardiac dysrhythmias.

DIAGNOSIS

The diagnosis of Lyme disease is often difficult because it mimics many other conditions. Viral infections, such as influenza and mononucleosis, also may manifest as a rash, aches, fever, and fatigue. Drug eruptions and insect bite reactions other than those caused by the *Ixodes* tick closely match the rash of early LB.

- **To diagnose early LB, it is important that**:
  - There is a history of tick exposure or bite in an area endemic for LB
  - The specific tick be identified as a potential vector of LB
  - The various presentations of EM be recognized
  - Laboratory tests are conducted
- **Laboratory testing**
  - Serologic testing, using enzyme-linked immunosorbent assay (ELISA) and Western Blot analyses for *B. burgdorferi*, are notoriously unreliable. At the early presenting stage of LB, serologic testing has been reported to be positive in only 25% of infected patients. After 4 to 6 weeks, approximately 75% of these patients test positive, even after antibiotic therapy. In fact, seroreactivity to *B. burgdorferi* may persist long after LB disease is cured.
  - The poor reputation of serologic testing is derived somewhat from the many false-negative tests of patients who have been treated very early in the course of the disease and from the many misdiagnosed cases of supposed LB.
- **Other diagnostic measures**, such as polymerase chain reaction (PCR) and cultures for *B. Burgdorferi* have met with some success; however, these techniques are time-consuming and expensive. Skin biopsies may give false-positive and false-negative results for *B. Burgdortari*.

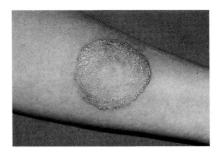

Figure 20.5.
Tinea corporis. Scaly border and KOH positive.

DIFFERENTIAL DIAGNOSIS

Tinea corporis (Figure 20.5; see Chapter 10, "Superficial Fungal Infections")
- There may be a history of exposure to fungus.
- Lesions are annular (ringlike) and clear in the center, with a scaly border.
- Lesions are KOH positive, or the fungal culture grows dermatophytes.
- Tinea corporis generally itches.

Urticaria (Figure 20.6; see Chapter 18, "Diseases of Vasculature")
- May be indistinguishable from LB
- Often annular or multiple
- Individual lesions disappear within 24 hours
- Generally itches
- Can resemble other hivelike conditions (e.g., a drug reaction)

Nontick insect bite reaction (see below)
- Generally itches
- Usually presents as wheals or papules with or without crusts
- Often grouped on exposed areas
- May be indistinguishable from LB when there is central induration or vesicles, or when annular

Less commonly: **granuloma annulare, erythema multiforme,** and **erythema annulare centrifugum**.

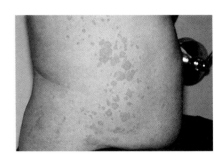

Figure 20.6.
Urticaria.

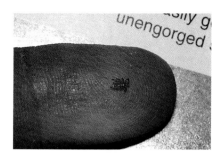

Figure 20.7.
Ixodes tick. Adult tick the size of the head of a match.

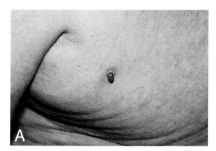

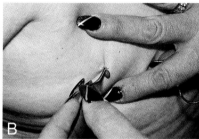

Figure 20.8.
(*A*)Dog tick. (*B*)An intact engorged adult dog tick being removed by the head.

MANAGEMENT

- **Tick recognition**
  - *Ixodes* ticks are much smaller than dog ticks.
  - In their larval and nymphal stages, they are no bigger than a pinhead.
  - Unengorged adult ticks are the size of the head of a match (Figure 20.7).
- **Tick removal**
  - An attached tick should be removed carefully by using a pair of tweezers.
  - The tick is grasped by the head (not the body) as close as possible to the skin to avoid force, which may crush it.
  - It should then be gently pulled straight out (Figure 20.8).
- **Treatment of EM (early LB)**
  - Doxycycline, 100 mg twice per day for 21 days (do not use in children under 10 years old or in pregnant women) or,
  - Amoxicillin, 500 mg three times per day for 21 days or,
  - Erythromycin, 250 mg four times per day for 21 days or,
  - Ceftriaxone or cefuroxime, 500 mg twice per day for 21 days (expensive; use if patient is unable to tolerate the other antibiotics)
- **Vaccines** have been used in dogs. Human vaccine is now available; however, its long-term efficacy has yet to be proved.

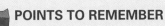

POINTS TO REMEMBER

- Serologic testing is usually negative early in the course of infection.
- Serologic testing should not be used to make a diagnosis, only to help confirm it.
- Patients can be reinfected. There is no lasting immunity to LB.

BASICS

- Insect bite reactions are also known as **papular urticaria** when lesions persist for more than 48 hours.
- Insects that **bite** include mosquitoes, fleas, flies, chiggers, and lice.
- Insects that **sting** include bees, wasps, hornets, and fire ants.
- Bites and stings often result in inflammatory reactions that are immunologically mediated. The reaction is caused by an acquired hypersensitivity to foreign chemicals and proteins injected into the skin. There is individual variability in the attraction of insects (possibly related to pheromones) and reactions (related to individual hypersensitivity). This may be the reason why in a group of people some members attract insects and have reactions to bites, while others do not.
- Stings generally cause immediate pain and are therefore usually remembered. Bites often go unnoticed, and the lesions that arise from them may not appear for hours to days after the bite because of what is often a delayed immune-mediated hypersensitivity reaction. Consequently, a patient may seek medical advice for unexplained itchy bumps or blisters.
- **Mosquito** and **fly bites** occur most often from outdoor exposures, particularly in the summer months.
- **Fleas bites** are most often acquired indoors from pets.

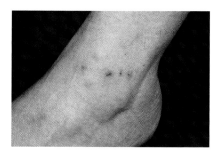

Figure 20.9.
Flea bites. "Breakfast, lunch, and dinner" lesions. Lesions are excoriated.

DESCRIPTION OF LESIONS

- May be indistinguishable from ordinary hives
- Generally seen on exposed areas
- Grouping of lesions, particularly flea bites ("breakfast, lunch, and dinner"; Figures 20.9 and 20.10)
- May have central punctum and crust; may also blister

DISTRIBUTION OF LESIONS

- Lesions are most often found on exposed areas of the body not covered by clothing.
- The papules of flea bites tend to be asymmetrical in distribution.
- Lesions are most likely seen on the lower legs, forearms, lower trunk, and waist; the axillary and anogenital areas are usually spared.

CLINICAL MANIFESTATIONS

- Insect bites may be an ongoing or a recurrent problem or simply a nuisance.
- Itching may be intense and persist for weeks.
- Secondary bacterial infection may occur.

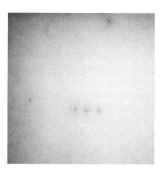

Figure 20.10.
Flea bites. Note the arrangement of lesions in groups of three ("breakfast, lunch, and dinner"); the fourth lesion probably represents a "midnight snack."

DIAGNOSIS

- Diagnosis is usually made on clinical appearance and history.
- Inquiry about household pets presently and formerly residing in the house may be a clue to the diagnosis of flea bites.
- If the residence was formerly host to a dog or cat infested with fleas, there is a possibility that the fleas left behind might have found new human hosts to live on.
- A skin biopsy is not diagnostic but may show suggestive findings consisting of a dense lymphocytic infiltrate (resembling lymphoma) with many eosinophils.

DIFFERENTIAL DIAGNOSIS

- **Urticaria** (unrelated to insect bite; see Chapter 18, "Diseases of the Vasculature")
  - Lacks central punctum
  - Often indistinguishable from insect bites
- **Scabies** (see below)
- **Fiberglass dermatitis**
  - Nonspecific itching
  - History of exposure (e.g., patient uses roofing materials)

MANAGEMENT

- Removal or destruction of the offending insect through fumigation and treating house pets will help to manage the situation.
- Insect repellents help to prevent against bites and stings (see Appendix 2, Patient Handouts, "Insect Repellents").
- Acute reactions to stings are treated symptomatically with topical steroids and oral antihistamines; people with severe reactions from stings may profit from desensitization therapy; anaphylactic reactions require epinephrine, systemic steroids, and antihistamines.

POINTS TO REMEMBER

- Patients who seek medical help generally do not consider insect bites to be the cause of their dermatosis or itching. A careful history and knowledge of the patient's environment and possible exposures should be sought and other diagnostic possibilities should always be kept in mind.
- Symptoms may persist weeks after the original bites.
- Other causes should be diligently sought if symptoms persist more than 4 to 6 weeks.

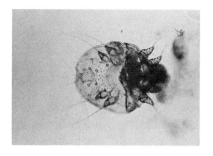

Figure 20.11.
Scabies. A fertilized female mite.

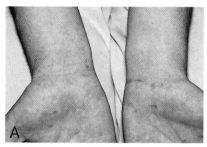

A

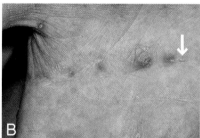

B

Figure 20.12.
Scabies. (*A*) Lesions on flexor wrists. (*B*) Close-up of a burrow (*arrow*) on the palm.

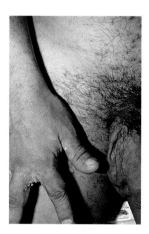

Figure 20.13.
Scabies. Finger web and groin lesions.

Mite infestation

BASICS

- **Scabies** is a skin infestation caused by the mite, *Sarcoptes scabiei*, var. *hominis*. It is usually spread by skin-to-skin contact, most frequently among family members and by sexual contact in young adults. Occasionally, epidemics occur in nursing homes and similar extended-care institutions, where the scabies is spread by person-to-person contact, and possibly by mite-infested clothing and bed linen. The diagnosis can be easily overlooked and treatment is often delayed for long time periods.
- The diagnosis of scabies should be considered when a patient presents with symptoms of intractable, persistent **pruritus**, especially when other family members, consorts, or fellow inhabitants of an institution, such as a nursing home or school, have similar symptoms.
- Although scabies is found more commonly in poor, crowded living conditions, it should be noted that scabies occurs worldwide and is not limited to the impoverished or those who practice poor personal hygiene.
- Blacks infrequently acquire scabies; the reason is unknown.
- **Etiology.** A fertilized female mite (Figure 20.11) excavates a burrow in the stratum corneum, lays her eggs, and deposits fecal pellets (scybala) behind her as she advances. The egg laying, scybala, or other secretions may act as irritants or allergens, which may account for the itching and subsequent hypersensitization reaction.

DESCRIPTION OF LESIONS

- The initial lesions of scabies include **tiny pinpoint vesicles**, and **erythematous papules**, some of which evolve into **burrows**, the classic tell-tale lesions of scabies (Figure 20.12).

The burrow
- Upon closer examination of a primary lesion, the burrow, may be seen. The burrow is a linear or S-shaped excavation that is pink–white in color and slightly scaly, which ends in a pinpoint vesicle or papule. This is where the mites may be found.
- Burrows are easiest to find on the hands, particularly in the finger webs and wrists in adults, and on the palms and soles in infants.
- Sometimes burrows can be highlighted by applying black ink with a felt-tipped pen to the suspected areas (the "burrow ink test").

DISTRIBUTION OF LESIONS

- They are most often located on the interdigital finger webs (Figure 20.13), sides of the hands and feet, flexor wrists, umbilicus, waistband area, axillae, ankles, buttocks, and groin. Insect bites, such as fleas, generally spare areas that are covered (e.g., the groin and axillae.)
- Children and immunocompetent adults rarely have lesions above the neck, whereas infants tend to have more widespread involvement including the face and scalp, and especially the palms and soles. This is an important diagnostic sign.

CLINICAL VARIANTS

- **Infants** have more **generalized involvement**. Frequently, intact vesicles are seen on the palms and soles. The typical clinical picture is that of an irritable infant doggedly pinching his or her skin (Figure 20.14).
- **Elderly** patients, particularly in an institutional setting, can have **intense pruritus** and few papular lesions, excoriations, or simply dry, scaly skin.
- **Norwegian scabies**, or **crusted scabies**, (Figure 20.15) occurs in people with varying degrees of immune deficiency such as that seen in Down's syndrome, leukemia, nutritional disorders, and in patients with AIDS. The lesions tend to involve large areas of the body. The hands and feet may be scaly and crusted with a thick keratotic material seen under nails. There may be wartlike vegetations on the skin, which are host to thousands of mites and their eggs.

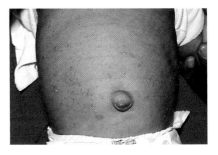

Figure 20.14.
Scabies infant with papular and vesicular lesions on the trunk.

CLINICAL MANIFESTATIONS

- Because the incubation period from initial infestation to the onset of pruritus is approximately 1 month, it is not uncommon for contacts to be asymptomatic, especially if they have recently been infested.
- Itching is most severe at night **(nocturnal pruritus)**; however, it should be kept in mind that pruritus, in general, tends to be more severe during the nighttime hours when people are inclined to be less distracted.

Course/secondary lesions

- Initially, itching is rather mild and focal, but when lesions begin spreading rapidly, usually after 4 to 6 weeks, it can sometimes reach an intolerable crescendo.
- This more generalized distribution of lesions is probably because of a hypersensitivity reaction. In this case, a more pleomorphic array of lesions, such as edematous papules and nodules, may be seen.
- Hemorrhagic crusts and ulcerations may replace the primary lesions.
- In men, **itchy papules and nodules**, particularly on the penis and scrotum, are almost pathognomonic for scabies (Figure 20.16).

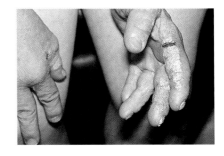

Figure 20.15.
Norwegian scabies. Child with Down syndrome has verrucous plaques on his hands and thickened dystrophic nails.

DIAGNOSIS

A conclusive diagnosis is made by finding scabies mites, eggs, or feces.

- A drop of mineral oil is applied to the most likely lesion (usually a vesicle or burrow on the finger web or wrist is chosen). The site is then scraped with a #11 or #15 blade (Figure 20.17); the scrapings are placed on a slide and a cover slip is then applied.
- Adults, who are more efficient scratchers than children, tend to remove the definitive evidence of scabies, (i.e., mite) with their fingernails. Because mites are few in number and particularly hard to find in adults, the time and effort spent searching for the mite may be better utilized by taking a good history and used to counsel the patient and his or her contacts. Thus, if scabies is strongly suspected on clinical grounds, scabicidal treatment should be initiated.

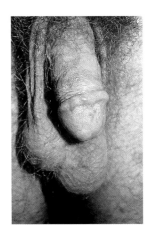

Figure 20.16.
Scabies. Pruritic papules and nodules on the penis and scrotum.

DIFFERENTIAL DIAGNOSIS

- Pruritus associated with systemic diseases, such as renal disease, hepatic disease, lymphomas, AIDS, leukemias, and Hodgkin's disease, should be excluded.
- Also included in the differential are:
  - Atopic dermatitis/dyshidrotic eczema
  - Drug eruptions
  - Other itchy rashes, including urticaria, tinea, xerosis, and contact dermatitis

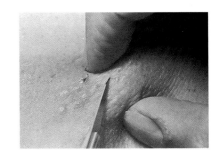

Figure 20.17.
Scraping for scabies.

MANAGEMENT

Treatment
- Treatment is directed at killing the mites with a scabicide.
- It is also aimed at affording rapid symptomatic relief with appropriate oral antihistamines and topical corticosteroids, if necessary.

Permethrin (Elimite Cream)
This is a safe and effective scabicide that is presently considered the treatment of choice for scabies. It comes in a 5% preparation and requires a prescription. Permethrin has not been proven to be safe in infants under 2 months of age and in pregnant and nursing women; however, it is probably the best treatment option in these situations.

Instructions for use
- After a warm bath, it is applied to all skin surfaces from head to toe (including the palms, soles, and scalp in small children) and is left on for 8 to 12 hours (usually overnight), and washed off the next morning.
- If indicated, other family members and contacts should be treated simultaneously. All bed linen and intimate undergarments should be washed in hot water after treatment is completed.
- Generally, only one treatment is necessary; however, a second treatment is often recommended in 4 to 5 days, especially in long-standing cases and for infants with scabies of the palms and soles.
- Patients should be advised that it is normal to continue itching for days or weeks after treatment, albeit, less intensely, and not to apply the medication repeatedly. Systemic antihistamines and a topical corticosteroid can be used for these symptoms.

Lindane (Kwell Lotion)
This is the generic name for gamma benzene hexachloride. Until recently, it was the mainstay of scabies treatment; now it is recommended as an alternative agent. It is available in a 1% formulation and also requires a prescription. It is also safe and effective, but controversy arose about its safety after several reports of neurotoxicity in infants. Ultimately, it was concluded that the drug was overused in these cases, leading to systemic absorption. Some resistance to lindane has been reported.

Instructions for use
- Used as an overnight treatment, it is applied from the neck to toes; the patient is instructed to wash it off in 8 to 12 hours.
- Treatment may be repeated in 4 to 5 days if there is little symptomatic improvement.
- Lindane is to be avoided in infants, pregnant or nursing women, or patients with a history of seizure disorders.

Precipitated sulfur ointment (6%)
Precipitated sulfur ointment is used in pregnant or lactating women and in infants less than 2 months of age. It should be administered nightly for 3 nights and can be messy and malodorous. However, it is considered safe and effective.

Ivermectin
Ivermectin is an antihelmintic that can be administered in a single oral dose. It has recently been used safely and effectively in patients who are HIV positive and in some patients with Norwegian scabies. This agent, in an oral dose of 200 μg/kg, used adjunctively with a topical scabicide may be helpful in treating large groups. (Now available as Stromectol, it is not yet approved for treatment of scabies.)

Crotamiton (Eurax Lotion and Cream)
This treatment is not very effective.

Management of institutional scabies
- Treatment must be conducted in an organized, cooperative fashion.
- Scabicide is applied to all patients, staff, family members, and frequent visitors.
- Laundering of all bed linen and clothes is necessary shortly after treatment.

POINTS TO REMEMBER
- Scabies mimics other skin diseases.
- Scabies rarely occurs above the neck in immune-competent adults.
- Treat contacts simultaneously to avoid "ping-ponging" (reinfection).
- Treatment failure may be the result of noncompliance (i.e., treating lesions only) or reinfection.
- Symptoms may persist after appropriate treatment.
- Lesions that resemble insect bites, an eczematous dermatitis, and so-called "neurotic excoriations" may confuse an unsuspecting diagnostician.

Think scabies when you see:
- An infant with palmar or plantar vesicles or pustules
- More than one family member, roommate, or sexual partner who is itching
- Pruritic scrotal or penile papules or nodules
- Vesicles in the finger webs

BASICS

There are two species of sucking lice, *Pediculosis humanus* and *Phthirus pubis*. *P. humanus* is further divided into two subspecies, *P. humanus capitis* (the head louse), and *P. humanus corporis* (the body louse).

Head lice (*Pediculosis capitis*)
- Head lice spread from human to human; epidemics of head lice are most commonly seen in schoolchildren.
- Head lice occur more often in females than in males; they are unusual in African Americans but are not unusual in African blacks.

Pubic lice or "crabs" (*Pediculosis pubis*)
Pubic lice are generally transmitted by sexual contact.

Body lice (*Pediculosis corporis*)
- Body lice are most often found in situations of poor personal hygiene, such as seen in homeless people.
- They are historically prevalent in war conditions.

DESCRIPTION OF LESIONS

Head lice
- There are no primary lesions; however, secondary crusts and eczematous dermatitis because of scratching may be present.
- Nits (louse eggs) are cemented to the hairs (Figure 20.18).
- It is difficult to find living lice.

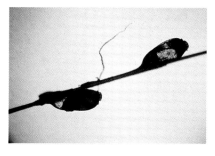

Figure 20.18.
Head lice. Nits attached to hair shaft. (Courtesy of Steven R. Cohen.)

Pubic lice

- Small brown lice and nits may be seen at the base of hairs (Figure 20.19).
- **Blue macules (maculae ceruleae)** may occur on nearby skin.

Body lice

Lesions begin as small papules. Later, secondary lesions develop because of scratching and may produce crusted papules, infected papules, and ulcerations.

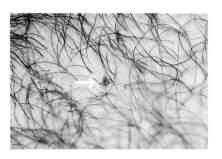

Figure 20.19.
Pubic lice. Small brown living crab louse at base of hairs (*arrow*).

DISTRIBUTION OF LESIONS

Head lice

Only the scalp is involved.

Pubic lice

Pubic hair, eyebrows, eyelashes, and axillary hair may be infested.

Body lice

Covered areas (under infested clothing) of the body may be affected.

CLINICAL MANIFESTATIONS

Head, pubic, and body lice

Itching is the predominant symptom.

There is a possibility of secondary infection from scratching.

With the exception of **body lice**, which has historically been known to carry epidemic typhus, trench fever, and relapsing fever, lice are not known to transmit any disease.

DIAGNOSIS

Head lice
- Knowledge of an epidemic at school generally alerts parents to look for evidence of lice.
- White nits may be obvious on a background of darker hair.
- A hair may be plucked and examined for nits using the low power of a microscope or hand lens. Nits are attached to the base of a hair shaft when the egg is first laid, and, as the hair grows, the egg remains cemented to it.

Pubic lice
- Lice and nits are present.
- Blue macules may be seen.
- Often, there is a sexual partner with "crabs."

Body lice
The diagnosis is not made from the patient but from the seams of his or her clothing where the lice are found.

DIFFERENTIAL DIAGNOSIS

Head, body, and pubic lice
- Atopic dermatitis of the scalp
- Atopic dermatitis or other eczematous dermatitis
- Scabies

MANAGEMENT

Head lice
Remove nits with a fine-tooth comb after soaking the hair in a vinegar solution; this helps to soften the cementing substance that attaches the nit to the hair.

Kwell Shampoo (lindane)
Shampoo, then repeat in 1 week to destroy remaining eggs, or

OTC Nix Creme Rinse (1% permethrin)
Shampoo, then repeat in 1 week to destroy remaining eggs.

Petrolatum
Petrolatum, such as Vaseline Petroleum Jelly, is messy and hard to remove but is an inexpensive and sometimes effective method that asphyxiates the lice and nits. It is applied to the entire scalp and left on overnight under a shower cap.

For resistant cases
- **Elimite Cream** (5% permethrin; a prescription is necessary) is applied to the entire scalp and left on overnight under an occlusive shower cap. Then it is repeated in 1 week to destroy the remaining eggs.
- **Oral Ivermectin**, which is not yet approved for treatment of head lice, can be administered in a single oral dose of 200 μg/kg and repeated in 10 days to destroy any remaining eggs.
- There have been recent reports of therapeutically recalcitrant cases of head lice responding to **trimethoprim-sulfamethoxazole**, which presumably destroys essential bacteria in the louse's gut, causing it to starve to death.

Pubic lice
- Kwell Shampoo is lathered and left on for 10 minutes.
- **Kwell, Rid,** and **Nix** Lotions are also effective.

Body lice
- A shower and clean clothing will generally cure body lice.
- Clothing should be washed at hot temperatures to kill the lice.
- Pediculocides are not necessary.

POINTS TO REMEMBER
- Shaving of pubic, scalp, or body hair is not necessary in order to treat lice.
- The body louse is the only louse that is known to transmit disease.

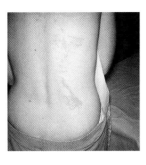

Figure 20.20.
Jelly fish sting. Note the curvilinear whiplike shape of the lesions.

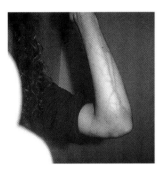

Figure 20.21.
Portuguese man-of-war sting. Note the linear shape of the lesions.

BASICS

- There are two types of stinging jellyfish seen floating in the coastal waters of North America: the smaller sea nettle and the more dangerous Portuguese man-of-war, whose poison may be fatal.
- The tentacles of jellyfish have many stinging nematocysts, which contain a hollow poisonous tip and hooks. The hooks hold the victim while the nematocysts discharge the toxic venom into their aquatic prey.

DESCRIPTION OF LESIONS

(Figures 20.20 and 20.21)
- The shape of the lesions, which are like linear welts that develop at the site of contact, often give the victim the appearance of having been whipped.
- Lesions may fade or blister and become necrotic, depending on the amount of injected venom and individual sensitivity.

DISTRIBUTION OF LESIONS

The distribution is unilateral.

CLINICAL MANIFESTATIONS

- Victims usually describe a stinging or burning sensation.
- There have been reported cases of anaphylactic reactions and fatalities.

DIAGNOSIS

Diagnosis is based upon the reported sting occurring in an endemic area and its characteristic eruption.

DIFFERENTIAL DIAGNOSIS

Other bites or stings

MANAGEMENT

- Mild stings may be treated symptomatically with cool soaks and topical steroids.
- For more severe reactions, the affected area should be washed with sea water, alcohol, or vinegar to remove nematocysts and inactivate any remaining toxins.

POINT TO REMEMBER

Severe stings that result in systemic reactions may require life-support measures.

Also known as "creeping eruption."

BASICS

- As the name suggests, cutaneous larva migrans is a cutaneous eruption that creeps or migrates in the skin. It is the result of the invasion and movement of various hookworm larvae that have penetrated the skin, having entered through the feet, lower legs, or buttocks.
- *Ancylostoma braziliense, A. caninum, A. ceylanicum, Uncinaria stenocephalia* (dog hookworm), *Bunostomum phlebotomum* (cattle hookworm), *A. duodenale,* and *Necator americanus* are the primary hookworms that cause cutaneous larvae migrans in the United States.
- The adult hookworm (nematode) lives in the intestines of dogs, cats, cattle, and monkeys. The feces of these animals contain hookworm eggs, which are deposited on sand or soil, hatch into larvae if conditions are favorable, then penetrate human skin, which serves as a "dead-end" host.
- At greatest risk are gardeners, sea bathers, plumbers, and farm workers.
- A distinct variant of cutaneous larvae migrans, known as larvae currens, caused by *Strongyloides stercoralis,* may produce visceral disease. Visceral larvae migrans is caused by *Toxocara canis, T. cati,* or *A. lumbricoides.*

DESCRIPTION OF LESIONS

- A thin curvilinear inflammatory erythematous and vesicular lesion is characteristic (Figure 20.22).
- Multiple larvae may produce multiple tracts.

DISTRIBUTION OF LESIONS

Areas that come into contact with the sand, most commonly the feet, are affected.

CLINICAL MANIFESTATIONS

A benign eruption occurs. It is usually pruritic and self-limited because the larvae die within 4 to 6 weeks.

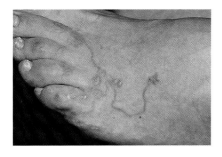

Figure 20.22.
Cutaneous larva migrans. Note the serpiginous, erythematous, raised, tunnel-like lesion.

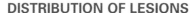

DIAGNOSIS

Based on clinical appearance

DIFFERENTIAL DIAGNOSIS

Granuloma annulare
- Annular
- Lacks scale and vesicles

Tinea pedis
KOH positive

Other bltes or stlngs
(e.g., jellyfish)

MANAGEMENT

- Superpotent topical steroids (e.g., clobetasol cream) for itching
- Topical thiabendazole suspension 500 mg/5 cc under occlusion three times daily for 1 week, or
- Oral thiabendazole (Mintezol) 50 mg/kg per day in two daily doses for 2 to 5 days, or
- Albendazole 400 mg per day for 3 days (has fewer side effects than thiabendazole), or
- LN_2, which is applied to the active, advancing end of lesion

POINT TO REMEMBER

- If the patient has been vacationing on the beach in an endemic area, consider cutaneous larva migrans as a cause of a focal itchy eruption on the feet.

CHAPTER 21

BENIGN SKIN NEOPLASMS

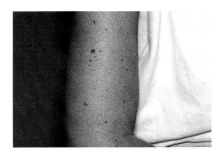

Figure 21.1.
Junctional melanocytic nevi (MN). Flat, round, uniformly pigmented, dark-brown macules.

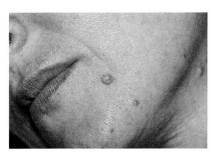

Figure 21.2.
Dermal melanocytic nevi (MN). Dome-shaped, flesh-colored papules.

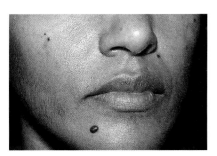

Figure 21.3.
Compound melanocytic nevi (MN). Pigmented papules.

BASICS

MELANOCYTIC NEVI (COMMON MOLES)

- **Nevi,** commonly called moles, are benign proliferations of normal skin components. **Melanocytic nevi (MN)** are comprised of nevus cells derived from melanocytes.
- MN may be congenital or acquired and are much more often seen in Caucasians than in blacks or Asians.
- The acquisition of MN is greatest in childhood and adolescence, with a tapering off of new lesions and a gradual involution and disappearance of older lesions during adulthood.
- Individuals with numerous MN, particularly if they are **dysplastic nevi** (see below), are at greater risk of developing a malignant melanoma.

DESCRIPTION OF LESIONS

Junctional melanocytic nevi
(Figure 21.1)
- Melanocytic nevus cells are located at the dermoepidermal junction.
- The nevi are macular, frecklelike lesions.
- Uniform in color, the nevi can range from brown to dark brown to black.

Dermal melanocytic nevi
(Figure 21.2)
- Melanocytic nevus cells are located in the dermis.
- The nevi are elevated, dome-shaped, warty-appearing, or pedunculated papules.
- The lesions are usually skin-colored, but they may be tan, brown, or dappled with pigmentation ("younger" lesions). They tend to loose pigmentation with age and become skin-colored.

Compound melanocytic nevi
(Figure 21.3)
- These lesions have **combined features of junctional and dermal nevi.**
- They are an elevated, dome-shaped papule or a papillomatous nodule.
- Uniform in color, the lesions can range from brown to dark brown or black, and they may contain hairs.

DISTRIBUTION OF LESIONS

- **Junctional nevi** can appear on the face, arms, legs, trunk, palms, and soles.
- **Dermal nevi** are most often seen on the face and neck.
- **Compound nevi** can appear on the face, arms, legs, and trunk.

CLINICAL MANIFESTATIONS

Junctional nevi
- Asymptomatic
- Rare transformation to malignant melanoma

Dermal nevi and compound nevi
- Asymptomatic unless irritated or inflamed
- Rare transformation to malignant melanoma

DIAGNOSIS

- Diagnosis is based upon clinical appearance or histopathology.
- Lesions are generally sent for histopathologic evaluation after removal.

DIFFERENTIAL DIAGNOSIS

Junctional nevus
A junctional nevus may be **clinically indistinguishable from a freckle, lentigo simplex, or a solar lentigo**.
- **Freckles (ephelides;** Figure 21.4)
  - Small, tan macules that appear on sun-exposed skin in fair-skinned people
  - Darken after sun exposure; lighten when no longer sun-exposed
- **Lentigo** (plural **lentigines**, "liver spots")
  - **Solar lentigines** (Figure 21.5)
    - Tan colored macules that arise on sun-exposed areas
    - Uniform in coloration
    - Acquired in middle age
  - **Lentigo simplex**
    - Uniform coloration
    - May be first noted in childhood
    - Not related to sun exposure

Dermal nevi and compound nevi
These are often **similar in appearance to one another** and to:
- Skin tags
- Seborrheic keratoses
- Dermatofibromas
- Neurofibromas
- Basal cell carcinomas
- Nodular melanoma
- Warts

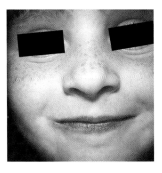

Figure 21.4.
Freckles (ephelides).

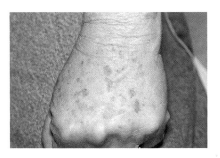

Figure 21.5.
Solar lentigines on sun-exposed area.

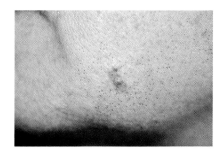

Figure 21.6.
Blue nevus. Note the characteristic bluish-gray coloration.

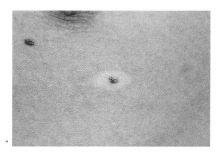

Figure 21.7.
Halo nevus. Compound nevus that is encircled by a white halo of depigmentation. Ultimately, the nevus may disappear and the area will repigment.

Blue nevus
(Figure 21.6)

- A **blue nevus** is a benign variant of a dermal MN.
  - Blue nevi are blue–gray or blue–black papules or nodules.
  - Blue nevi are rarely malignant.
  - The lesion may resemble a dermatofibroma or a nodular malignant melanoma. If there is any suspicion of malignancy, a biopsy should be performed.
- **Halo nevus** (Figure 21.7)
  - Halo nevus is a form of MN that is encircled by a white halo of depigmentation.
  - It is seen in adolescents, usually on the trunk.
  - The halo represents a regression of the nevus caused by a lymphocytic infiltrate.
  - The entire nevus frequently depigments and then repigments to the patient's usual color of skin without residual trace of the original nevus.
  - If the nevus appears to be clinically atypical, a biopsy should be performed.
  - If a halo nevus occurs in an adult, the rare possibility of malignancy of the lesion or a melanoma elsewhere on the body should be considered.
- **Congenital melanocytic nevus** (Figures 21.8–21.10)
  - Congenital nevi are of the greatest concern when they are large, measuring greater than 20 cm in diameter.
  - So-called giant pigmented hairy nevi (otherwise known as "garment" or "bathing trunk nevi" because their appearance suggests an article of clothing) are associated with a lifetime risk of developing melanoma in 5 to 10 % of cases.
  - The malignant potential of smaller or midsize congenital MN is a controversial issue; however, congenital nevi should be carefully examined and considered for biopsy, particularly if there is any clinical suggestion of atypia.

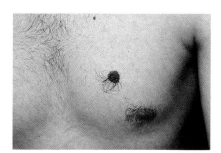

Figure 21.8.
Small congenital hairy melanocytic nevus.

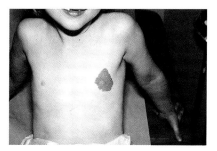

Figure 21.9.
Medium-size congenital melanocytic nevus.

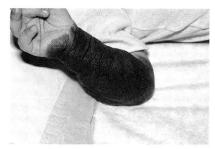

Figure 21.10.
Giant congenital hairy melanocytic nevus. Giant hairy "garment nevus."

MANAGEMENT

For the vast majority of MN, a biopsy is not indicated.

Indications for removal:
- Uncertain diagnosis
- Cosmetic reasons
- Repeated irritation by clothing (e.g., a bra strap)
- If lesion persistently itches, hurts, or bleeds

Methods of removal (see Chapter 26, "Basic Procedures")
- **Biopsy.** Use a **shave excision/biopsy** method often followed by **electrodesiccation**.
  - **Advantages**. This method is fast and economical with generally satisfactory cosmetic results.
  - **Disadvantages.** The procedure often results only in partial removal of lesions.
- **Excision.**
  - Advantages. This method is performed with the intent of completely removing lesions. Surgical margins can be identified.
  - **Disadvantages** This method is slower, requires suturing and suture removal, and results in linear scars.

DYSPLASTIC NEVUS (ATYPICAL MOLE, CLARK'S NEVUS)

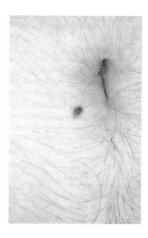

Figure 21.11.
Dysplastic nevus (DN). Raised center, indistinct border, "sunny-side up–egg" lesion.

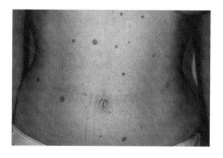

Figure 21.12.
Multiple dysplastic nevi in a characteristic distribution on the trunk.

BASICS

- The dysplastic nevus (DN) is a controversial and confusing lesion. There is no consensus among dermatopathologists regarding the histopathologic criteria for its diagnosis.
- It is accepted, however, that DN, when numerous and found in other family members in addition to the patient, are **considered markers for potential melanoma** in that family.
- DN are also regarded as potential precursors of melanoma.
- In the **DN syndrome**, in which there is a family history of malignant melanoma, virtually all family members with DN may develop a malignant melanoma in their lifetime.
- When DN are seen as a few isolated lesions and there is no family history of melanoma or familial DN syndrome, the risk of developing melanoma is probably only minimally greater than would be expected in the general population.

DESCRIPTION OF LESIONS

Clinically, DN have some or all of the following features:
- Larger than 5 mm (Figure 21.11)
- Irregular, indistinct borders
- Macular, but may have a raised center ("sunny-side up–egg" lesions)
- Irregular coloration of tan, brown, black, pink, or red

DISTRIBUTION OF LESIONS

Lesions occur primarily on sun-protected areas, on the trunk, legs, and arms. The face is spared (Figure 21.12).

CLINICAL MANIFESTATIONS

Unlike common nevi, lesions often continue to appear into adulthood.

DIAGNOSIS

Excisional or shave biopsy may be performed on several lesions to establish the diagnosis.

DIFFERENTIAL DIAGNOSIS

- Other MNs
- Malignant melanoma
- Pigmented basal cell carcinoma

MANAGEMENT

- Annual follow-up examinations are strongly recommended.
- In patients with a family history of melanoma, more frequent examinations are advised.
- Removal and biopsy of changing or suspicious lesions are also advised.
- The method chosen for removing the lesion depends on the purpose of removal.
  - If a melanoma is suspected, complete excision should be performed.
  - If a lesion is thought to be a DN, individual judgment may be made as to whether shave or elliptical excision is performed.

POINTS TO REMEMBER

- Any pigmented lesion with a rapid change in size or color, or one that has an atypical appearance, should be removed for biopsy.
- People with DN, who have a personal and/or family history of melanoma, have a much greater risk of developing a melanoma than those with DN who do not have a personal or family history of melanoma.
- Once the diagnosis of DN is established, other family members should be examined.
- Patients with DN should be advised to use sunscreens and to avoid sunbathing.
- Advise and teach self-examination of the skin.

SKIN TAGS (ACROCHORDONS)

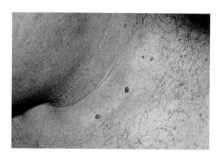

Figure 21.13.
Skin tags. Pigmented and flesh-colored papules around the neck.

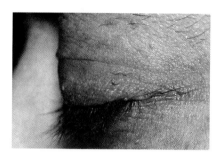

Figure 21.14.
Skin tags on the eyelids.

BASICS

- **Skin tags** are common, benign skin lesions.
- They are sometimes referred to as **acrochordons, fibroepithelial polyps (FEPs)**, and, if large in size, **soft fibroma** or **pedunculated lipofibroma**.
- They are commonly seen in the intertriginous areas of obese individuals.
- Skin tags were suspected by several investigators to be markers for intestinal polyps or possibly internal malignancies; however, current evidence suggests that this association is not justifiable.

DESCRIPTION OF LESIONS

(Figure 21.13)
- Generally, 1- to 10-mm, fleshy papules
- Skin-toned, tan, or darkly pigmented in color
- Polypoid, sessile, or pedunculated in shape

DISTRIBUTION OF LESIONS

They are most often found on the neck, the axillae, the inframammary area, the groin (especially the inguinal creases), the upper thighs, and the eyelids (Figure 21.14).

CLINICAL MANIFESTATIONS

- Skin tags are primarily of cosmetic concern; however, they may become a nuisance from the irritation of necklaces or underarm shaving.
- In pregnant women, they tend to grow larger and more numerous over time.
- They are often seen in association with **acanthosis nigricans** (see Chapter 25, "The Cutaneous Manifestations of Systemic Disease").

DIAGNOSIS

Skin tags are easy to recognize, and a skin biopsy is rarely necessary.

DIFFERENTIAL DIAGNOSIS

- Pedunculated seborrheic keratoses
- Compound or dermal nevi
- Neurofibromas

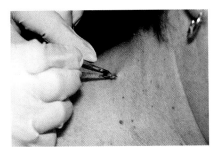

Figure 21.15.
Scissor excision of a skin tag.

MANAGEMENT

- Skin tags are easily removed by simply snipping them off at their base using iris scissors, with or without local anesthesia. The crushing action of the scissors results in very little bleeding or pain (Figure 21.15).
- Skin tags, if disregarded, have been known to spontaneously self-destruct. Following torsion, they may become necrotic and auto-amputate.

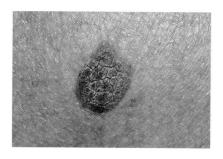

Figure 21.16.
Seborrheic keratosis (SK). Warty-, stuck-on–appearing lesion.

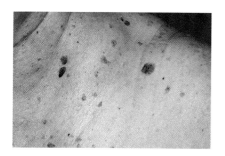

Figure 21.17.
Seborrheic keratosis (SK). Multiple lesions demonstrating various colors and sizes.

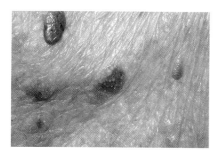

Figure 21.18.
Seborrheic keratosis (SK). Note white pseudo-horncysts on the surface of the lesions.

BASICS

- **Seborrheic keratoses (SKs)** are extremely common, benign skin growths that become apparent in people older than age 40. They represent the most common tumor in the elderly, and they have virtually no malignant potential. Patients often report a positive family history of SKs, with men and women being equally affected.
- SKs have been whimsically described by some observers as "barnacles in the sea of life," which serves as a metaphor intended to allay patients' anxiety.

DESCRIPTION OF LESIONS

(Figure 21.16)
- The typical SK has best been described as a lesion that appears warty and stuck-on, ranging in color from tan to dark brown to black.
- The dry, crumbly, keratotic surface of some lesions are occasionally rubbed or picked off, only to recur later.
- The use of the word "seborrheic," a misnomer, stems from an occasional greasy or shiny appearance; however, SKs are actually epidermal in origin, having no sebaceous derivation.
- The appearance of individual lesions tends to vary considerably, even on the same person.
- Lesions may be warty, scaly, flat, or small skin tag–like pigmented papules (Figure 21.17).

DISTRIBUTION OF LESIONS

- SKs are most often located on the back, chest, and face, particularly along the frontal hairline and scalp, but are also frequently found on the arms, legs, and abdomen.
- Smaller skin tag–like lesions can be seen around the neck, under the breast, or in the axillae.
- When many SKs are present, distribution is usually bilateral and symmetrical.

CLINICAL MANIFESTATIONS

- SKs are mainly a cosmetic concern, except in instances when they are inflamed or irritated, when they can be an annoyance.
- The health care provider must distinguish them from skin cancer, particularly malignant melanoma.

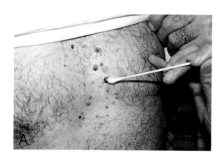
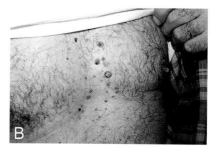

Figures 21.19.
(*A* and *B*) Accentuation of pseudo-horn-cysts by freezing a seborrheic keratosis with LN$_2$.

Figures 21.19. (continued)

DIAGNOSIS

With experience, SKs are easily recognized.

- The diagnosis can be confirmed by the presence of pseudo-horncysts, which appear as white or dark dots of keratin plugs that are sometimes noted on the surface of the lesions (Figure 21.18). They are often visible with a hand lens and can be accentuated by freezing the lesion with LN_2, which turns the surrounding SK whiter than the pseudo-horncyst (Figure 21.19).
- If necessary, a shave biopsy using #15 scalpel blade or a curettage (see Chapter 26, "Basic Procedures") may be performed for histologic confirmation.

DIFFERENTIAL DIAGNOSIS

- Malignant melanoma (Figure 21.20)
- Pigmented basal cell carcinoma (Figure 21.21)
- Verruca vulgaris (wart)
- Solar lentigo
- Pigmented solar keratosis (actinic keratosis)
- Melanocytic nevus
- Dysplastic nevus

CLINICAL VARIANTS OF SEBORRHEIC KERATOSIS

Stucco keratosis

(Figure 21.22)

- Stucco keratosis is probably a nonpigmented variant of SK.
- The lesions are commonly noted on the distal lower leg, particularly around the ankles, and are also located on the dorsal forearms in the elderly.
- Stucco keratoses are flesh-colored or whitish papules that become whiter and scalier when scratched. They typify the dry, stuck-on type of SK.

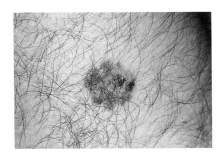

Figure 21.20.
Malignant melanoma (MM). Note the variegation in color and the irregular notched border.

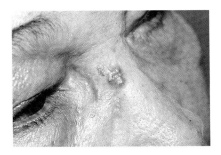

Figure 21.21.
Pigmented basal cell carcinoma (BCC). Note the pearly color and rolled border.

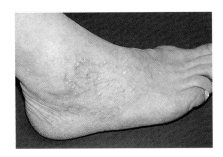

Figure 21.22.
Stucco keratosis. Whitish, stuck-on–appearing lesions.

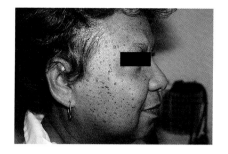

Figure 21.23.
Dermatosis papulosa nigra. The lesions appear as small pigmented seborrheic keratosis–like papules on the face.

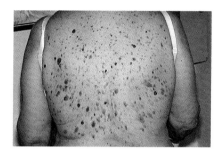

Figure 21.24.
The sign of Leser-Trelat. Multiple seborrheic keratoses (SKs) that rapidly increased in number.

Dermatosis papulosa nigra
(Figure 21.23)

- DPN is found particularly in African Americans, Afro-Caribbeans, and sub-Saharan black Africans; it is also seen in darker-skinned persons of other races.
- DPNs start appearing in adolescence and progress into adulthood.
- The lesions are generally seen on the face, especially the upper cheeks and lateral periorbital areas.
- They are darkly pigmented and, in contrast to typical SKs, have minimal, if any, scale.
- They are histopathologically identical to SKs and are considered to be of autosomal dominant inheritance.

The sign of Leser-Trélat
(Figure 21.24)

- This refers to the sudden appearance of multiple SKs in a short period of time and/or a rapid increase in their size.
- It is a rare phenomenon presumed by some observers to be a cutaneous sign of leukemia or internal malignancy, especially of the gastrointestinal tract, prostate, breast, ovary, uterus, liver, and lung.
- In light of the frequency of malignancy in the elderly, and the ubiquitous presence of SKs in this age group, the relationship may be fortuitous in nature.

MANAGEMENT

- Patients with SKs are frequently referred to dermatologists with the presumptive diagnosis of warts or moles or to have the lesion(s) evaluated to rule out skin cancer.
- A biopsy, generally a shave biopsy, is performed if necessary to confirm the diagnosis or to distinguish it from a basal cell carcinoma, a melanocytic nevus, or a wart.

- Because numerous lesions are frequently observed in some patients, it is an impractical expenditure of time and money to perform multiple biopsies of the remaining clinically typical SK lesions; however, an excisional biopsy should be performed if a malignant melanoma is suspected.

TREATMENT

- Light electrocautery and curettage is performed. Treating the base of the lesion helps prevent recurrence.
- Cryosurgery with LN_2 spray or Q-tip application is another method of treatment.
- Excisional surgery, which results in scar formation, is unnecessary unless a biopsy of a completely removed lesion is required to rule out malignancy.

POINT TO REMEMBER

SKs may be numerous on some individuals. All lesions should be carefully examined because they may be confused with melanomas.

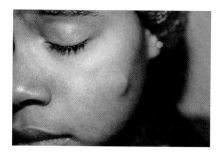

Figure 21.25.
Epidermoid cyst. Smooth, discrete, freely moveable, bluish-tinted dome-shaped nodule.

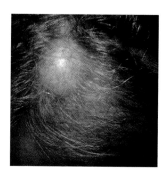

Figure 21.26.
Pilar cyst.

BASICS

- A cyst is a sac containing semisolid or liquid material. A true cyst has an epithelial lining, while pseudocysts do not.
- **Epidermoid cysts** are the most common type.
- **Pilar** or **trichilemmal cysts** ("wen" and "sebaceous cyst" are obsolete terms) are the type most frequently seen on the scalp. Both types tend to be familial, begin in adulthood, and may occur as multiple lesions.

DESCRIPTION OF LESIONS

- Lesions appear as smooth, discrete, freely moveable, dome-shaped nodules (Figure 21.25).
- Cysts that have previously been infected, ruptured, drained, or scarred may be more firm and less freely moveable.
- Lesions range from 0.5 to 5.0 cm in diameter.
- Often, there is a central punctum (seen in epidermoid cysts), from which cheesy-white, malodorous, keratin material can be expressed.

DISTRIBUTION OF LESIONS

- Epidermoid cysts occur most often on the face, behind the ears, and on the neck, trunk, scrotum, and labia.
- Pilar cysts are found on the scalp (Figure 21.26).

CLINICAL MANIFESTATIONS

- Cysts are usually asymptomatic, unless inflamed or infected.
- Scrotal and pilar cysts may calcify (idiopathic scrotal calcinosis).
- Pilar cysts are generally devoid of overlying scalp hair.

DIAGNOSIS

Upon compression, an intact epidermoid or pilar cyst feels like an eyeball.

DIFFERENTIAL DIAGNOSIS

Lipomas (see below)

Lipoma should be considered when cystlike lesions are found on the neck, upper back, and thighs.

- The consistency is rubbery and softer than that of cysts.
- The shape is irregular.

CLINICAL VARIANT

Milia

- Milia are epidermal cysts that contain keratin. They are 1.0 to 2.0 mm in size and white to yellow in color (Figure 21.27).
- They can occur at any age and are most commonly seen on the face, especially around the eyes and on the cheeks and forehead.
- They may arise in traumatic scars or in association with certain scarring skin conditions, such as **porphyria cutanea tarda**.
- In contrast to closed comedones, which they resemble, milia must first be incised (usually with a #11 blade) before their contents can be expressed.

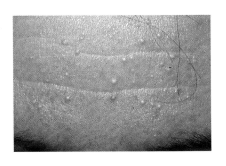

Figure 21.27.
Milia. Small white cysts.

MANAGEMENT

- Complete excision is performed, with the attempt to remove the entire cyst wall to prevent recurrence.
- Alternatively, incision and drainage may be used, followed by removal of the cyst wall with a curette or forceps.

Infected or inflamed cysts

- A fluctuant, infected cyst may be incised with a #11 blade and drained, and then packed with iodoform gauze.
- Alternatively, oral antibiotics may be given to decrease inflammation before incising or excising the lesion (*Staphylococcus aureus* is the most common pathogen found in infected cysts).
- Inflamed, noninfected cysts may sometimes regress after intralesional steroid injections; thus excision or incision and drainage may be avoided.

POINT TO REMEMBER

- Incision and drainage of cysts do not always prevent recurrence.
- Even excision does not always prevent recurrence.

BASICS

A dermatofibroma (DF), also known as fibrous histiocytoma and sclerosing hemangioma, is a common dermal fibrous tumor of unknown cause.

DESCRIPTION OF LESIONS

- The lesion may be a papule or a nodule, be elevated and dome-shaped, flat, or depressed below the plane of the surrounding skin.
- The color can vary, even in a single lesion, from flesh-colored to red, chocolate-brown, or purple.
- The borders are often ill-defined, fading into normal skin. The surface can be smooth or scaly, depending if the lesion has been traumatized (e.g., by shaving).

DISTRIBUTION OF LESIONS

DFs occur most commonly on the legs, trunk, and arms, especially in women older than 20 years.

CLINICAL MANIFESTATIONS

- They are benign growths that are brought to medical attention usually to rule out a skin cancer.
- DFs are mainly a cosmetic concern.
- Lesions may be pruritic or traumatized by repeated shaving of legs.

DIAGNOSIS

Typically, a DF feels like a firm pea or a button that is fixed to the surrounding dermis (accounting for the dimple, or collar button sign). It is freely movable over deeper adipose tissue (Figure 21.28).

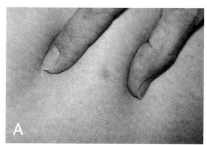
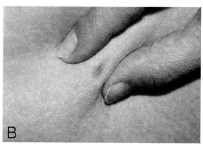

Figure 21.28.
(*A*) Dermatofibroma (DF). (*B*) Note the dimple or collar-button sign.

DIFFERENTIAL DIAGNOSIS

Malignant melanoma

Malignant melanoma is more variable in shape and size than a DF. The lesion should be biopsied if suspicious.

Pigmented and nonpigmented basal cell carcinoma

* May closely resemble DF
* Pearly and telangiectatic
* Biopsy, if suspicious

Melanocytic nevus

Not as firm as DF

MANAGEMENT

No treatment is necessary; however, local excision can be performed for biopsy confirmation, cosmetic concerns, or if the lesion is symptomatic.

POINTS TO REMEMBER

* If there is any doubt about the diagnosis, a biopsy should be performed.
* The scar, after removal of a lesion, may look worse than the original lesion.

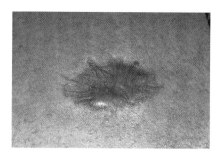

Figure 21.29.
Treated hypertrophic scar. A shiny hypertrophic scar that shows the effects of intralesional steroid injections: atrophy, telangiectasias, and perilesional hypopigmentation.

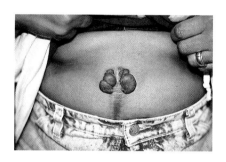

Figure 21.30.
Keloid growing well beyond the border of a surgical scar.

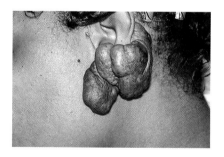

Figure 21.31.
Keloid on a common location, the earlobes.

BASICS

- **Hypertrophic scars** represent an exaggerated formation of scar tissue in response to skin injuries such as lacerations, insect bites, ear piercing, and surgical wounds. They may also result from healed inflammatory lesions of acne or varicella. Hypertrophic scars tend to regress over time.
- A **keloid** is a scar whose size far exceeds that which would be expected from the extent and margins of injury. Keloids do not regress without treatment. They are much more common in blacks than in whites and Asians.

DESCRIPTION OF LESIONS

- Lesions are firm, shiny, hairless, papules, nodules, or tumors (Figure 21.29).
- They may be flesh-colored, tan, or brown. If lesions are inflamed or are of recent onset, they may be red or purple.

DISTRIBUTION OF LESIONS

Hypertrophic scars and keloids can occur on the earlobes, chest, shoulders, and upper back (Figures 21.30 and 21.31).

CLINICAL MANIFESTATIONS

- There is cosmetic disfigurement.
- Lesions may itch, be tender, or painful.

DIAGNOSIS

Diagnosis for hypertrophic scars and keloids is made on clinical appearance.

DIFFERENTIAL DIAGNOSIS

- Nevus
- Dermatofibroma

MANAGEMENT

Hypertrophic scars
- Intralesional steroid injections
- Pulsed-dye lasers, which have been used successfully on some persistent lesions

Keloids
Intralesional steroid injections
Surgical ablation followed by compression dressings
Silicone gel sheeting
Irradiation alone, or following surgery

POINTS TO REMEMBER
- Counsel predisposed patients to avoid trauma.
- Wound care should be meticulous.
- Treat infections early.
- Surgery of keloids may result in larger keloids.

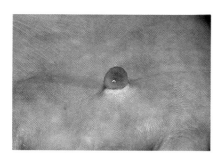

Figure 21.32.
Pyogenic granuloma (PG). Solitary nodule surrounded by a collarette of skin.

BASICS

- A pyogenic granuloma (PG) is a benign, rapidly developing, red, purple, or red–brown dome-shaped papule or nodule (Figure 21.32).
- PGs occur more often in young children and adolescents and during pregnancy (**granuloma gravidarum**).

DESCRIPTION OF LESIONS

- PGs are generally solitary papules or nodules.
- They resemble hemangiomas or granulation tissue (proud flesh).
- Size ranges from a few millimeters to 3- to 4-centimeter nodules.
- The color is red, dusky red, purple or brown.
- The base of the lesions are often surrounded by a collarette of skin.

DISTRIBUTION OF LESIONS

- Usually at sites of minor trauma
- Fingers, toes, and the trunk
- Lips and gums during pregnancy

CLINICAL MANIFESTATIONS

- PGs present as asymptomatic lesions that tend to bleed after minor trauma.
- Spontaneous resolution may occur after childbirth.

DIAGNOSIS

- Typical clinical appearance
- History of rapid growth
- Bleeding after minimal trauma
- Biopsy

DIFFERENTIAL DIAGNOSIS

The following diagnoses should be considered in the proper clinical setting and biopsied accordingly:
- Nodular malignant melanoma
- Kaposi's sarcoma
- Squamous cell carcinoma
- Bacillary angiomatosis

MANAGEMENT

- A biopsy should be performed.
- The lesion is generally destroyed either by electrocautery, laser, cryosurgery, or excisional surgery. Recurrences are not uncommon.

POINT TO REMEMBER

The clinical presentation of a rapidly developing, friable, vascular lesion in a child or pregnant woman suggests a PG.

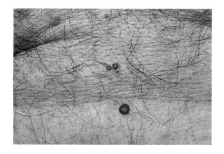

Figure 21.33.
Cherry angiomas. Cherry- and plum-colored papules.

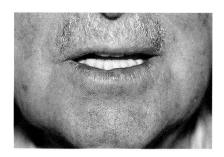

Figure 21.34.
Venous lake.

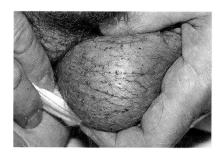

Figure 21.35.
Angiokeratomas. Caviarlike lesions on scrotum.

CHERRY ANGIOMA, VENOUS LAKE, AND ANGIOKERATOMA

BASICS

- **Cherry angiomas,** also known as Campbell De Morgan spots, ruby spots, and senile angiomas, are common, benign, vascular neoplasms that occur in fair-skinned adults older than the age of 40.
- **Venous lake** is also a vascular neoplasm; it occurs in an older population of patients, usually older than the age of 60.
- **Angiokeratomas** (Fordyce spots) are usually noted on the scrotum or vulvae, first in young adulthood.

DESCRIPTION OF LESIONS

- Cherry angiomas are cherry- to plum-colored papules (Figure 21.33).
- A venous lake is generally a dark blue to purple macule or papule (Figure 21.34).
- Angiokeratoma consist of multiple red–purple papules.

DISTRIBUTION OF LESIONS

- Cherry angiomas occur primarily on the trunk.
- A venous lake may be seen on the lower lip, face, and eyelids.
- Angiokeratomas are most commonly seen on the scrotum (Figure 21.35) or vulvae.

CLINICAL MANIFESTATIONS

- Asymptomatic
- Occasionally of cosmetic concern

DIAGNOSIS

Typical **clinical appearance**

DIFFERENTIAL DIAGNOSIS

There should be little reason to confuse these lesions with pyogenic granulomata and nodular malignant melanoma.

MANAGEMENT

- The patient should be reassured as to the benign nature of these lesions.
- Electrocautery or laser destruction may be performed, if desired.

BASICS

- A spider angioma (nevus araneus) is a cluster of telangiectasias, or dilated capillaries, that radiate from a central arteriole.
- It is more commonly seen in women and may be associated with pregnancy and oral contraceptives. Spider angiomata are also seen in hyperestrogenic conditions such as chronic liver disease. They are also found in normal children.

DESCRIPTION OF LESIONS

(Figure 21.36)
Lesions appear as spokelike capillaries radiating from a central arteriole.

DISTRIBUTION OF LESIONS

Spider angiomata occur on the face and trunk.

CLINICAL MANIFESTATIONS

- Spider angiomas are asymptomatic and are usually only a cosmetic concern.
- On occasion, lesions may regress spontaneously.

DIAGNOSIS

Compression of central arteriole completely blanches the lesion (Figure 21.37).

DIFFERENTIAL DIAGNOSIS

Other types of telangiectasias may serve as a clue to an underlying collagen vascular disease, such as the periungual telangiectasias of systemic lupus and dermatomyositis, or the matlike telangiectasias seen in scleroderma and CREST syndrome (see Chapter 25, "The Cutaneous Manifestations of Systemic Disease").

MANAGEMENT

Light electrocautery or laser destruction of the spider angioma may be performed.

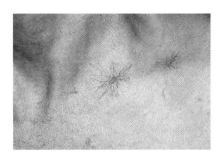

Figure 21.36.
Spider angioma. Spokelike capillaries radiating from a central arteriole.

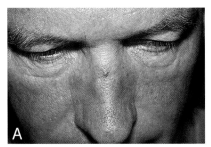

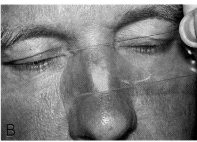

Figures 21.37.
(A) Spider angioma. (B) Compression of central arteriole completely blanches the lesion.

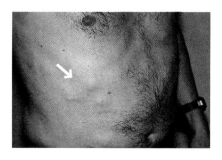

Figure 21.38.
Lipomas. Rubbery nodules (*arrow*).

BASICS

- Lipomas are benign, subcutaneous tumors composed of fat cells.
- **Dercum's disease** is a syndrome of multiple tender lipomas occurring in middle-age women.

DESCRIPTION OF LESIONS

(Figure 21.38)
- Rubbery nodular to tumor-sized masses
- Usually irregular in shape
- May be greater than 7.0 cm

DISTRIBUTION OF LESIONS

Lipomas most commonly occur on the trunk, back of neck, and forearms.

CLINICAL MANIFESTATIONS

- Lipomas generally are asymptomatic.
- Angiolipomas may be tender or painful.

DIAGNOSIS

Diagnosis is made on **clinical** grounds.

DIFFERENTIAL DIAGNOSIS

Epidermoid cyst (see above)
- Feels like an eyeball
- Regular dome shape

MANAGEMENT

- Excision
- Removal by liposuction
- Reassurance that the lesion is benign and no treatment is necessary

SEBACEOUS HYPERPLASIA

BASICS

- Sebaceous hyperplasia refers to small, benign papules on the face of adults representing hypertrophy of the sebaceous glands.
- They are fairly common lesions that are often confused with basal cell carcinomas.

DESCRIPTION OF LESIONS

(Figure 21.39)
- Yellow papules, often donut-shaped (with a dell in the center)
- Small in diameter (1 to 3 mm)
- Telangiectasias on a raised border

DISTRIBUTION OF LESIONS

Lesions occur on the forehead and cheeks.

CLINICAL MANIFESTATIONS

- Asymptomatic
- May be of cosmetic concern

DIAGNOSIS

- **Clinical appearance**
- Biopsy, if basal cell carcinoma is suspected

DIFFERENTIAL DIAGNOSIS

Basal cell carcinoma (see Chapter 22, "Premalignant and Malignant Neoplasms")

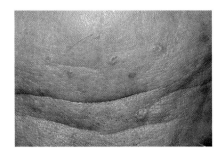

Figure 21.39.
Sebaceous hyperplasia. Multiple yellow papules. Note the central dell and telangiectasias.

MANAGEMENT

- The patient should be reassured as to the benign nature of this condition.
- Light electrocautery may be performed to remove lesions, if desired.

POINT TO REMEMBER

A simple shave biopsy can be performed if the diagnosis is in doubt.

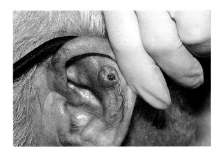

Figure 21.40.
Keratoacanthoma. Dome-shaped nodule with a central keratin core.

BASICS

- A keratoacanthoma is a unique lesion with a characteristic clinical appearance. At one time, it was considered to be a variant of squamous cell carcinoma, which it resembles histologically; however, it is now believed to be a benign lesion (possibly an abortive, self-healing, squamous cell carcinoma). In fact, lesions often regress spontaneously.
- These lesions generally occur in individuals older than 65 years of age.

DESCRIPTION OF LESIONS

- Keratoacanthoma usually occurs as a single dome-shaped erythematous or skin-colored nodule with a central keratin core with an overlying crust (Figure 21.40).
- It attains a diameter of 1.0 to 2.5 cm.

DISTRIBUTION OF LESIONS

Lesions appear on the face, ears, neck, dorsa of hands, and forearms.

CLINICAL MANIFESTATIONS

- Lesions arise quickly, usually taking 3 to 4 weeks.
- There is infrequently a history of trauma at the site of the lesion.
- Spontaneous regression may result in significant scarring.

DIAGNOSIS

An excisional or incisional biopsy is recommended so that the complete architecture of the lesion can be evaluated histologically. (An insufficient biopsy, such as a shave biopsy, may result in a histology that is indistinguishable from a squamous cell carcinoma).

DIFFERENTIAL DIAGNOSIS

- Squamous cell carcinoma
- Verruca
- Cutaneous horn

MANAGEMENT

- Excisional removal
- Intralesional 5-fluorouracil

CHAPTER 22

PREMALIGNANT AND MALIGNANT NEOPLASMS

This chapter is intended to help health care providers distinguish skin cancers from precancers and benign growths. Therapy of lesions should **only** be undertaken by persons experienced in skin cancer therapy. Specific techniques are described in Part IV, "Dermatologic Procedures."

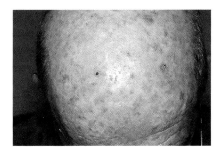

Figure 22.1.
Solar keratoses. Rough, scaly papules on the scalp.

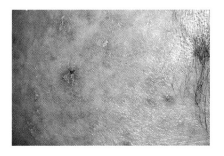

Figure 22.2.
Closer view of solar keratoses.

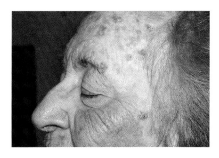

Figure 22.3.
Patient with vitiligo has solar keratoses primarily in areas of unprotected vitiliginous skin.

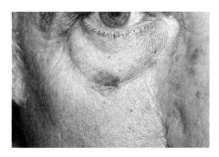

Figure 22.4.
Pigmented solar keratosis.

BASICS

- Solar (actinic) keratoses are **common premalignant neoplasms** that are caused by the cumulative effects of sun exposure on **fair-skinned people** who are genetically predisposed (e.g., those of Celtic origin).
- Typically, solar keratoses are most often seen on a background of **sun-damaged skin**. They are rare in dark-skinned individuals.
- Solar keratoses are precursors of a type of **squamous cell carcinoma** (SCC), which is slow growing, indolent, not highly invasive, and rarely metastatic. The percentage of solar keratoses that undergo malignant degeneration and become SCC is small. Among dermatologists, there is an ongoing debate regarding the need to be aggressive or somewhat laissez-faire in the approach to these lesions.
- Solar keratoses are **more common in men**, particularly those who work in outdoor occupations, such as farmers, sailors, and gardeners and those who participate in outdoor sports.

DESCRIPTION OF LESIONS

(Figures 22.1–22.3)
- Lesions are discrete, rough, scaly papules or plaques.
- They are generally 1 to 5 mm in diameter.
- Lesions have a red base with an overlying white or yellowish scale or crust.
- Sometimes, they are yellow, tan, or dark brown in color **(pigmented solar keratosis)**.
- Lesions sometimes become thick and hypertrophic and may develop an overlying **cutaneous horn**.

DISTRIBUTION OF LESIONS

Lesions occur on sun-exposed areas (e.g., the **face** [especially on the nose, temples, and forehead], **bald scalp** and **top of ears** in men, **dorsa of forearms and hands, V of neck, neck below the hairline**).

CLINICAL MANIFESTATIONS

- Lesions are usually asymptomatic, but they may itch, become tender, or irritated.
- They are of cosmetic concern.
- They may regress spontaneously.
- Solar keratoses of the lower lip is known as **actinic cheilitis**.

DIAGNOSIS

- **Clinically**, small lesions are often better discovered by palpation than by sight, revealing gritty, sandpaperlike papules.
- **A shave biopsy** is performed if the diagnosis is in doubt.
- It is necessary to shave more deeply under a cutaneous horn.

CLINICAL VARIANTS

- **Pigmented solar keratosis** (Figure 22.4)
- **Hypertrophic (hyperkeratotic) solar keratosis** (Figure 22.5)
- **Solar keratosis with an overlying cutaneous horn** (Figure 22.6). A cutaneous horn represents a nail-like keratinization produced by the solar keratosis. Besides solar keratoses, **warts** and **SCC in situ** (Bowen's disease) also can form a cutaneous horn.

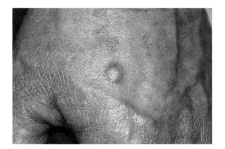

Figure 22.5.
Hypertrophic solar keratosis.

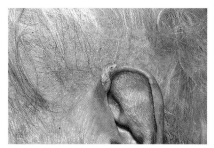

Figure 22.6.
Cutaneous horn produced by an underlying solar keratosis.

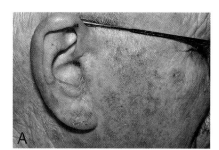

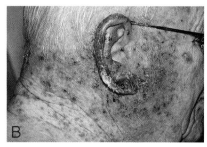

Figure 22.7.
Multiple solar keratoses. (*A*)Before treatment; (*B*) 2 weeks after treatment with topical 5-fluorouracil (5-FU).

DIFFERENTIAL DIAGNOSIS

Squamous cell carcinoma
- May be indistinguishable from an actinic keratosis
- Untreated, it becomes indurated, with a tendency to ooze, ulcerate, or bleed.

Seborrheic keratosis (see Chapter 21, "Benign Skin Neoplasms")
- Seborrheic keratosis may be indistinguishable from a solar keratosis.
- Seborrheic keratosis has a stuck-on appearance.

Verruca (wart)
May also be indistinguishable from a solar keratosis

MANAGEMENT

- **Prevention** is achieved by avoiding the sun, using sunscreens, and wearing protective clothing (Appendix 2).
- **Treatment** (see Chapter 26, "Basic Procedures") is by destruction of solar keratoses.
- **Liquid nitrogen** (LN$_2$) is applied to individual lesions.
- **Biopsy** can be performed followed by **electrocautery**, or electrocautery is used alone.
- Topical application of **5-fluorouracil** (5-FU) is a method that may be used when lesions are too numerous to treat individually (Figure 22.7).
- **Topical tretinoin** (Retin-A) has been shown to reverse mild actinic damage to the skin.

POINTS TO REMEMBER

- If a lesion persists despite treatment, it should be biopsied.
- Recent evidence suggests a diet low in fat appears to reduce the incidence of solar keratoses.
- Sunscreens should also be applied to the lower lip to prevent actinic cheilitis.

BASICS

- SCC occurs in several forms:
  - **In situ** SCC (Bowen's disease)
  - SCC arising in a **solar keratosis**
  - SCC arising **de novo**
  - SCC occurring on **mucous membranes**
- The risk for **metastasis of SCC depends on its degree of differentiation, depth of penetration, and location.**
  - Lesions on mucous membranes have the highest risk for metastasis.
  - Tumors that are induced by ionizing radiation or those that arise in old burn scars or in inflammatory lesions are also more likely to metastasize.
- SCC is seen much less frequently than basal cell carcinoma (BCC) and occurs in an older age group.
- As with solar keratoses and BCC, SCC is related to sun exposure and develops more frequently in those with a greater degree of outdoor activity.
- Although rare in dark-skinned individuals, SCC may occur because of reasons other than sun exposure. For example, it may arise in an old burn scar, at the site of radiation therapy, or in a lesion of chronic cutaneous lupus erythematosus.

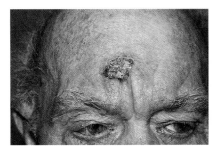

Figure 22.8.
Ulcerated squamous cell carcinoma (SCC). Compare with Figure 22.12.

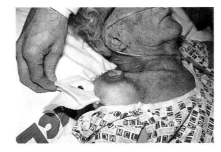

Figure 22.9.
Squamous cell carcinoma. Neglected tumor has ulcerated.

DESCRIPTION OF LESIONS

- Lesions may be papules, plaques, nodules, or tumors that are slow growing.
- Lesions may be scaly or ulcerated with crust (Figure 22.8).
- SCC may be pearly and indistinguishable from BCC.
- Tumors may develop in neglected lesions (Figure 22.9).

DISTRIBUTION OF LESIONS

- As in solar keratoses, lesions occur on sun-exposed areas (e.g., **face, bald scalp** and **top of ears in men, dorsa of forearms and hands, "V" of neck, neck below the hairline**).
- Lesions may occur on **legs in women.**

CLINICAL MANIFESTATIONS

- Slow-growing, firm papules with the ability to produce scale (keratinization) tend to be more differentiated and less likely to metastasize.
- Softer, nonkeratinizing lesions are less well-differentiated and are more likely to spread.

DIAGNOSIS

- An early lesion is difficult to distinguish from a precursor solar keratosis.
- Diagnosis is generally made by **shave or excisional biopsy**.

CLINICAL VARIANTS

- **Bowen's disease** (in situ SCC; Figure 22.10) is a solitary lesion that resembles a scaly psoriatic or eczematous plaque; the lesion often arises in non–sun-exposed sites such as the trunk or extremities. When it occurs on the penis, it is known as **erythroplasia of Queyrat**.
- SCC may **arise in an old scar** (Figure 22.11).

DIFFERENTIAL DIAGNOSIS

- **Solar keratosis**, which is often indistinguishable from SCC
- **BCC** (Figure 22.12)
  - Often indistinguishable from SCC, particularly if the lesion is ulcerated
  - Generally pearly, telangiectatic
  - More common than SCC and is noted in a younger age group
- **Keratoacanthoma**
  - Often indistinguishable from SCC (Figure 22.13)
  - Fast growing
  - Usually has a typical central crater

MANAGEMENT (see Chapter 27, "Highly Specialized Procedures)

- **Electrodesiccation** and **curettage** for small lesions and Bowen's disease
- **Excision**, which is the preferred method of therapy for SCC, permitting histologic diagnosis of the tumor margins
- **Micrographic** (Mohs') **surgery** for recurrent or large lesions and for lesions on the nose, the nasolabial area, around the lips, around the eyes, behind the ears, in the ear canal, and on the scalp
- **Radiation therapy** for elderly patients or for those who are physically unable to undergo excisional surgery

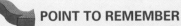

POINT TO REMEMBER

SCC arising on a mucous membrane such as the lip or glans penis, one arising from a chronic ulcer, or one arising in an immunocompromised patient should be regarded as potentially metastatic.

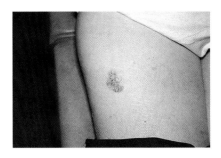

Figure 22.10.
Bowen's disease (in situ squamous cell carcinoma) resembles a scaly psoriatic or eczematous plaque.

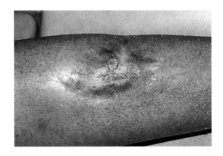

Figure 22.11.
Squamous cell carcinoma arising in a burn scar.

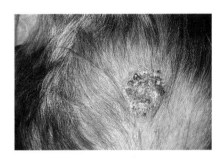

Figure 22.12.
Basal cell carcinoma (BCC). Ulcerated lesion may be indistinguishable from squamous cell carcinoma. Note the pearly border.

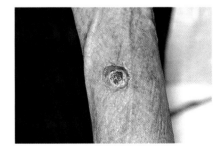

Figure 22.13.
Keratoacanthoma.

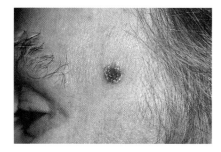

Figure 22.14.
Nodular basal cell carcinoma (BCC). Pearly papule with ulceration (rodent ulcer).

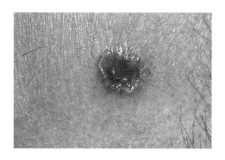

Figure 22.15.
Close-up view of Figure 22.14. Rolled borders with telangiectasias.

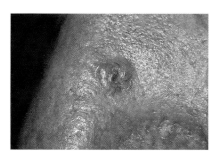

Figure 22.16.
Typical location of basal cell carcinoma (BCC). Note the central crust, telangiectasias, and pearly, rolled border.

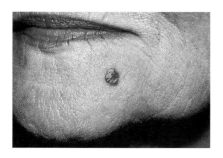

Figure 22.17.
Pigmented basal cell carcinoma (BCC). Note the pearly, waxy surface.

BASICS

- Skin cancer is the most common cancer in the United States, and basal cell carcinoma (BCC) is, by far, the **most common type of skin cancer**.
- A BCC is locally invasive and destructive, but it is **rare for one to metastasize**.
- As with SCCs and solar keratoses, BCCs are **induced by ultraviolet radiation** in susceptible individuals.
- **Risk factors** for BCC include the following:
  - Age older than 40 years
  - Male sex
  - Positive family history of BCC
  - Light complexion with poor tanning ability
- As with SCC and solar keratoses, BCCs are **rare in blacks and Asians**.

DESCRIPTION OF LESIONS

- **Nodular BCC** is the most common type (Figures 22.14 and 22.15).
- The lesion may be a pearly papule or nodule, often with ulcer and scale crust (rodent ulcer).
- There may be rolled borders with telangiectasias (Figure 22.16).
- The lesion may be waxy, semitranslucent, or pink in color, or
- Brownish to blue–black in **pigmented BCC** (Figure 22.17).

DISTRIBUTION OF LESIONS

- Lesions occur on the **head and neck** in 85% of all affected patients.
- Lesions occur on sun-exposed areas (e.g., **face** [cheeks, forehead, lower face, and especially on the nose], **periorbital area**, and **back of neck**).

CLINICAL MANIFESTATIONS

- Lesions are often ignored, asymptomatic, slow growing, and may bleed.
- In time, lesions may ulcerate (e.g., the "sore that will not heal").
- Pigmented BCC occurs more commonly in darkly pigmented individuals.

DIAGNOSIS

- Diagnosis is generally made by **shave or excisional biopsy.**

CLINICAL VARIANTS

- **Superficial BCC** (Figure 22.18) occurs as a scaly erythematous patch with a threadlike border.
  - The lesions tend to be indolent, asymptomatic, and the least aggressive of BCCs.
  - Lesions are often multiple, occurring primarily on the trunk and proximal extremities.
  - When solitary, a lesion of superficial BCC may resemble psoriasis, eczema, seborrheic keratosis, or Bowen's disease (SCC in situ).
  - There is no clear association between superficial BCC and sun exposure.

- **Morpheaform BCC** is the least common and most aggressive form of BCC.
  - Lesions appear as whitish, scarred atrophic plaques with surrounding telangiectasia (Figure 22.19).
  - The margins of these lesions are often difficult to evaluate clinically; similar to icebergs, what is seen on the surface is not always what lies under the surface. Consequently, morpheaform BCCs are generally more difficult to treat than other BCCs.

DIFFERENTIAL DIAGNOSIS

- **SCC**
- **Solar keratosis**
- **Sebaceous hyperplasia** (see Chapter 21, "Benign Skin Neoplasms")
- **Angiofibroma** (fibrous papule of the nose; Figure 22.20), which may be clinically indistinguishable from BCC
- **Nodular melanoma** or **seborrheic keratosis**, which may be difficult to distinguish from pigmented BCC

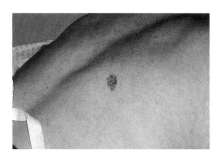

Figure 22.18.
Superficial basal cell carcinoma (BCC) resembles a psoriatic plaque and Bowen's disease.

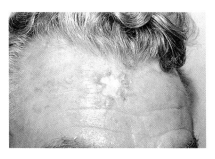

Figure 22.19.
Morpheaform basal cell carcinoma (BCC). Whitish atrophic plaque with surrounding telangiectasias and pearly papules surrounding the telangiectasias.

MANAGEMENT

- **Prevention** (see Appendix 2) is achieved by sun avoidance, use of sunscreens with a sun protection factor (SPF) of at least 15, and wearing protective clothing. Patients should learn skin self-examination and have annual skin examinations by a physician.
- **Treatment** (see Chapter 27, "Highly Specialized Procedures") is achieved by the following:
  - **Electrodesiccation** and **curettage**
  - **Cryosurgery with LN₂**, which is excellent for selected eyelid lesions
  - **Excision**, permitting histologic diagnosis of margins
  - **Micrographic** (Mohs') **surgery** for morpheaform, recurrent, or large lesions and for lesions in danger zones (e.g., the nasolabial area, around the eyes, behind the ears, in the ear canal, on the scalp)
  - **Radiation therapy** for elderly patients or for those who are physically unable to undergo excisional surgery
  - **Topical 5-FU** therapy for multiple superficial BCCs

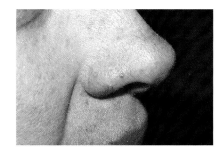

Figure 22.20.
Angiofibroma (fibrous papule of the nose). Note small papules with telangiectasias.

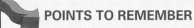

POINTS TO REMEMBER

- Almost 50% of patients with BCC have another BCC within 5 years.
- Patients with BCC have an increased risk for melanoma.
- Patients should always be undressed for adequate examination of the skin.

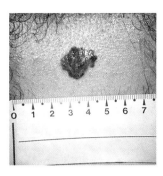

Figure 22.21.
Superficial spreading melanoma (SMM). Note "ABCD" features: **a**symmetry, notched **b**order, varied **c**olors, and almost 2 cm in **d**iameter. Compare with Figure 22.30.

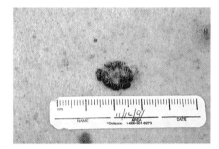

Figure 22.22.
Superficial spreading melanoma (SMM). Note central area (whitish-gray) of regression.

BASICS

- Malignant melanoma (MM) is one of the few skin diseases that **can be fatal** if it is neglected. Consequently, early recognition and prompt removal of a melanoma can save a life.
- MM is a **cancer of pigment-producing cells** (melanocytes).
- The incidence of melanoma has markedly increased over the past several decades, representing 1 to 2% of all cancer-related deaths.
- MM is rare in dark-skinned persons; however, when it does occur, it tends to occur on acral areas (hands and feet).
- Individuals at greatest risk for melanoma have the following **characteristics**:
  - Age older than 15 years
  - Light complexion, with an inability to tan and a history of sunburns
  - Numerous moles, changing moles, or atypical moles (dysplastic nevi)
  - Personal or family history of melanoma
  - Personal or family history of BCC or SCC
- **Warning signs** of MM include the following:
  - New, changing, or unusual moles
  - Symptomatic moles (e.g., pain, itching, burning)
- **Superficial spreading melanoma (SSM)**, the most common type, may arise de novo or in a preexisting nevus.

DESCRIPTION OF LESIONS

(Figures 22.21 and 22.22)
- The SSM lesions may conform to some or all of the **"ABCD"** criteria for melanoma in which the primary lesion is a **macular lesion** or an **elevated plaque** that displays:
  - A = Asymmetry
  - B = **Border** that is irregular or notched
  - C = **Color** is that is varied (brown, black, pink, blue–gray, white, or admixtures of these colors)
  - D = **Diameter** that is greater than 6 mm (diameter of a pencil eraser)

DISTRIBUTION OF LESIONS

- The most common sites are the **upper back, lower legs,** and **trunk.**
- The **arms and legs** are more common sites **in women.**
- The **trunk** is the more common site **in men.**

DIAGNOSIS

- Clinical diagnosis is based on **ABCD criteria**.
- **Elliptical excisional biopsy** should include all of the visible lesion.
- The use of **skin surface microscopy** (epiluminescent microscopy) increases the sensitivity for clinical diagnosis of pigmented lesions, but it is no substitute for biopsy of suspicious lesions.

CLINICAL MANIFESTATIONS

- MM is generally asymptomatic, unless inflammation or invasion occurs.
- SSM often begins with a slow horizontal growth phase, which in months or years, if left untreated, is followed by a vertical growth phase, which indicates invasive disease and potential metastasis.

DIFFERENTIAL DIAGNOSIS

- **Seborrheic keratosis** (See Chapter 21, "Benign Skin Neoplasms")
  - ▪ Frequently mistaken by nondermatologists as being a potential melanoma (particularly, if the lesion is darkly pigmented) (Figures 22.23–22.25).
  - ▪ Biopsy is sometimes required.
- **Pigmented BCC**
  - ▪ Pigmented BCC may be indistinguishable from MM.
  - ▪ Biopsy is necessary.
- **Dysplastic nevi** or clinically **atypical-appearing melanocytic nevi**
  - ▪ This lesion may be indistinguishable from MM.
  - ▪ Biopsy is always necessary; excisional biopsy is recommended when MM is suspected.
- **Angiokeratomas** (particularly thrombosed lesions)
  - ▪ Angiokeratomas may be indistinguishable from MM. Excisional biopsy is necessary.

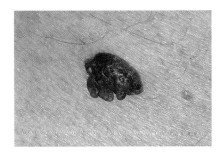

Figure 22.23.
Seborrheic keratosis. Note pseudo-horncysts.

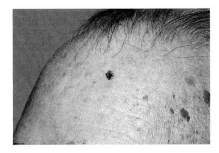

Figure 22.24.
In situ malignant melanoma. Note lesion showing jet-black coloration. Compare to surrounding brown-colored seborrheic keratoses.

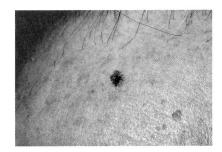

Figure 22.25.
Close-up of Figure 22.24.

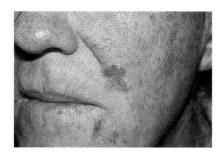

Figure 22.26.
Lentigo maligna. Malignant melanoma (MM) in situ.

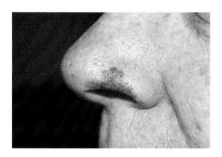

Figure 22.27.
Lentigo maligna melanoma.

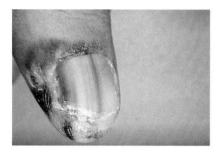

Figure 22.28.
Acral lentiginous melanoma. Hutchinson's sign, showing pigmentation spreading beyond the nail into surrounding skin.

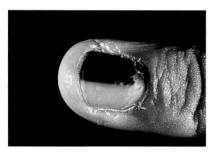

Figure 22.29.
Junctional nevus. Note even pigmentation.

CLINICAL VARIANTS

- **Lentigo maligna** (Figure 22.26) is a type of lentigo that is considered a MM in situ.
  — It occurs most often on the face in elderly, fair-complexioned individuals.
  — It has irregular color and border.
  — When a lentigo maligna becomes papular and invades the dermis, it is then referred to as a **lentigo maligna melanoma** (Figure 22.27).
- **Acral lentiginous melanoma** (Figure 22.28) occurs in blacks and Asians on non–hair-bearing areas such as the palms, soles, and periungual areas. Early metastases is a feature of this melanoma, which may be confused with a **subungual hematoma** or **junctional nevus** (Figure 22.29).
  — A nodular melanoma may be indistinguishable from a pigmented BCC or a pyogenic granuloma.

- **Nodular melanoma** arises de novo as a nodule or plaque (Figure 22.30).
- **Metastatic melanoma** (Figures 22.31 and 22.32) is blue or blue–black, or nonpigmented **(amelanotic melanoma)**. Color is more uniform than that seen in SSMs.
  — Early invasion results from a rapid vertical growth phase, and it may occur anywhere on the body.

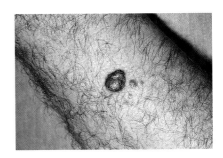

Figure 22.30.
Nodular malignant melanoma. Nodule with surrounding satellite lesions representing local metastasis.

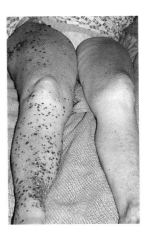

Figure 22.31.
Metastatic malignant melanoma (MM). Lymphedema and multiple metastatic nodules on the leg.

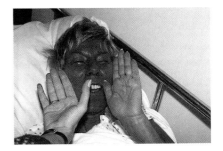

Figure 22.32.
Metastatic malignant melanoma (MM). Unusual brown–blue coloration presumably from widespread melanin pigmentation in the tissues.

Prognosis

- Five-year survival is based on tumor thickness, known as **Breslow's measurement** (Table 22.1).
- Other important prognostic factors include whether there is ulceration and whether there is regional or distant spread. Grading tumor location in the dermis using **Clark's levels** (Table 22.2) is also helpful.

Table 22.1 Breslow's Measurement

TUMOR THICKNESS (MM)	5-YEAR SURVIVAL (%)
0.75	98–99
0.76–1.50	94
1.51–2.25	83
2.26–3.00	72–77
3.00	50

Table 22.2 Clark's Levels

LEVEL	LOCATION IN DERMIS
I	In situ, disease confined to the epidermis
II	Melanoma cells in papillary dermis
III	Melanoma cells filling papillary dermis
IV	Melanoma cells in reticular dermis
V	Melanoma cells in subcutaneous fat

MANAGEMENT

- Patients with MM of less than 0.75 mm in thickness should be followed up every 6 months for 2 years, then annually. At each visit, the patient's total skin should be examined.
  - Patients with MM greater than 0.75 mm are followed up more frequently. Lymph nodes as well as skin should also be examined.
- Patients with invasive disease require an annual chest radiograph examination, complete blood count, and liver function studies.
- **Treatment options** include the following:
  - **Elliptical excision** should include all of the visible lesion down to the subcutaneous fat. For lesions smaller than 1 mm thick, a 1-cm margin of normal skin is usually adequate. Greater than 1-cm margins are needed for thicker lesions (margin size is based on histologic type and the anatomic location of the lesion).
  - Elective lymph node dissection is not recommended for lesions smaller than 1 mm thick, unless lymph nodes are palpable. The decision whether to perform elective lymph node dissection on thicker lesions (1 to 4 mm) is controversial.
  - The technique of **sentinel node dissection** (the lymph node closest to the site of the primary melanoma) allows for a less invasive procedure than a regional lymphadenectomy. This procedure uses radioisotopic imaging (lymphoscintigraphy) to determine if the sentinel node is free of melanoma; if so, a surgeon may conclude that the more distal lymph nodes are melanoma free as well.
  - **Amputation, regional lymph node dissection, or regional chemotherapy perfusion** is often necessary for acral lentiginous melanomas.
  - For more advanced stages of MM, chemotherapy and radiation therapy have not been very effective for achieving metastatic disease remission.
  - **Vaccines, arterial limb perfusion,** and **immunotherapy** are more promising adjuvants to surgery; in fact, an injectable recombinant interferon α-2b has been shown to yield a significant improvement in the 5-year survival rate in patients with thick lesions and/or lymph node involvement.

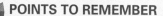

POINTS TO REMEMBER

- Anyone with a history of melanoma needs lifelong skin surveillance because a second MM will develop in 3% of these patients within 3 years.
- Patients may develop recurrences after 10 years or more of being disease free. Sun protection should be stressed. Although there is some controversy regarding the long-term application of sunscreens and melanoma prevention, The American Academy of Dermatology has reaffirmed its position that sunscreen is beneficial when used regularly as part of an overall sun-protection program.
- Patients should be taught skin self-examination.
- All family members should be examined.
- Any lesion that looks suspicious must be biopsied.
- Removal of thin lesions (less than 0.76 mm) results in cure in almost all patients.
- Beginning at an early age, children should be protected from excessive sun exposure.
- Trauma from rubbing or irritation does not cause malignant degeneration of moles.
- An **amelanotic melanoma** is easily overlooked because of its lack of pigmentation.

CHAPTER 23

CUTANEOUS MANIFESTATIONS OF PREGNANCY

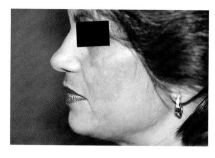

Figure 23.1.
Melasma, the "mask of pregnancy."

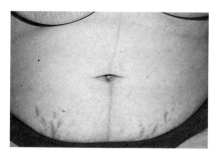

Figure 23.2.
Striae gravidarum and linea nigra.

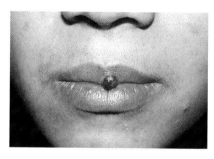

Figure 23.3.
Pyogenic granuloma.

BASICS

During pregnancy, there are many physiologic changes that become evident in the skin.

Hyperpigmentation

Hyperpigmentation is secondary to increased levels of melanocyte-stimulating hormone (MSH) and estrogens, resulting frequently in:
- The linea nigra and the darkening of the areolae.
- Melasma (mask of pregnancy; Figure 23.1; see also Chapter 14, "Pigmentary Disorders") occurs in more than 50% of pregnant women; it is worsened by exposure to the sun.
- Darkening of freckles and nevi that usually regresses following the termination of pregnancy

Connective tissue changes
- Striae gravidarum (striae distensae; Figure 23.2)
- Growth of keloids
- Skin tags, which may develop or increase in number

Vascular phenomena
- Spider telangiectasias
- Palmar erythema, flushing

Pyogenic granulomas

(Figure 23.3)

Pyogenic granulomas often occur on the lips and gums and usually regress shortly postpartum.

Acne

Acne may improve or worsen during pregnancy.

Telogen effluvium

Hair loss may occur from 1 to 5 months postpartum and is generally followed by total regrowth.

Other findings

Other possible findings include increased nail fragility, leg edema, increased eccrine sweating, hirsutism, and marked enlargement of condyloma acuminata.

DERMATOSES OF PREGNANCY

There is a group of cutaneous eruptions that are unique to pregnancy. Historically, there has been a vast array of classification of these eruptions, resulting in overlapping and confusing terminology. Few laboratories will clinch the diagnosis of these dermatoses. The following short list is an effort to help simplify the approach to these entities.

Pruritic urticarial papules and plaques of pregnancy (PUPPP)

This is a fairly common dermatosis of late pregnancy.

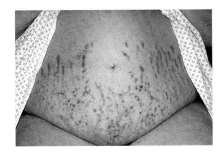

Figure 23.4.
Pruritic urticarial papules and plaques of pregnancy (PUPPP). Lesions are located in the stretch marks. Note periumbilical sparing.

- As the name suggests, PUPPP is an eruption consisting of urticarial papules that coalesce into plaques. Papules are initially found in the striae distensae, or stretch marks of the abdomen. They are often characteristically centered around the umbilicus (Figure 23.4), but later can be found on the thighs and buttocks, coalescing to form plaques.
- The itching, which can become intense, generally begins in the last few weeks of the third trimester of pregnancy. Itching can be so extraordinary as to require potent topical, and sometimes oral, corticosteroids for relief.
- Fortunately, the natural history of PUPPP is generally spontaneous resolution, in most cases, within a few days of delivery. There appears to be no increased incidence of infant morbidity.

Pruritus gravidarum

Pruitus gravidarum is a benign generalized itching that begins in the later stages of pregnancy. There are no primary skin lesions, and the condition clears after delivery. (This may be a variation of PUPPP, without lesions.)

Recurrent cholestasis of pregnancy (prurigo gravidarum)

This is characterized by generalized itching and jaundice, which is secondary to bile salt accumulation in the skin. It occurs in the second or third trimester of pregnancy, clears after delivery, but may recur in future pregnancies. There are no primary lesions; however, excoriations may result from the intense pruritus.

Poorly defined papular and vesicular eruptions, as well as pruritus without lesions

These conditions, which may occur at any time during pregnancy, have been described with no clear diagnostic consensus.

Herpes gestationis

Herpes gestationis is a rare vesicobullous autoimmune dermatitis, which may be confused with PUPPP.

Impetigo herpetiformis

This is an extremely rare dermatosis, which resembles a form of pustular psoriasis.

MANAGEMENT

Management of these various conditions should be aimed at symptomatic control of pruritus with the use of bland emollients and topical antipruritic agents. Oral antihistamines are sometimes effective.

POINT TO REMEMBER

Many common skin diseases unrelated to pregnancy should always be kept in mind when evaluating a pregnant patient with a skin disorder.

CHAPTER 24

CUTANEOUS MANIFESTATIONS OF HIV INFECTION

Mary Ruth Buchness

Overview

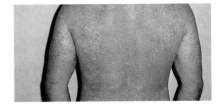

Figure 24.1.
Acute HIV infection characterized by a measleslike rash.

- The first organ that may be affected in HIV infection is the skin. HIV infection is often suspected initially when a patient has a skin disease known to be associated with HIV or when the patient has a common skin disease that presents more severely than expected or is recalcitrant to treatment. **Acute HIV infection** is characterized by a papular or measleslike rash (Figure 24.1), fever, lymphadenopathy, sore throat, and malaise. As the number of CD4 cells decreases during the course of infection, other rashes appear.

- Recent therapeutic advances in antiretroviral therapy have resulted in a dramatic decrease in many of the opportunistic infections described in this chapter. This includes molluscum contagiosum, genital warts, oral hairy leukoplakia, mucosal candidiasis, and Kaposi's sarcoma. Psoriasis and herpes zoster also appear to clear more quickly when patients are taking antiviral protease inhibitors.

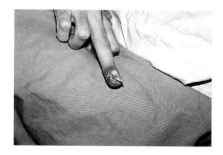

Figure 24.2.
HIV-associated chronic, ulcerated herpes simplex resistant to acyclovir. Patient is receiving intravenous foscarnet.

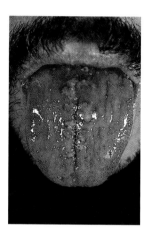

Figure 24.3.
Herpes simplex. Mucosal papules.

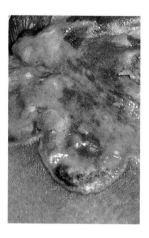

Figure 24.4.
Herpes simplex. Centrifugally expanding ulceration with scalloped borders (slide courtesy of Janet Moy, MD).

BASICS

- Herpes simplex is caused by herpes simplex virus **HSV-1** and **HSV-2**.
- HSV-1 most commonly affects the skin and mucous membranes above the waist, and HSV-2 most commonly affects the skin below the waist.
- **Immunocompetent hosts**
  - In immunocompetent hosts, primary HSV infection causes a severe outbreak of vesicles on the oral and genital mucous membranes. The lesions evolve into pustules and superficial erosions that last an average of 10 to 14 days.
  - Because the virus becomes latent in the dorsal root ganglia, reactivation of the virus leads to localized recurrences, which affect cutaneous but not mucosal surfaces. Recurrences last an average of 3 to 5 days.
- **Immunocompromised hosts**
  - The clinical manifestations and course of herpes simplex differ in patients with defective cell-mediated immunity, as seen in HIV infection.
  - Recurrent lesions may affect mucous membranes, possibly developing into chronic, centrifugally expanding ulcerations. These ulcerations last 1 month or more in an HIV-positive patient and are an AIDS-defining diagnosis.
  - Lesions may become resistant to acyclovir, or they may develop into chronic keratotic papules. Because acyclovir resistance is associated with previous treatment of suboptimal doses, it is important not to undertreat HIV-positive patients with HSV.

DESCRIPTION OF LESIONS

- Grouped vesicles on an erythematous base (see Chapter 7, "Superficial Viral Infections")
- Vesicular lesions, which evolve into pustules, erosions, and crusts
- Chronic digital ulceration (Figure 24.2)
- Mucosal erosions or papules (Figure 24.3)
- Centrifugally expanding ulcerations with scalloped borders (Figure 24.4)
- Keratotic (or wartlike papules) or plaques (Figure 24.5)

DISTRIBUTION OF LESIONS

- May be similar to those in immunocompetent hosts (see Chapter 7, "Superficial Viral Infections" and Chapter 19, "Sexually Transmitted Diseases")
- Intraoral areas: tongue, buccal mucosa, palate, and gingivae
- Chronic ulcerative lesions in perianal areas, especially in male homosexuals, possibly extending into intergluteal cleft (see Figure 19.11)
- Keratotic lesions in any location

CLINICAL MANIFESTATIONS

- The symptom of pain should alert the clinician to the possibility of HSV infection in a clinically atypical lesion.
- Lesions may be more severe and more extensive than in immunocompetent hosts.
- Erosions may progress to deep ulcerations.

DIAGNOSIS

- Clinically, diagnosis is made by appearance and the presence of prominent pain or itch.
- Tzanck smear shows multinucleate giant cells (see Chapter 26, "Basic Procedures").
- Viral culture takes 1 week.
- Tissue culture using monoclonal antibodies or polymerase chain reaction is sensitive but expensive.
- Antiviral susceptibility testing is not readily available.
- Serologic testing for HSV is not helpful.

DIFFERENTIAL DIAGNOSIS

Herpes zoster
- Lesions of herpes zoster may involve only part of a dermatome and may be clinically indistinguishable from HSV lesions.
- Culture can distinguish between herpes zoster and HSV lesions.
- When in doubt, sufficient doses of antiviral medications are recommended for herpes zoster infection. Avoid underdosing.

Chronic perianal ulcerative type of HSV
- **Decubitus ulcer** affects bony prominences in debilitated patients and does not extend to the intergluteal cleft.
- In **cutaneous cytomegalovirus** (CMV) infection, perianal ulcers develop as an extension of gastrointestinal involvement. Skin biopsy shows characteristic viral inclusion bodies.

Oral mucosal type of HSV
Aphthous stomatitis is distinguishable from HSV by a negative Tzanck smear and no growth on viral culture.

Disseminated *Mycobacterium avium-intracellulare complex*
- Patients may present with oral and cutaneous ulcerations.
- This infection is associated with severe systemic disease and fever in HIV-infected patients.

Disseminated histoplasmosis
- Patients may present with oral and cutaneous ulcerations.
- Disseminated histoplasmosis is associated with systemic disease.
- Chest radiograph is abnormal.

Keratotic type of CMV
- Disseminated CMV (Figure 24.6) is associated with retinal CMV, so an ophthalmologic examination is essential.
- Skin biopsy shows characteristic viral inclusions.

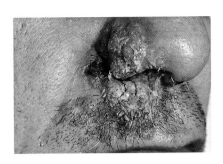

Figure 24.5.
Herpes simplex. Crusted wartlike papules.

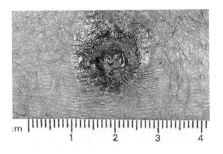

Figure 24.6.
Disseminated lesion of cytomegalovirus.

MANAGEMENT

Topical therapy
- Topical antivirals are ineffective.
- Symptomatic relief is achieved with **cold compresses, viscous lidocaine, EMLA** (an eutectic mixture of lidocaine and prilocaine), **and oral analgesics.**
- Superinfection is prevented with **topical antibacterial ointments**.

Systemic therapy
- **Acyclovir**, 400 mg, is given by mouth 5 times per day.
- **Famciclovir**, 250 mg, is given by mouth 3 times per day.
- Valacyclovir is not recommended in patients with HIV to avoid associated thrombotic thrombocytopenic purpura.
- Lesions are treated until they are completely resolved to prevent early recurrence and the need for retreatment.
- If the patient has malabsorption or if lesions do not respond, acyclovir, 5 to 10 mg/kg every 8 hours, is infused over 1 hour. The dosage interval should be increased in patients with renal failure.

Acyclovir resistance
- Failure to respond to intravenous acyclovir indicates acyclovir resistance.
- Foscarnet, 40 mg/kg intravenously every 8 hours, is used in acyclovir-resistant patients.
- Strains that recur after treatment with foscarnet are usually acyclovir sensitive.

 POINTS TO REMEMBER

- Chronic suppressive therapy with acyclovir has been associated with acyclovir resistance.
- Treatment should continue until clinical lesions resolve completely.
- Clinicians should be careful not to underdose with antiviral agents.

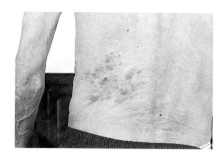

Figure 24.7.
Herpes zoster affecting a dermatome.

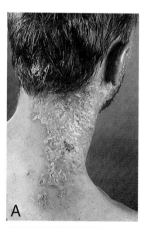

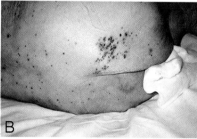

Figure 24.8.
(*A*) Herpes zoster with severe scarring.
(*B*) Disseminated herpes zoster. Note initial dermatomal involvement on buttock (slide courtesy of Herbert A. Hochman, MD).

BASICS

- Herpes zoster is caused by a reactivation of the **varicella-zoster virus** (VZV), usually in a single, dorsal root ganglion in the spinal cord.
- It is a sign of decreasing immunity to VZV, which most people acquire in childhood as chickenpox.
- Herpes zoster is most common in the elderly and immunocompromised persons.

DESCRIPTION OF LESIONS

- Grouped vesicles or bullae on an erythematous base affect all or part of a dermatome (Figure 24.7).
- Lesions evolve into pustules and crusts and may erode.
- Chronic ulcerations and crusted or verrucous lesions may occur.
- Severe scarring may result (Figure 24.8; see Figure 24.8*A*).

DISTRIBUTION OF LESIONS

- Any dermatome can be affected.
- Occasional dissemination may lead to 25 or more lesions outside the primary lesion and two contiguous dermatomes (disseminated herpes zoster; see Figure 24.8*B*), in which case the eruption may be indistinguishable from varicella.

CLINICAL MANIFESTATIONS

- Prodromal symptoms of pain and itching may be severe enough to lead to suspicion of a serious illness. For example, the prodromal pain of thoracic zoster has led to critical care unit admission to rule out myocardial infarction.
- Regional adenopathy may occur.
- Varicella pneumonia may develop.
- Cutaneous lesions may become chronic in HIV patients.

DIAGNOSIS

- Clinically, diagnosis is made based on characteristic appearance and distribution of lesions.
- Tzanck preparation shows characteristic multinucleated giant cells.
- Viral culture takes 2 weeks.
- Serologic testing is not helpful.

DIFFERENTIAL DIAGNOSIS

HSV

- Infection occasionally occurs dermatomally.
- History of recurrences at the same site indicates HSV infection.
- Culture distinguishes between HSV and herpes zoster virus, but treatment should be initiated immediately.
- When in doubt, doses of antiviral agents appropriate for VZV should be given.

MANAGEMENT

Topical therapy
- Topical antivirals are ineffective.
- Symptomatic relief is achieved with **cold compresses, calamine lotion, pramoxine,** or **oral analgesics.**
- **Narcotics** may be needed for severe pain.

Systemic therapy
- **Acyclovir,** 800 mg, is given 5 times per day for 10 to 14 days.
- **Famciclovir,** 500 mg, is given 3 times per day for 10 to 14 days.
- **Intravenous acyclovir,** 10 mg/kg every 8 hours, is given for 10 to 14 days.
- Dosage is reduced in patients with renal failure.
- If lesions improve but persist beyond 10 to 14 days, treatment is continued until all lesions resolve.
- If lesions fail to resolve, the virus may be acyclovir-resistant.
- Acyclovir-resistant VZV responds to **foscarnet,** 40 mg/kg every 8 hours, which is used until lesions resolve.

 POINTS TO REMEMBER

- Undertreatment may lead to viral resistance.
- Valacyclovir is not recommended in patients with HIV.
- Patients with herpes zoster can transmit the virus as chickenpox to nonimmune persons.

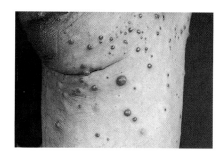

Figure 24.9.
Bacillary angiomatosis (BA). Dome-shaped papules and nodules.

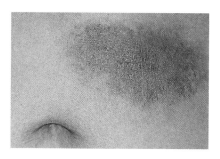

Figure 24.10.
Bacillary angiomatosis (BA). Flatter, violaceous lesions.

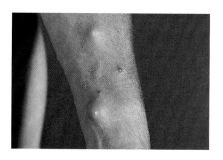

Figure 24.11.
Bacillary angiomatosis (BA). Subcutaneous nodules.

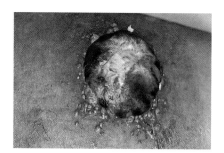

Figure 24.12.
Bacillary angiomatosis (BA). Necrotic tumors.

BASICS

- Bacillary angiomatosis (BA), which was first reported in 1983, is seen almost exclusively in HIV-positive patients.
- BA is caused by the bacilli *Bartonella henselae* and *Bartonella quintana*.
  - *B. henselae* is one of the causative agents of cat-scratch disease, and the only known predisposing factor in patients with BA is a cat scratch or bite.
  - *B. quintana* is the cause of trench fever, transmitted to humans by the body louse. Up until now, *B. quintana* was not known to cause skin lesions.
- BA is a systemic infection, and lesions have been described in nearly every organ of the body.
- **Untreated BA can be fatal.**

DESCRIPTION OF LESIONS

- Erythematous dome-shaped papules and nodules (Figure 24.9)
- Occasional flatter, violaceous lesions (Figure 24.10)
- Subcutaneous nodules (Figure 24.11)
- Rare necrotic tumors (Figure 24.12)

DISTRIBUTION OF LESIONS

BA can occur on any location of the skin or internally.

CLINICAL MANIFESTATIONS

- There may be associated fever.
- Untreated lesions can lead to respiratory obstruction, gastrointestinal bleeding, and local or systemic infection.
- Deaths have been reported from laryngeal obstruction and disseminated intravascular coagulopathy.

DIAGNOSIS

- Skin biopsy
- Culture, which is available only in research centers

DIFFERENTIAL DIAGNOSIS

Pyogenic granuloma
(Figure 24.13)
- May be clinically identical to lesions of BA
- Usually solitary
- May affect immunocompetent hosts and HIV patients
- Occurs at sites of trauma

Epidemic Kaposi's sarcoma (HIV-associated)
(Figure 24.14)
- Lesions are usually less elevated and more violaceous.
- Lesions are more often acrally distributed.
- Male homosexuals with HIV are most frequently affected.

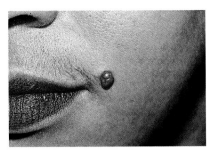

Figure 24.13.
Pyogenic granuloma.

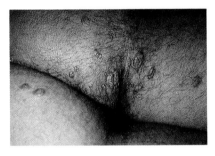

Figure 24.14.
Epidemic Kaposi's sarcoma (KS).

MANAGEMENT

- **Doxycycline**, 100 mg twice per day
- **Erythromycin**, 250 to 500 mg 4 times per day
- Treatment until lesions have resolved (usually 3 to 4 weeks)

POINTS TO REMEMBER

- Diagnosis requires biopsy.
- Treatment should continue until lesions have completely resolved.

BASICS

- *S. aureus* is the most common bacterial pathogen to affect the skin in immunocompetent and immunocompromised individuals.
- The presence of pruritic dermatoses predisposes patients to cutaneous colonization by *S. aureus*. Colonization of the skin has been shown to exacerbate itching, leading to a vicious cycle of chronic itching and scratching.
- The most common sites colonized are the nasal mucosa, weeping skin lesions, and insertion sites of intravenous catheters.

DESCRIPTION OF LESIONS

- Pustules
- Abscesses
- Excoriations
- Cellulitis
- Erythroderma (staphylococcal scalded-skin syndrome [SSSS])

DISTRIBUTION OF LESIONS

- Any body site
- Follicular sites
- At sites of minor trauma (e.g., from scratching or from fissures in toe webs secondary to tinea pedis)
- Scalp or nasal mucosa

CLINICAL MANIFESTATIONS

- Pain and/or itching at sites of lesions
- Regional adenopathy
- Fever and leukocytosis in severe cases
- **SSSS**
  - Generalized erythema and scale secondary to staphylococcal exotoxins
  - Syndrome analogous to a second-degree burn affecting 100% of the body
  - Temperature dysregulation
  - Fluid and electrolyte imbalances
  - Shock

DIAGNOSIS

- **Gram's stain** of pus
- **Culture** and sensitivity of lesions, nasal mucosa, intravenous insertion sites
- **Blood culture** in systemically ill patients

MANAGEMENT

- Incise and **drain abscesses**.
- **Mupirocin Ointment** can be applied twice per day to nasal mucosa for 5 days for staphlococcal colonization (repeated or chronic treatment for patients with HIV).
- Mupirocin Ointment can be applied twice per day for 10 to 14 days for minor skin infections.
- **Systemic antibiotics** may be taken according to bacterial sensitivity and history of patient allergy.
- In non–penicillin-allergic patients, **dicloxacillin**, 250 to 500 mg, may be taken orally four times per day for 14 days; **Rifampin**, 300 mg twice per day for 14 days, is synergistic and may help to eliminate the carrier state.
- **Intravenous antibiotics** may be taken for more serious infections.
- Implement more intensive treatment in patients with SSSS to prevent fluid and electrolyte imbalance and shock.

 POINTS TO REMEMBER

- *S. aureus* may be a cause of chronic itching in HIV patients.
- Incision and drainage of abscesses are necessary.
- HIV patients are susceptible to SSSS.
- Frequently hospitalized patients may have methicillin-resistant *S. aureus* infection and may require treatment with intravenous vancomycin.

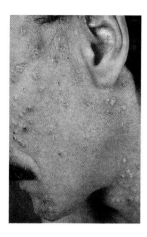

Figure 24.15.
Molluscum contagiosum
(MC).

(See Chapter 7, "Superficial Viral Infections.")

BASICS

- Molluscum contagiosum (MC) is caused by a pox virus and is most commonly seen in immunocompetent children and less commonly in healthy adults.
- In children, lesions develop on areas of the skin in contact with other infected children during play.
- In adults, lesions develop most often on the genitals and thighs because the virus is transmitted during sexual activity.
- A typical lesion is a skin-colored, yellowish or reddish dome-shaped papule measuring 2 to 4 mm in size, with a central umbilication.
- Lesions are superficial and are easily treated by topical salicylic acid preparations, curettage with a sharp instrument, electrodesiccation, or LN_2 cryosurgery.
- Multiple and extensive facial lesions and lesions with atypical morphology should alert the practitioner to the possibility of HIV infection.

DESCRIPTION OF LESIONS IN HIV PATIENTS

- Papules may be dome-shaped or, more commonly, are atypical in appearance.
- Size may be up to, or greater than, 1 cm (**giant MC**).
- Lesions may lack central umbilication or may have several umbilications.
- Lesions on hairy areas tend to penetrate into hair follicles.

DISTRIBUTION OF LESIONS

- All areas of the body, most commonly **face and genitals**
- In men, possible extensive involvement of the beard area from shaving (Figure 24.15)

CLINICAL MANIFESTATIONS

There is occasional tenderness or inflammation.

DIAGNOSIS

- **Clinical appearance**
- **Crush preparation**, which is performed by removing a lesion, crushing it between two glass slides, and staining it with any dye to show characteristic viral inclusions called molluscum bodies (see Figure 7.17)
- **Skin biopsy**
- **Culture** is unavailable for the pox virus.

DIFFERENTIAL DIAGNOSIS

Disseminated cryptococcosis
- Cutaneous lesions may be clinically identical to MC (Figure 24.16).
- Affected patients are usually systemically ill, although cutaneous involvement may be the first sign of illness.
- Crush preparation with India ink shows encapsulated yeast.
- When in doubt, lesions can be identified by biopsy.
- Patients with cutaneous dissemination have neurologic involvement, and a more rapid diagnosis can be made by a CSF examination.

Disseminated histoplasmosis
- Less common cause of MC-like lesions than cryptococcosis
- Always indicative of systemic infection

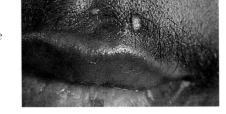

Figure 24.16.
Disseminated cryptococcosis.

MANAGEMENT

- Treatment is individualized for each patient.
- Topical tretinoin is a useful adjunctive treatment in cases of beard MC.
- **Surgical treatment** is with curettage or LN$_2$ cryosurgery.
- **Trichloroacetic acid** 25 to 75% may be applied to individual lesions.
- **Podofilox** 5% may be applied to lesions twice per day, 3 days per week.
- Treatment is chronic and unlikely to eradicate all lesions unless the patient's immunity improves.

POINTS TO REMEMBER
- Cutaneous lesions of disseminated cryptococcosis and histoplasmosis may be identical in appearance to MC.
- Primary skin infections with *Cryptococcus neoformans*, *Coccidioides immitis*, *Histoplasma capsulatum*, and *Toxoplasma gondii* are exceedingly rare. The presence of these organisms in the skin indicates a systemic infection caused by these organisms.

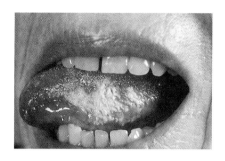

Figure 24.17.
Oral hairy leukoplakia (OHL).

(See Chapter 12, "Disorders of the Mouth, Lips, and Tongue.")

BASICS

Oral hairy leukoplakia (OHL) is a marker of HIV infection, which is thought to be caused by Epstein-Barr virus infection of the oral mucosa.

DESCRIPTION OF LESIONS

- White plaques with the appearance of "corrugated cardboard" (Figure 24.17)
- Fixed, not friable, lesions

DISTRIBUTION OF LESIONS

Lesions most often appear on the lateral aspects of the **tongue**.

CLINICAL MANIFESTATIONS

- Usually asymptomatic
- Occasionally burning

DIAGNOSIS

Diagnosis is made on **clinical grounds**.

DIFFERENTIAL DIAGNOSIS

Oral candidiasis
(Figure 24.18)
- Lesions are more common on the dorsal aspect of the tongue and buccal mucosa.
- White plaques scrape off easily with a tongue blade.
- KOH preparation shows yeast.

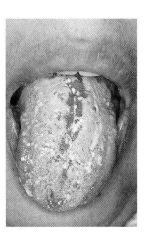

Figure 24.18.
Oral candidiasis.

MANAGEMENT

- Treatment is necessary **only in symptomatic cases**.
- **Surgical excision** can be performed, but lesions recur at the margins.
- **Acyclovir**, 3.2 g/day, is given with recurrence of lesions upon cessation of treatment.
- **Topical tretinoin**, 0.05% solution for 15 minutes daily, is applied with a gauze sponge.
- **Podophyllin** 25% solution is applied sparingly to one side of the tongue at a time and allowed to air dry. This is repeated once weekly.

POINT TO REMEMBER

OHL is a marker of HIV infection, and affected patients should be tested accordingly.

BASICS

- Drug eruptions are common in the HIV-infected population because of the large number of medications that are taken by these patients. The most commonly implicated medications are **sulfamethoxazole-trimethoprim**, to which at least 60% of AIDS patients develop an allergy, followed by the aminopenicillins.

- When the drug allergy is a typical morbilliform eruption, it is possible to continue the offending medication and treat the patient's symptoms with antihistamines and topical steroids. More serious drug eruptions require prompt discontinuation of the offending medication. These are characterized by urticaria, mucosal involvement, target lesions, erythroderma, and tenderness of the skin.
- Mucosal involvement and target lesions are indicative of erythema multiforme/Stevens-Johnson syndrome, whereas erythroderma and skin tenderness are seen in toxic epidermal necrolysis. The non–nucleoside reverse transcriptase inhibitor, nevirapine, has been associated with severe cases of Stevens-Johnson syndrome (Figure 24.19). For a complete discussion of drug eruptions, see Chapter 17 "Drug Eruptions."

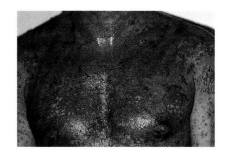

Figure 24.19.
Drug eruption. Toxic epidermal necrolysis resulting from treatment with nevirapine.

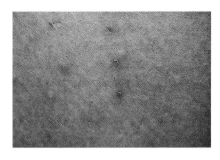

Figure 24.20.
HIV-associated eosinophilic folliculitis (EF). Lesions resemble insect bites.

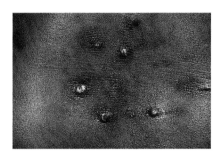

Figure 24.21.
HIV-associated eosinophilic folliculitis (EF). Note lichenification.

BASICS

- HIV-associated eosinophilic folliculitis (EF), also known as **eosinophilic pustular folliculitis**, is an extremely pruritic rash that is seen in the later stages of HIV infection.
- EF appears to be a hypersensitivity reaction because of the large numbers of eosinophils that are seen in the skin, but no consistent association with specific allergens has been seen.
- Very few patients with EF respond to antihistamines.
- HIV-infected patients have high circulating levels of interleukin 4 and 5, the cytokines that are chemotactic for eosinophils, so a seemingly allergic manifestation such as EF may be a result of the general immunologic derangement in these patients.

DESCRIPTION OF LESIONS

- Primary lesions are urticarial papules measuring 3 to 5 mm, which look like insect bites (Figure 24.20).
- Pustules may be present, but they are not the predominant lesions.
- In many cases, only excoriations are present because of the intense pruritus.
- Patients with long-standing EF may have lichenification (Figure 24.21).

DISTRIBUTION OF LESIONS

Lesions may occur anywhere, but they are prominent on the "seborrheic areas" of the skin (e.g., scalp, face, chest, upper back).

CLINICAL MANIFESTATIONS

- Severe pruritus may interfere with the patient's ability to function.
- Pain may occur in secondarily infected lesions.

DIAGNOSIS

- **Skin biopsy** showing perifollicular and follicular infiltration by eosinophils
- Occasional **peripheral eosinophilia**

DIFFERENTIAL DIAGNOSIS

Bacterial folliculitis
- Bacterial folliculitis may be clinically indistinguishable from EF.
- Gram's stain and bacterial culture should be performed.

Pityrosporum folliculitis
- Pityrosporum folliculitis may be clinically indistinguishable from EF.
- KOH preparation of pus shows yeast and hyphae.
- Periodic acid-Schiff (PAS) stain of skin biopsy specimen shows yeast and hyphae.

Arthropod bite reaction
- Arthropod bite reaction may be clinically and histologically indistinguishable from EF.
- Lesions are less likely to be folliculocentric.
- History should include possible exposure to arthropods (e.g., fleas, lice, scabies, bed bugs, mosquitoes).

MANAGEMENT

- Topical steroids, antihistamines, and antibiotics are usually ineffective.
- **Ultraviolet B phototherapy** is effective. Patients should be referred to a qualified phototherapy center. Sunlight is effective in the summer months.
- **Isotretinoin**, 40 mg/day, is effective in some patients. Treatment must be continued for at least 3 months. Cholesterol and triglyceride levels require monitoring on a monthly basis.
- **Itraconazole**, 200 mg twice per day, may be effective.

POINT TO REMEMBER

EF, as it is described herein, is almost always associated with HIV infection.

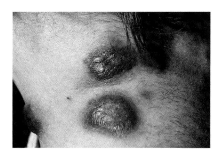

Figure 24.22.
Epidemic Kaposi's sarcoma (KS). Violaceous nodules.

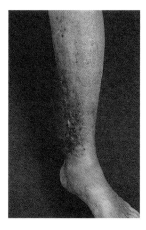

Figure 24.23.
Epidemic Kaposi's sarcoma (KS). Multiple papules and nodules.

BASICS

- Epidemic Kaposi's sarcoma (KS) is an **AIDS-defining diagnosis**.
- Because it is found almost exclusively in men who have had homosexual contact, it is thought to be sexually transmitted.
- KS is exceedingly **rare in women**, and women with KS are presumed to have had sexual contact with bisexual men.
- KS is associated with infection of **human herpes virus 8** (HHV-8), which has been detected in saliva and in semen of affected patients.
- Lesions may resolve spontaneously as immunity improves. A similar phenomenon has been observed in immunocompromised renal transplant recipients.

DESCRIPTION OF LESIONS

- Violaceous macules, papules, or nodules (Figure 24.22)
- Limb edema with subtle violaceous discoloration of the skin (Figure 24.23)

DISTRIBUTION OF LESIONS

- Acrally, on **nose, penis,** and **extremities**
- **Mucous membranes**

CLINICAL MANIFESTATIONS

- Lesions are most commonly asymptomatic.
- Edema usually occurs in extremities but sometimes in the face.
- Oral lesions can cause pain, difficulty with eating, and loss of teeth.

DIFFERENTIAL DIAGNOSIS

Bacillary angiomatosis
- More erythematous, than violaceous
- Often dome-shaped

Disseminated *M. avium-intracellulare* complex

- Violaceous nodules may resemble KS (Figure 24.24).
- Diagnosis is made by a skin biopsy showing granulomatous inflammation and acid-fast bacilli.
- Culture of tissue is positive for *M. avium-intracellulare*.

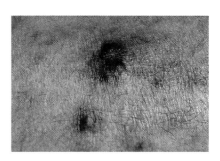

Figure 24.24.
Disseminated *Mycobacterium avium-intracellulare* complex. Nodules resemble Kaposi's sarcoma (KS).

MANAGEMENT

Disseminated cutaneous KS
Requires **systemic chemotherapy**.

Lymphangitic KS
- Requires **chemotherapy**
- **Intermittent sequential compression boots** to decrease edema

Localized cutaneous or mucosal KS
- **Radiation therapy** is used particularly for facial lesions.
- **Intralesional vinblastine** is given at doses of 0.1 to 0.6 mg/cc.
- **LN$_2$ cryosurgery** is used for macular lesions.
- A **retinoid gel**, which is useful for macular lesions, is currently in trials.

POINTS TO REMEMBER

- KS in an HIV-infected patient is an AIDS-defining diagnosis.
- Treatment of individual lesions does not prevent the occurrence of new lesions.
- Lesions may resolve spontaneously in patients on effective antiretroviral therapy.

(See Chapter 19, "Sexually Transmitted Diseases.")

- Condyloma acuminata is **caused by a cutaneous infection with human papillomavirus** (HPV).
- Lesions most commonly occur perianally and intra-anally, on the penis of men, on the oral mucosa, and on the vulva and cervix of women.
- HIV-infected patients appear to have an increased susceptibility to **malignant degeneration** (the development of anal cancers in homosexual men and cervical cancer in women) when infected with oncogenic subtypes of HPV.

- Condylomata are difficult to eradicate in immunocompromised hosts. A cause of recurrent perianal warts is the presence of internal condylomata, and affected patients should be referred to a rectal surgeon. For a detailed discussion of the diagnosis and management of condyloma acuminata.

BASICS

- Pruritus is a common and troubling symptom in HIV-infected patients. It is often multifactorial in etiology.
- Many patients use **antibacterial or deodorant soaps** with the mistaken belief that they will decrease the risk of infection. In fact, these soaps dry the skin and make the patients itchy, making them more susceptible to cutaneous infection because of the excoriations that result.
- Patients may become itchy because of subclinical **drug eruptions** or as a side effect of protease inhibitors.

MANAGEMENT

- Careful history and physical examination **rule out dermatologic disease** as the cause.
- Patients should discontinue use of deodorant and antibacterial soaps; superfatted soaps are the least drying.
- Patients should be instructed to **limit bathing** to once per day.
- **Emollients** should be applied after the patient has bathed and pats dry; ointments are more emollient than creams, which are more emollient than lotions.
- Patients need to try different preparations to find which is most cosmetically acceptable and effective.
- Patients who do not obtain relief with over-the counter moisturizers often do well with **ammonium lactate 12% lotion**.
- **Anti-itch preparations** containing calamine, pramoxine, menthol, camphor, and oatmeal may be soothing.
- **Sedating antihistamines** are useful, especially before bedtime.
- **Topical steroids** should be prescribed for dermatitis, which may result from dry skin.
- **Ultraviolet B phototherapy** is palliative.
- For further discussion of pruritus, see Chapter 15, "Pruritus, the "Itchy" Patient."

(See Chapter 5, "Eruptions of Unknown Cause.")

BASICS

- Seborrheic dermatitis is a **scaly skin** condition that affects up to 5% of the human population.
- In immunocompetent patients, it may be associated with an overgrowth of saprophytic *Pityrosporum* yeast on the scalp and face; it is not known whether the same is true in HIV-infected patients.
- The frequency and severity of seborrheic dermatitis are increased in HIV-infected patients, for unknown reasons.
- Seborrheic dermatitis appears commonly in hospitalized patients, probably because of the changes in hygiene (e.g., inability to shampoo the hair) experienced during illness.

DESCRIPTION OF LESIONS

- Erythematous patches and papules
- Characteristic greasy, yellow scale

DISTRIBUTION OF LESIONS

- Scalp
- Retroauricular skin
- Glabella and eyebrows
- Nasomalar and nasolabial folds (Figure 24.25)
- Beard area in men
- Sternal and interscapular areas in men
- Axillae
- Genital skin

CLINICAL MANIFESTATIONS

- Burning, itching
- Dandruff
- Oozing lesions

DIAGNOSIS

- **Clinical appearance** and distribution
- Rapid **response to treatment**

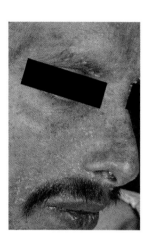

Figure 24.25.
Seborrheic dermatitis in a patient with AIDS.

DIFFERENTIAL DIAGNOSIS

Psoriasis
(See Chapter 4, "Psoriasis.")
- There is often psoriatic involvement on the elbows, knees, and sacrum.
- Psoriasis, in the distribution of seborrheic dermatitis, is called "sebopsoriasis."

Systemic lupus erythematosus
(See Chapter 25, "Cutaneous Manifestations of Systemic Disease.")
- Lupus affects the malar areas, not skin folds.
- Antinuclear antibodies (ANAs) and double-stranded deoxyribonucleic acid (ds-DNA) are positive.
- The disease occurs most commonly in immunocompetent women.

MANAGEMENT

- Shampoos with **tar, zinc pyrithione, selenium sulfide,** or **salicylic acid** may be helpful.
- **Nonfluorinated topical steroid creams** may be applied twice per day to the face.
- **Ketoconazole cream 2%** can be used as an adjunctive treatment.
- **Topical steroid lotions** or solutions can be used for the scalp.
- **Ultraviolet B phototherapy** is used for resistant cases.
- **Advise the patient** that the condition is chronic and recurrent and should be treated as needed.

POINTS TO REMEMBER

- Seborrheic dermatitis is common in HIV-infected patients, and the sudden onset of severe, recalcitrant, seborrheic dermatitis should lead to an inquiry regarding risk factors and HIV testing.
- It is a chronic, recurrent condition.

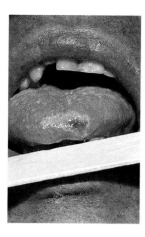

Figure 24.26.
Aphthous ulcer in an AIDS patient.

(See Chapter 12, "Disorders of the Mouth, Lips, and Tongue.")

BASICS

- Aphthous ulcers may be severe in HIV-infected patients.
- The pain may interfere with the patient's ability to eat.

DESCRIPTION OF LESIONS

(Figure 24.26)
- Punched-out mucosal ulceration
- Yellow, fibrinous bases
- A few millimeters to more than 1 centimeter in size

DISTRIBUTION OF LESIONS

- Buccal and labial mucosa
- Tongue

CLINICAL MANIFESTATIONS

- Pain
- Inability to eat and drink, possibly leading to dehydration

DIFFERENTIAL DIAGNOSIS

Herpes simplex
- HSV causes mouth ulcers in first episodes in immunocompetent hosts.
- It can cause recurrent painful ulcers on the oral mucosa in immunocompromised hosts.
- Diagnosis of HSV is by Tzanck smear and viral culture.

Disseminated *Mycobacterium avium-intracellulare*
- The infection is associated with fever.
- There is evidence of involvement of other organs.
- Blood cultures are sometimes positive.

Cytomegalovirus
- Diagnosis is by mucosal biopsy.
- CMV has characteristic inclusion bodies.

Autoimmune blistering diseases (pemphigus vulgaris, bullous pemphigoid)
- These diseases are rare in HIV patients.
- They may be accompanied by cutaneous blisters.
- Diagnosis is by skin biopsy for histopathologic and direct immunofluorescence examinations.
- Serum autoantibodies can be found to the intercellular cement substance or to the basement membrane zone.

MANAGEMENT

- **Topical steroids** applied directly to the ulcerations
- **Stomatitis elixir**, consisting of equal parts of magnesium carbonate or magnesium hydroxide suspension, viscous lidocaine, diphenhydramine elixir 12.5 mg/5 cc, and 1 g of tetracycline powder, to be swished and spit out of the mouth as needed for pain
- **Thalidomide**, 100 mg by mouth twice per day, with notable toxic effects of sedation, neutropenia, and peripheral neuropathy

---

(See Chapter 4 "Psoriasis.")

BASICS

- Psoriasis is a **scaly skin** disease that affects 1 to 2% of the general population.
- It is not more common in HIV-infected patients, but it may present in a more severe or unusual form and may be recalcitrant to the usual treatments.
- The most severe manifestation is Reiter's disease, with psoriatic lesions, arthritis, urethritis, and conjunctivitis (see Chapter 25, "Cutaneous Manifestations of Systemic Disease).

DESCRIPTION OF LESIONS

- Erythematous papules and plaques with silvery or "micaceous" scale
- Intertriginous lesions that lack scale, possibly appearing white from maceration
- Periungual erythema and edema
- Onychodystrophy (nail pits, "oil spots," onycholysis)
- Erythroderma
- Pustules, most common in patients given systemic steroids
- Erythema and swelling of joints, with eventual deformity

DISTRIBUTION OF LESIONS

- Scalp
- Extensor aspects of the extremities
- "Inverse psoriasis," which involves intertriginous areas
- Palms, soles
- Nails
- Joints

CLINICAL MANIFESTATIONS

- May be asymptomatic
- Itching
- Pain in skin or joints
- With more extensive involvement, temperature dysregulation and fluid and electrolyte imbalance

DIAGNOSIS

- **Clinical appearance**
- **Skin biopsy**
- **Gram's stain** and culture of pustules
- **KOH examination** of pustules

MANAGEMENT

Limited plaque–type psoriasis
- **Keratolytic agents** to remove scale and allow penetration of other therapeutic agents
- **Tar baths** and oils for antipruritic and antipsoriatic effects
- **Topical steroids** for rapid relief of symptoms—these lose effectiveness with time and lead to recurrence (tachyphylaxis)
- **Anthralin** cream or ointment applied to affected areas for 20 minutes per day
- **Calcipotriene** ointment, cream, or scalp solution applied twice per day
- **Tazarotene** topical gel 0.05 to 0.1% applied at bedtime
- **Ultraviolet B phototherapy**
- **PUVA** (psoralen plus ultraviolet A)
- **Sulfasalazine**

Erythroderma, or pustular, psoriasis
- **Acitretin**, 10 to 50 mg per day
- **Ultraviolet B phototherapy** or **PUVA** as adjunctive treatment
- **Topical treatment** for limited psoriasis

Scalp psoriasis
- **Keratolytic solutions**, containing salicylic acid to remove scales
- **Olive oil** applied to the scalp overnight with shower-cap occlusion
- Shampoos containing **tar, salicylic acid, selenium sulfide,** and **zinc pyrithione**
- **Anthralin, calcipotriene, and topical steroids** in scalp preparations

Intertriginous psoriasis
- Most medications used for psoriasis are too irritating for skinfold areas.
- **Mild (nonfluorinated) topical steroids** in conjunction with **topical antifungals** may be effective.
- If genital psoriasis is debilitating, consider **systemic treatment**.

POINTS TO REMEMBER

- Psoriasis may be more severe and recalcitrant to treatment in patients with HIV.
- New onset of severe psoriasis in a patient at risk for HIV should lead to HIV testing.
- The combination of treatment with methotrexate and sulfonamides can lead to **fatal bone marrow suppression**.
- The use of systemic steroids for treatment of psoriasis may result in **life-threatening pustular psoriasis**.

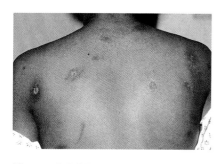

Figure 24.27.
Syphilis in an AIDS patient. Note necrotic lesions.

(See Chapter 19 "Sexually Transmitted Diseases.")

BASICS

- Syphilis is a sexually transmitted disease caused by the spirochete *Treponema pallidum*.
- An intact cell-mediated immune system is necessary to "cure" the infection.
- Unusual manifestations of syphilis have been reported in patients with co-infection with HIV. These include negative serologic examination for syphilis in the face of active secondary syphilis; relapse after treatment that should have been adequate; fulminant, cutaneous lesions with induration and necrosis (Figure 24.27); and fulminant neurosyphilis resulting in permanent neurologic deficits.

POINTS TO REMEMBER

- If syphilis is suspected in an HIV-infected patient and the serology is negative, then a **skin biopsy** should be performed.

The only medication for the treatment of syphilis that adequately penetrates the blood-brain barrier is **intravenous aqueous penicillin**, which should be given at a dose of 2 to 4 million units every 4 hours for 10 to 14 days in cases of suspected or proven neurosyphilis. Penicillin-allergic patients should undergo desensitization.

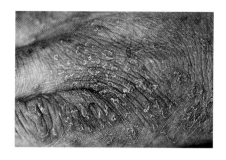

Figure 24.28.
Norwegian scabies in an AIDS patient. Note white linear burrows.

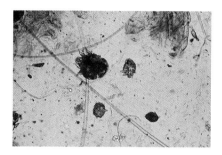

Figure 24.29.
Scabies. Mites, ova, and fecal pellets.

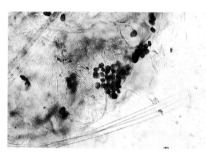

Figure 24.30.
Scabies. Mites, ova, and fecal pellets.

(See Chapter 20, "Bites, Stings, and Infestations.")

BASICS

- Norwegian scabies is an infestation with *Sarcoptes scabiei* var. *hominis* in an immunocompromised host.
- Immunocompetent hosts are able to limit the number of mites (10 to 12) that remain in the epidermis.
- The rash and itching are the result of a delayed hypersensitivity response to the mite, its eggs, and its fecal products.
- Immunocompromised hosts are not able to contain the population of mites and may be infested with millions of mites. These patients may not itch because of their defective cell-mediated immunity.
- HIV-infected patients with Norwegian scabies infestation pose a significant risk of transmission of scabies to household contacts and medical personnel.

DESCRIPTION OF LESIONS

- Fine white linear lesions from female mites burrowing into the skin (Figure 24.28)
- Excoriations
- Crusted, keratotic plaques

DISTRIBUTION OF LESIONS

- Finger webs
- Axillae
- Nipples
- Waist
- Genitals
- Atypical acral lesions in HIV patients

CLINICAL MANIFESTATIONS

- Intense itching, which may not be present in Norwegian scabies
- Secondary infection

DIAGNOSIS

Mineral oil preparation is performed by scraping the epidermal surface of a burrow with a scalpel that has been dipped in mineral oil. It is examined with low-power microscopy. Mites, ova, or fecal pellets are seen (Figures 24.29 and 24.30).

DIFFERENTIAL DIAGNOSIS

Psoriasis
- Psoriatic lesions tend to be located on extensor aspects of the extremities.
- Predominance of scale in the finger webs should lead to suspicion of Norwegian scabies.
- Mineral oil preparation distinguishes Norwegian scabies.

Solar keratoses
Norwegian scabies on sun-exposed areas in elderly patients can mimic solar keratoses (Figure 24.31).

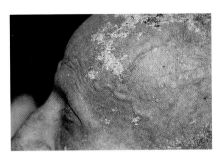

Figure 24.31.
Norwegian scabies in AIDS patient. Lesions resemble solar keratoses.

MANAGEMENT

- **Scabicides**
  - **Elimite Cream** (5% permethrin) is applied to all skin surfaces from head to toe (including palms, soles, and scalp in small children) after a warm bath and is left on for 8 to 12 hours (usually overnight) and washed off the next morning.
  - **Kwell Lotion** (lindane) is applied from head to toe after bathing. Treatment should be continued once weekly until there is no evidence of residual lesions.
- **Keratolytic agents**, such as 10 to 40% salicylic acid, remove crusts and allow penetration of the scabicides.
- **Ivermectin**, 0.6 mg by mouth, has been shown to be effective in eradicating infection. It is not approved by the Food and Drug Administration (FDA) for this use.
- Household contacts and medical staff who come into contact with the patient or the patient's bedclothes should undergo treatment as for scabies in an immunocompetent host, regardless of symptoms.

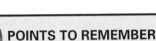

POINTS TO REMEMBER

- Norwegian scabies is an infestation with millions of scabies mites and is highly contagious. Failure to treat promptly has led to epidemics affecting dozens of people.
- Prolonged treatment may be necessary because of the immunodeficiency in patients with Norwegian scabies.

CHAPTER 25

CUTANEOUS MANIFESTATIONS OF SYSTEMIC DISEASE

Peter G. Burk and Herbert P. Goodheart

NEUROCUTANEOUS SYNDROMES

Neurocutaneous syndromes are diseases in which skin lesions provide clinically useful markers of diseases with neurologic manifestations.

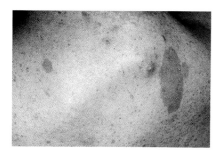

Figure 25.1.
Neurofibromatosis (NF). Multiple light-brown, macules (café au lait spots).

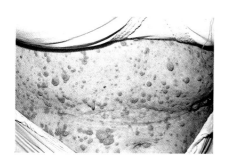

Figure 25.2.
Neurofibromas. Soft, rubbery, flesh-colored papules and nodules.

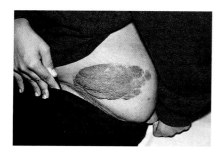

Figure 25.3.
Neurofibromatosis (NF). Plexiform neuroma feels like a "bag of worms."

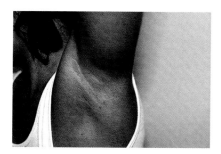

Figure 25.4.
Neurofibromatosis (NF). Crowe's sign (axillary "freckles").

BASICS

- Neurofibromatosis (NF), or **von Recklinghausen's disease**, is an autosomally inherited disease, in which macular pigmented skin lesions **(café au lait spots)** and skin tumors **(neurofibromas)** occur in patients in whom a wide range of central nervous system (CNS) or spinal cord lesions may ultimately develop.
- The incidence of NF is 4 per 10,000 births. Fifty percent of cases are thought to be inherited in an **autosomal dominant** fashion; the remainder are the result of spontaneous new mutations.
- **Type 1** NF is caused by a mutation in a gene on **chromosome 17**. This gene has been isolated and may act as a tumor-suppressor gene.
- **Type 2** disease, which is localized to **chromosome 22**, is characterized by bilateral acoustic neuromas and fewer skin manifestations.

DESCRIPTION OF LESIONS

- Multiple, light-brown, macules (café au lait spots; Figure 25.1)
- Cutaneous neurofibromas, which are soft, rubbery, flesh-colored or tan-colored papules and nodules (Figure 25.2)
- Plexiform neuromas manifesting as large, drooping tumors, which, on palpation, feel like a "bag of worms" (Figure 25.3)
- **Axillary or inguinal freckling** (Crowe's sign) in some patients, which is considered to be **pathognomonic** for NF (Figure 25.4)

DISTRIBUTION OF LESIONS

- Café au lait spots most often appear on the **trunk** and **extremities**.
- Neurofibromas may appear on the **face, trunk,** and **extremities**.

CLINICAL MANIFESTATIONS

- Café au lait spots usually present at birth, or shortly thereafter.
- Cutaneous neurofibromas may first develop in adolescence, and new lesions may continue to emerge during the patient's lifetime. Up to 5% of skin tumors may develop into neurofibrosarcomas.
- **Ocular lesions** (Lisch nodules) are asymptomatic, pigmented iris hamartomas seen in 80% of NF cases.
- CNS tumors, optic gliomas, and spinal cord tumors may develop at any age.
- **CNS involvement** usually consists of benign lesions such as optic gliomas, acoustic neuromas, and meningiomas. CNS lesions may become astrocytomas.
  - CNS involvement may occur in up to 10% of patients with NF.
  - Spinal cord tumors may produce cord damage and paraplegia.
  - Many patients with NF have seizure disorders and mental retardation.
  - Macrocephaly may be present in up to 16% of patients.
- **Musculoskeletal disorders** are uncommon but **pseudoarthrosis of the tibia and kyphoscoliosis may be diagnostic** in some patients with NF.
- **Gastrointestinal symptoms** may occur in some patients with NF in whom intussusception and obstruction of the small intestine develop from intraabdominal neurofibromas.
- **Endocrine disorders** are unusual, but pheochromocytomas characterized by life-threatening severe hypertension can occur in less than 1% of patients with NF.

DIAGNOSIS

- Isolated neurofibromas are not uncommon.
- Café au lait spots are seen in 10 to 20% of the normal population; however, **6 or more café au lait spots** that are **greater than 0.5 cm in diameter in infants or greater than 1 cm in diameter in adults** are supportive of the diagnosis of NF.
- A **first-degree relative with NF** supports the diagnosis.
- Other findings that are supportive of the diagnosis include the following:
  - **Crowe's sign**
  - **Lisch nodules**
  - **Bilateral optic nerve gliomas**
  - Distinctive **osseous lesions**

Laboratory evaluations
- Skin biopsies of café au lait macules may show macromelanosomes on electron microscopy, but these findings are not diagnostic.
- **Biopsies of neurofibromas** show characteristic **Schwann cells** and **neuronal cells**.

DIFFERENTIAL DIAGNOSIS

McCune-Albright syndrome
- Pigmented macular lesions
- Polyostotic fibrous dysplasia
- Precocious puberty

Segmental neurofibromatosis
- Café au lait macules localized to one area of the body
- Cutaneous localized neurofibromas
- No CNS tumors
- Rarely inherited (somatic mutation)

MANAGEMENT

- **Surgical removal** of symptomatic or disfiguring neurofibromas
- **Follow-up** for the development of neurofibrosarcomas, optic gliomas, acoustic neuromas, and pheochromocytomas
- **Genetic counseling** for patients and their families

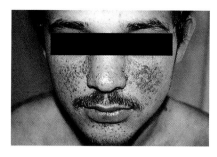

Figure 25.5.
Tuberous sclerosis (TS). Adenoma sebaceum (angiofibromas).

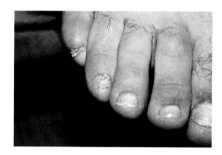

Figure 25.6.
Tuberous sclerosis (TS). Periungual fibromas (Koenen's tumors).

BASICS

- Tuberous sclerosis (TS) (**Bourneville's disease**) is a disease in which cutaneous lesions may be seen in association with CNS and other organ manifestations. The **classic triad** of TS includes the following:
  - **Adenoma sebaceum**
  - **Epilepsy**
  - **Mental retardation**, although at least 50% of affected persons show no evidence of mental retardation
- TS, which is inherited in an autosomal dominant fashion, is found in less than 1 per 10,000 births.

DESCRIPTION OF LESIONS

- **Ash-leaf macules**, which are hypopigmented, characteristically oval, and sometimes linear or "confetti-shaped" macular lesions
- So-called adenoma sebaceum (actually **angiofibromas**), which are pink to reddish-brown, dome-shaped papules (Figure 25.5)
- **Periungual fibromas** (**Koenen's tumors**), which are smooth, firm, flesh-colored papules (Figure 25.6)
- Pebbly, flesh-colored "peau d'orange" or "pigskinlike" dermal plaque (**Shagreen patch**), with fine confettilike hypopigmentation

DISTRIBUTION OF LESIONS

- Ash-leaf spots are more common on the **trunk** and **proximal extremities**.
- Adenoma sebaceum papules are symmetric in distribution and are most commonly located on the **nose, nasolabial folds,** and **cheeks**. More widespread distribution involves the **forehead, ears,** and **scalp**.
- Periungual fibromas occur around and under the nails on the **periungual areas of the fingers and toes**.
- Shagreen patches appear on the trunk, most often in the **lumbosacral region**.

CLINICAL MANIFESTATIONS

- Ash-leaf macules and Shagreen patches are usually present at birth.
- Adenoma sebaceum may begin to develop in late childhood and adolescence.
- **CNS lesions** consist of the following:
  - Gliomatous brain tumors (tubers), which may calcify in 50% of patients
  - Seizure disorders in 60 to 70% of patients, with less than 50% showing evidence of mental retardation
  - Retinal and optic nerve gliomas
- **Systemic organic involvement** includes the following:
  - Cardiac rhabdomyomas of the atrium in 30% of patients, which rarely cause cardiac obstructive disease
  - Renal hamartomas
  - Renal tumors (angiomyolipomas) and polycystic kidneys in approximately 15% of patients, which must be differentiated from renal carcinoma

DIAGNOSIS

- **Retinal gliomas** are **pathognomonic** of TS.
- **Adenoma sebaceum** is **pathognomonic** of TS.
- **Periungual fibromas** are **pathognomonic** of TS.
- **Ash-leaf macules** are best visualized with a Wood's light.
- **Shagreen patches, seizure disorder,** and **a family history of cutaneous lesions and seizure disorder** support the diagnosis of TS.

Laboratory evaluations
- **Magnetic resonance imaging (MRI)** of the head (for infants)
- Posteroanterior and lateral **skull films** (for adults) to demonstrate calcifications of gliomas of the brain
- **Skin biopsy** of cutaneous lesions

DIFFERENTIAL DIAGNOSIS OF ADENOMA SEBACEUM

Acneiform papules
- Often resemble adenoma sebaceum
- Waxing and waning course
- Biopsy necessary only if diagnosis is in doubt

MANAGEMENT

- **Follow-up** of infants with ash-leaf spots for the development of seizure disorder or mental retardation
- **Follow-up** of patients with TS for development of cardiac and/or renal lesions
- Removal of cosmetically objectionable or disfiguring adenoma sebaceum by **excision, electrocautery, dermabrasion,** or **laser resurfacing**
- **Surgical removal** of painful periungual fibromas
- **Genetic counseling** of patients with TS and their families after CT scanning is performed on the parents and siblings of the affected patient (CT studies have demonstrated CNS lesions in asymptomatic parents of patients with TS)

ENDOCRINE DISEASES

A wide variety of skin lesions are seen in conjunction with endocrine diseases. Some of these cutaneous lesions are directly related to the degree of endocrine dysfunction and may be caused by an excess or lack of a hormone acting on a specific tissue (e.g., warm and moist skin associated with hyperthyroidism; dry, cool skin associated with hypothyroidism). Other skin lesions may be seen in association with a specific endocrine disease such as diabetes, but it may be difficult to link these skin findings to a specific degree of endocrine dysfunction (e.g., necrobiosis lipoidica diabeticorum with hyperglycemia).

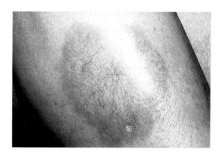

Figure 25.7.
Necrobiosis lipoidica diabeticorum (NLD). Translucent plaque with epidermal atrophy and telangiectasias.

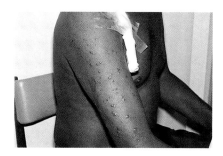

Figure 25.8.
Perforating folliculitis (Kyrle's disease). Hyperkeratotic papules on extensor areas of upper extremity.

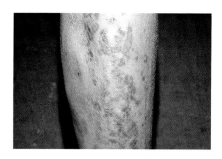

Figure 25.9.
Diabetic dermopathy. Small, brownish, atrophic, scarred, hyperpigmented plaques.

BASICS

- Diabetes mellitus (DM) is a disease characterized by a **disturbance in the production of insulin** or **resistance to insulin activity**, which results in abnormal glucose metabolism.
- The clinical results of diabetes include cellular changes, such as microangiopathy of small blood vessels. This causes organ damage, producing retinal disease, renal dysfunction, and possibly cutaneous lesions.
- DM can also affect immune function, resulting in increased fungal and yeast infections. It is currently believed that well-controlled diabetics suppress bacterial infections normally.

DESCRIPTION OF LESIONS

- **Necrobiosis lipoidica diabeticorum (NLD)** is characterized by yellow–brown, translucent plaques with epidermal atrophy and telangiectasias (Figure 25.7).
- **Perforating folliculitis (Kyrle's disease)** consists of firm, rough hyperkeratotic papules, which are often hyperpigmented in dark-skinned people (Figure 25.8).
- **Diabetic dermopathy** is characterized by small (less than 0.5 cm), brownish, atrophic, scarred, hyperpigmented plaques (Figure 25.9).
- **Diabetic bullous disease** manifests as large, tense subepidermal blisters (Figure 25.10).
- **Acanthosis nigricans** (AN) sometimes occurs in insulin-resistant diabetes (see below).
- **Cutaneous candidiasis** (see Chapter 10, "Superficial Fungal Infections")
- **Disseminated granuloma annulare** consists of annular dermal papules (see Chapter 5, "Eruptions of Unknown Cause") and occurs in patients with clinical diabetes and in nondiabetics.
- **Staphylococcal skin infections** may occur.
- **Diabetic neuropathic ulcers** (**mal perforans;** Figure 25.11) may occur.
- **Scleredema of Buschke-Lowenstein** (rare) is a sclerotic, thickened plaque seen on the upper back.

DISTRIBUTION OF LESIONS

- NLD is seen most commonly on the **pretibial areas** but may be seen on other sites.
- Perforating folliculitis is found most commonly on the **extensor surfaces** of the lower extremities.
- Diabetic dermopathy occurs primarily on the **anterior lower legs**.
- Bullous diabetic lesions most often occur on the lower extremities, especially the **ankles and feet**.
- Diabetic neuropathic ulcers are noted at sites of pressure (e.g., the heel) in areas of poor sensory function and poor circulation.

CLINICAL MANIFESTATIONS

- NLD is seen more frequently in juvenile- than in adult-onset diabetes and may occur before the onset of clinical diabetes. Lesions may ulcerate. A minority of patients have no clinical evidence or family history of diabetes; hence, the term "**necrobiosis lipoidica**" is used.
- Perforating folliculitis, which can itch intensely, is seen primarily in patients with long-standing severe diabetes who have microangiopathy and neuropathy. There is a high incidence of perforating folliculitis in patients with diabetes who are on chronic hemodialysis.
- Diabetic dermopathy occurs in juvenile- and adult-onset diabetes. It is typically a late manifestation of diabetes and usually asymptomatic.
- Bullous diabetic lesions occur most frequently in patients with severe neuropathy.
- Diabetic neuropathic ulcers are usually painless because of peripheral neuropathy.

DIAGNOSIS

- Diagnosis for most of these entities is generally made on **clinical grounds**.
- **Skin biopsy** is performed to confirm the diagnosis.

Laboratory evaluations
- **Serum glucose levels** and **glucose tolerance tests** are performed to confirm the diagnosis of DM.
- Skin biopsies of necrobiosis lipoidica and granuloma annulare demonstrate **palisading granulomas with degeneration of collagen**.
- Skin biopsy of perforating folliculitis demonstrates **basophilic material in the dermis** with transepidermal elimination.
- Skin biopsies of diabetic dermopathy show **thickening of blood vessels and mild perivascular infiltrate**.
- Diabetic bullous lesions have **subepidermal blistering** on hematoxylin and eosin staining of skin biopsy tissue; direct immunofluorescence of skin biopsies in these lesions is negative for immunoglobulins.
- Diabetic neuropathic ulcers are rarely biopsied.

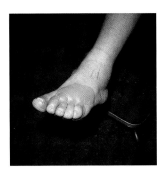

Figure 25.10.
Diabetic bullous disease. Large, tense blister.

DIFFERENTIAL DIAGNOSIS

- NLD lesions can be similar to **morphea and other localized sclerosing lesions**.
- Perforating folliculitis can be differentiated from other **keratotic papules** by the size and distribution of lesions.
- Diabetic dermopathy must be differentiated from **lesions caused by trauma**.
- Bullous diabetic lesions can be differentiated from **bullous pemphigoid** by the localized lesions and negative direct immunofluorescence of skin biopsies.
- Diabetic neuropathic ulcers are diagnosed clinically.

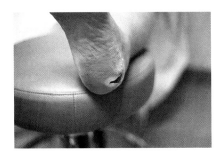

Figure 25.11.
Diabetic ulcer of heel (mal perforans).

MANAGEMENT

- **Long-term clinical control of glucose levels** in DM reduces microangiopathy and subsequent organ damage, which leads to retinopathy, nephropathy, neuropathy, and other tissue damage.
- **High-potency topical steroids** or **intralesional steroid injections** are used in the management of NLD and granuloma annulare lesions.
- **Oral antihistamines** are used to control pruritus in patients with cutaneous folliculitis lesions that are resistant to therapy.
- **Topical antibiotic therapy** is recommended for bullous diabetic lesions until the blisters heal. Recently, **Regranex Gel** (becaplermin), a recombinant human platelet-derived growth factor, has become available as a topical therapy (in conjunction with good ulcer care) to promote healing of diabetic neuropathic foot ulcers.

POINTS TO REMEMBER

- Careful consideration should be given before performing a skin biopsy on a patient with diabetes, particularly on areas such as the lower extremities.
- Rule out osteomyelitis in patients with prolonged, purulent, nonhealing ulcers.

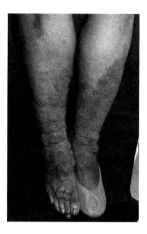

Figure 25.12.
Pretibial myxedema.

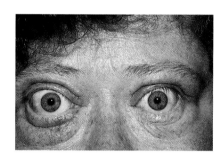

Figure 25.13.
Exophthalmos.

BASICS

- Thyroid hormones profoundly influence the growth and differentiation of epidermal and dermal tissues.
- **Abnormal levels of thyroid hormone produce striking changes in the texture of the skin, hair, and nails.**
- Some of the associated skin alterations in thyroid disease are the result of a deficiency or a high toxic level of tissue thyroid hormone; other skin changes seen with thyroid disease such as vitiligo and alopecia areata are associated clinical findings, which are not directly related to thyroid hormone function but are seen frequently in patients with thyroid disease.
- Findings such as pretibial myxedema may be correlated with a circulating autoimmune γ-globulin, which stimulates fibroblasts to produce mucin.
- Hyperthyroidism may be caused by Graves' disease (85%), subacute thyroiditis, toxic goiter, and thyroid carcinoma (rare). Hypothyroidism may be caused by iodine deficiency (cretinism), Hashimoto's thyroiditis, pituitary dysfunction with thyroid-stimulating hormone deficiency, and surgical or radiation ablation of the thyroid.
- Patients with thyroid disease may be hyperthyroid at one point in their clinical course and hypothyroid at another time.

DESCRIPTION OF LESIONS

Hyperthyroid skin lesions
- Warm, moist, and velvety skin
- Alopecia with diffuse hair loss
- Nail changes with onycholysis (Plummer's nails)
- Hyperpigmentation

Hyperthyroid systemic findings
- Nervousness and tremor
- Weight loss
- Tachycardia with atrial fibrillation
- Proximal muscle weakness

Graves' disease
- Pretibial myxedema lesions—flesh-colored, waxy infiltrated translucent plaques (Figure 25.12)
- Exophthalmos with protruding eyes (Figure 25.13)

Hypothyroid skin lesions
- Myxedema of the skin with generalized thickening and a dry coarse feel; yellow skin secondary to carotenemia
- Hair changes—coarse, sparse hair; lateral third of eyebrows lost

Associated skin lesions in thyroid disease
Alopecia areata in up to 8% of patients
Vitiligo
Anemia
Bullous disorders
Connective tissue diseases
Multiple endocrinopathy syndrome
Urticaria

DISTRIBUTION OF LESIONS

- Hyperthyroid and hypothyroid skin lesions are **diffuse**.
- Pretibial myxedema (Graves' disease) lesions are found most frequently on the **lower legs**.

CLINICAL MANIFESTATIONS

- Hyperthyroid skin changes that result from the hypermetabolic state (e.g., warm, moist, and flushed skin) occur during the active thyrotoxic stage of thyroiditis, during active Graves' disease, and in patients with toxic goiters. These skin changes may gradually resolve when the patient returns to a euthyroid state.
- Graves' disease lesions (pretibial myxedema) occurs in up to 4% of these patients. The skin lesions and eye lesions usually do not resolve even after treatment of the thyroid disease brings a return to a euthyroid state.
- Hypothyroid skin changes (e.g., cool, dry skin) are related to length and severity of the clinical hypothyroid state. These skin lesions gradually improve some months after a return to euthyroid state.

DIAGNOSIS

- Diagnosis of hyperthyroid and hypothyroid disease is made by specific **thyroid function tests**.
- Graves' disease is diagnosed **clinically** and with confirmatory thyroid function tests and **skin biopsy**.

Laboratory evaluations
- **Thyroid serum hormone levels** can be most accurately measured by obtaining free thyroxine and free triiodothyronine levels.
- Elevated **thyroid-stimulating hormone levels** are found in patients with hypothyroidism.
- **Antithyroglobulin antibodies** and **antithyroid microsomal antibodies** are often positive in Graves' disease and Hashimoto's thyroiditis.
- **Skin biopsies** in Graves' disease show increased staining of hyaluronic acid with mucin stains.

DIFFERENTIAL DIAGNOSIS

Graves' disease must be differentiated from other skin diseases with increased mucin production, such as **papular mucinosis** and **scleredema**.

MANAGEMENT

- Functional symptoms (e.g., increase or decrease of sweating, dry skin, hair and nail changes) of hyper- and hypothyroidism may improve after appropriate treatment of thyroid disease and **return to a euthyroid state**.
- Treatment of Graves' disease lesions can be attempted with **high-potency topical steroids** and **intralesional steroids**, although the response is poor.

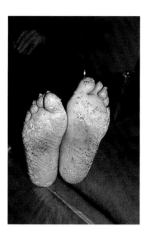

Figure 25.14.
Keratoderma blennorrhagica. Scaly, red-brown, inflammatory, pustular psoriasislike lesions on the soles.

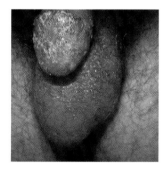

Figure 25.15.
Circinate balanitis. Psoriasiform lesions on the glans penis and scrotum.

BASICS

- Reiter's syndrome (RS) is an idiopathic inflammatory process affecting the skin, joints, and mucous membranes. The **classic triad** of **urethritis, conjunctivitis,** and **arthritis** is found in only 40% of cases at the time of clinical presentation.
- RS is seen most commonly in young white men of European origin.
- Initial symptoms often occur following a nongonococcal urethritis (e.g., chlamydial infection) or infection with an enteric pathogen (e.g., *Shigella*).
- HLA-B27 is frequently positive in patients with RS and portends a poorer prognosis.

DESCRIPTION OF LESIONS

- Skin lesions are often indistinguishable from psoriasis; however, RS often manifests certain characteristic findings.
  - **Keratoderma blennorrhagica** (Figure 25.14) consists of scaly, red, inflammatory psoriasislike lesions on the palms and soles. The lesions may have a thick scale and be pustular.
  - Similar scaling red plaques or erosions may be found on the glans penis (**circinate balanitis**; Figure 25.15).
- Nail changes may include findings such as those seen in psoriasis: onycholysis and subungual hyperkeratosis; furthermore, subungual pustules with resultant shedding of nails may occur.
- Oral lesions are painless, irregularly shaped, white plaques on the tongue that resemble geographic tongue.

DISTRIBUTION OF LESIONS

- Keratoderma blennorrhagica is most often noted on the **palms and soles**.
- Psoriasislike plaques may be seen on the **scalp, elbows, knees, buttocks, shaft of penis,** and **scrotum**.

CLINICAL MANIFESTATIONS

- RS is a multisystem disease that may present with fever, malaise, dysuria, arthralgias, and red irritated eyes with accompanying cutaneous lesions.
- **Arthritis** is an asymmetric oligoarthritis that commonly involves large joints (elbows, knees); it may also involve smaller joints. A sacroiliitis and ankylosing spondylitis may occur.
- **Ocular disease** may include conjunctivitis and, less commonly, iritis and keratitis.
- **Urethritis** is a nonspecific urethral inflammation.
- During initial or recurrent episodes, most patients with RS do not manifest the complete triad of urethritis, conjunctivitis, and arthritis.
- Frequently RS has a self-limited course, but it may become a chronic, relapsing condition.

DIAGNOSIS

Diagnosis is generally made on **clinical grounds**.

Laboratory evaluations
- HLA-B27 is positive in 75% of patients.
- Antinuclear antibody (ANA) and rheumatoid factor are usually negative.
- The histopathology of skin lesions in RS is indistinguishable from that of psoriasis.

DIFFERENTIAL DIAGNOSIS

Psoriasis with arthritis
- Psoriasiform skin lesions
- Arthritis similar to RS
- No ocular symptoms
- No urethritis

Behçet's syndrome
- Painful oral ulcers
- Arthritis
- Iritis
- Vasculitic skin lesions

Candidal balanitis
Positive KOH

MANAGEMENT
- **Mild cases**
  - RS may be treated with **topical steroids** for the skin lesions.
  - **Nonsteroidal antiinflammatory drugs** (NSAIDs) are prescribed for pain.
- **Severe cases**
  - **Oral methotrexate** is sometimes used on a weekly basis for severe cases.
  - **Oral steroids** may be necessary; however, tapering of steroids can produce an extreme flare of the pustular lesions.
  - **Oral retinoids** (e.g., Accutane) have also been used to treat skin lesions.

BASICS

- Exfoliative dermatitis (ED), also known as **erythroderma**, refers to a total, or almost total, redness and/or scaling of the skin. It is an uncommon disorder seen more often in men; 50 years is the average age of occurrence. When seen in children, ED most often is secondary to severe atopic dermatitis. In adults, psoriasis is the most frequently associated skin disease (see Chapter 4 "Psoriasis").
- ED may appear suddenly or gradually, occasionally accompanied by fever, chills, and lymphadenopathy. It may be seen in the following situations:
  - As a stage in the natural history of the following skin disorders:
    — Severe eczematous and atopic dermatitis
    — Psoriasis
  - Less commonly, as a finding in the following skin disorders:
    — Allergic contact dermatitis
    — Stasis dermatitis with secondary autoeczematization
    — Pityriasis rubra pilaris (a rare disorder of keratinization)
    — Graft-versus-host disease
    — Seborrheic dermatitis (Leiner's disease) in infants
    — Pemphigus foliaceus
    — Lichen planus
    — Papulosquamous dermatitis of AIDS
  - As a reaction to the following drugs: sulfonamides, penicillins, antimalarials, lithium, phenothiazines, barbiturates, gold, allopurinol, NSAIDs, aspirin, captopril, codeine, and diphenylhydantoin.
  - As a complication or presenting symptom of the following malignancies:
    — Mycosis fungoides (cutaneous T-cell lymphoma)
    — Sézary syndrome (leukemic variant of mycosis fungoides)
    — Hodgkin's disease
    — Non-Hodgkin's lymphoma
- As an idiopathic phenomenon in 20 to 30% of cases without any preceding dermatosis or systemic disease

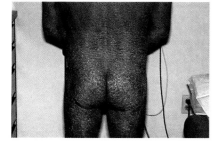

Figure 25.16.
Severe generalized exfoliative dermatitis (ED).

DESCRIPTION OF LESIONS

- Erythema followed by scaling (Figure 25.16)
- Pruritus
- Edema and increased warmth of skin
- Lymphadenopathy, usually a reactive type (dermatopathic lymphadenopathy)

DISTRIBUTION OF LESIONS

ED usually begins in a limited area; however, it may rapidly become generalized.

CLINICAL MANIFESTATIONS

- The course of ED depends on the underlying etiology. ED as a result of a drug eruption may clear in days to weeks, whereas, in some cases, the disease may persist for many years, with exacerbations and remissions and with no diagnosis ever having been made. The prognosis of acute, severe episodes, particularly in elderly persons or in persons with preexisting heart disease, is more guarded
- Unlike toxic epidermal necrolysis, ED spares mucous membranes. Unless there is a known preexisting skin condition or concurrent physical evidence of a skin disease such as psoriasis, the clinical appearance and symptoms of most cases of ED tend to be similar, consisting of the following.
  - Erythema may occur followed by scaling.
  - Pruritus may develop.
  - Edema and increased warmth of skin are usually present.
  - Lymphadenopathy, usually a reactive type (dermatopathic lymphadenopathy), secondary to the marked inflammatory changes in the skin may be seen; however, lymphoma should be considered, particularly if the nodes are large or unilateral.
  - Thermoregulatory disturbances manifested by fever or hypothermia. If widespread inflammation occurs, the barrier efficiency of the skin may be impaired secondary to extensive vasodilatation.
  - Protein loss secondary to a massive shedding of scale may occur, with resultant hypoalbuminemia.
  - Rarely, high-output cardiac failure may develop, particularly in patients with a history of cardiac disease.

Chronic changes
- Scaling of palms and soles (keratoderma)
- Thickening and lichenification of the skin
- Scalp involvement, occasionally producing a nonscarring alopecia
- Nail dystrophy, onycholysis (separation of the nail plate from the nail bed), or nail shedding
- Pigmentary changes (postinflammatory hypopigmentation or hyperpigmentation)
- Persistent generalized erythema
- Conjunctivitis, keratitis, or ectropion

DIAGNOSIS

- Diagnosis of ED is made on a **clinical basis**. Diagnosis of the underlying cause is often elusive. Clinical findings, such as the characteristic lichenification and crusting of atopic dermatitis or nail pitting that suggests psoriasis, may be found.
- Eliciting a **history** of drug ingestion or a preexisting dermatosis may be valuable.
- **Laboratory testing** can provide serologic evidence of Sézary syndrome or leukemia.
- **Patch testing** during a period of remission may uncover a contact allergen.

Histopathology

Histologic findings of the various etiologies are similar and are generally nondiagnostic; however, a diligent search for lymphoma, particularly mycosis fungoides, must be pursued with repeated skin biopsies.

Possible laboratory findings

- Anemia (usually the anemia of chronic disease)
- Decreased serum levels of protein and albumin
- Leukocytosis
- Eosinophilia
- Elevated sedimentation rate
- Elevated immunoglobulin E level (possibly supporting the diagnosis of atopic dermatitis)
- Leukemia (found by peripheral blood smear)

DIFFERENTIAL DIAGNOSIS

Toxic epidermal necrolysis in which the mucous membranes are usually involved

MANAGEMENT

(See Chapter 4, "Psoriasis.")

- **Treatment is directed toward the underlying cause**, if it is known. For example, suspected etiologic drugs or contactants should be eliminated.
- **Bed rest, cool compresses, lubrication with emollients, antipruritic therapy with oral antihistamines**, and low to intermediate strength **topical steroids** are used.
- In severe cases, the patient frequently requires hospitalization, where measures such as **fluid replacement, temperature control, expert topical skin care**, and **systemic corticosteroids** may be used.

Management of ED secondary to psoriasis

- **Avoidance** of possible precipitating factors (e.g., ultraviolet exposure) or avoidance of suspected drugs that may provoke ED (e.g., antimalarials).
- **Systemic and topical steroids** are helpful, except that they may worsen psoriasis and have been known to precipitate ED or an acute fulminant form of pustular psoriasis, which is known as pustular psoriasis of Von Zumbusch. This worsening of psoriasis tends to occur after rapid steroid withdrawal.
- If conservative therapy fails, **methotrexate, cyclosporine,** or **retinoids** (e.g., acitretin) are additional therapeutic options.

POINT TO REMEMBER

In its more severe manifestations, ED is a medical/dermatological emergency. Consultation and ongoing management, using the expertise of both disciplines, are often necessary.

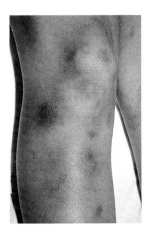

Figure 25.17.
Erythema nodosum (EN).
Red, tender nodules.

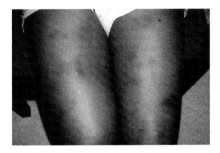

Figure 25.18.
Erythema nodosum (EN) "contusiform"
lesions.

BASICS

- Erythema nodosum (EN) is an acute inflammatory reaction of the subcutaneous fat.
- EN is three times more common in women than men and has a peak incidence between 20 and 30 years of age.
- Sarcoidosis, streptococcal infections, pregnancy, and the use of oral contraceptives are the most common causes of EN in the United States.
- In children, streptococcal pharyngitis is the most likely agent. Generally, EN indicates a better prognosis in patients who have sarcoidosis.
- EN is associated with a variety of agents and conditions: poststreptococcal; pregnancy; drugs, including oral contraceptives and sulfonamides; sarcoidosis; deep fungal infections (in endemic areas), including coccidioidomycosis, histoplasmosis, and blastomycosis; tuberculosis; *Yersinia enterocolitica*; inflammatory bowel disease, including ulcerative colitis and Crohn's disease; malignant disease, including lymphoma and leukemia; postradiation therapy; and Behçet's syndrome. Approximate 40% of cases are idiopathic.

DESCRIPTION OF LESIONS

- Lesions begin as bright-red, deep, tender nodules (Figure 25.17).
- During resolution, lesions become dark brown, violaceous, or bruiselike macules ("contusiform"; Figure 25.18).

DISTRIBUTION OF LESIONS

EN tends to occur in a bilateral distribution on the **anterior shins, thighs, knees, and arms**.

CLINICAL MANIFESTATIONS

- Malaise, fever, arthralgias, and ankle swelling may be present.
- Other symptoms, depending on the etiology of EN
- Spontaneous resolution of lesions in 3 to 6 weeks, regardless of the underlying cause

DIAGNOSIS

Diagnosis is generally made on **clinical grounds**.

Laboratory evaluations
- Usually, a **complete blood count, erythrocyte sedimentation rate, throat culture, antistreptolysin titer, purified protein derivative skin test,** and **chest film** are all that are necessary.
- Further tests, such as gastrointestinal tract evaluation and serum angiotensin-converting enzyme can be performed if suggested by the review of systems and physical examination.

MANAGEMENT

- **Treatment is symptomatic**, consisting of bed rest, leg elevation, NSAIDs, or iodides (SSKI).
- **Systemic corticosteroids**, which often bring dramatic improvement, can be used if an infectious cause is excluded.
- Treatment or avoidance of the underlying etiology, if discovered, should be attempted.

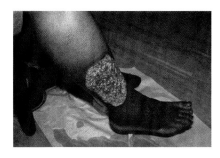

Figure 25.19.
Pyoderma gangrenosum (PG). Lesion beginning to heal with craterlike (cribriform) scar.

BASICS

Pyoderma gangrenosum (PG) is a painful, inflammatory, ulcerative process of the skin. It is often seen in association with a number of systemic diseases; however, it is believed to be a distinct disease by some authors.

DESCRIPTION OF LESIONS

- PG skin ulcers are 2 to 10 cm in diameter.
- They are deep ulcerations with an erythematous to violaceous border. The border is often undermined (a probe can be placed under the overhanging edge of the lesion).
- Lesions may be multiple.
- Lesions heal with scarring (Figure 25.19).

DISTRIBUTION OF LESIONS

PG skin ulcers are most commonly found on the **lower extremities** (pretibial and ankles).

CLINICAL MANIFESTATIONS

- PG lesions can appear as a rapidly expanding, painful, skin ulcer.
- There is often an associated oligoarticular arthritis.
- Diseases associated with PG include the following:
  - Ulcerative colitis
  - Regional enteritis (Crohn's disease)
  - Rheumatoid arthritis
  - Myelogenous leukemia
  - Myeloma (IgA)
- Fifty percent of patients with PG do not have an underlying systemic disease.

DIAGNOSIS

Diagnosis of PG is made by **clinical evaluation** and by **ruling out other causes** of skin ulcers, such as stasis ulcers and carcinoma.

Laboratory evaluations

- **Skin biopsy** of the edge of the ulcer may be performed to rule out other causes of skin ulcers, such as infections or malignancy; however, the pathological findings for PG are nonspecific.
- **Bacterial, fungal,** and **viral cultures** of the ulcer are performed if clinically indicated.
- **Workup for systemic disease** should include complete blood count with differential, sedimentation rate, sequential multichannel autoanalyzer (SMA) 20, ANA, rheumatoid factor, and chest film.
- A **gastrointestinal series** for inflammatory bowel disease should be performed if clinically indicated.

DIFFERENTIAL DIAGNOSIS

Cutaneous malignancies
- Basal cell carcinoma
- Squamous cell carcinoma

Infectious processes
- Bacterial infections
- Deep fungal infections
- Herpes simplex infections

Inflammatory processes
- Collagen vascular diseases
- Polyarteritis nodosa
- Behçet's disease

MANAGEMENT

- **Local compresses, antiseptic washes,** and **topical antibiotics** may be used on the ulcer.
- **Oral steroids** may be administered for several weeks to several months (starting at 60 to 80 mg of prednisone daily, tapering the steroid slowly). They may be administered alone or in combination with dapsone, azathioprine, or chlorambucil. In patients with steroid-resistant PG, oral cyclosporine has been proven to be effective.
- **Intralesional steroid injections** (triamcinolone acetonide 10 mg/ml) should be administered into the edge of the ulcer.
- Diagnosis and **treatment of underlying associated diseases** does not necessarily promote the healing of PG.

BASICS

- Systemic lupus erythematosus (SLE) is a chronic, idiopathic, **multisystem, autoimmune disease**. Fibrinoid degeneration of connective tissue and the walls of blood vessels associated with an inflammatory infiltrate involving various organs may result in arthralgia or arthritis, kidney disease, liver disease, CNS disease, gastrointestinal disease, pericarditis, pneumonitis, myopathy, splenomegaly, and skin disease.
- The cutaneous manifestations of SLE result from the production of multiple autoantibodies that deposit immune complexes at the dermal–epidermal junction.
- SLE is seen in a 9:1 female to male ratio; it is more common in blacks and Hispanics.
- Approximately 10% of patients with SLE have a first-degree relative with the disease.
- An SLE-like syndrome can be induced by certain drugs (hydralazine, procainamide, phenytoin, INH (isoniazid), sulfonamides, and methyldopa).

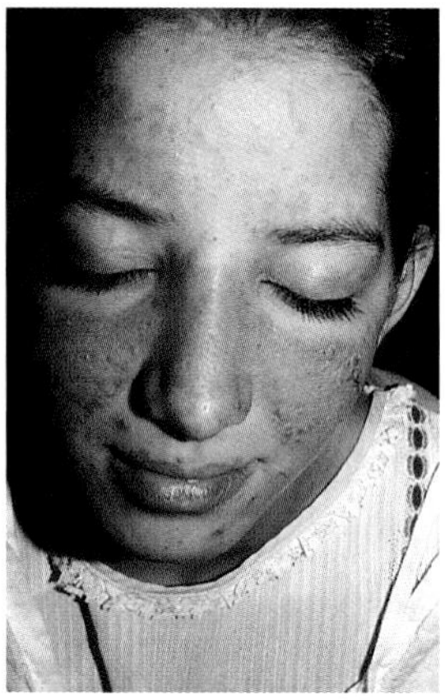

DESCRIPTION OF LESIONS

- Four of the eleven American Rheumatologic Association criteria for SLE are related to the skin and are **lupus specific**:
  - The classic **malar, or "butterfly rash"** (Figure 25.20)
    - Persistent **erythema over the cheeks** tends to spare the nasolabial creases.
    - Sometimes, this is the initial symptom of lupus, often occurring after sun exposure.
  - **Photosensitivity** (Figure 25.21)
    - Photosensitivity occurs as an exaggerated or unusual reaction to sunlight.
    - The reaction may resemble a drug eruption.
  - **Discoid lesions** (chronic cutaneous lupus erythematosus [CCLE]; Figure 25.22)
    - Erythematous plaques evolve into scaly, atrophic scarring plaques.
    - Discoid lesions affect 10 to 15% of patients with SLE.
  - **Oral ulcerations** (Figure 25.23) develop, often on the hard palate or nasopharynx (see Chapter 12, "Disorders of the Mouth, Lips, and Tongue?")
- **Lupus-nonspecific lesions** that may be seen in SLE and other connective tissue diseases include the following:
  - **Telangiectasias**
    - Macular (matlike) telangiectasias that usually occur more often in scleroderma
    - Periungual telangiectasias are seen in dermatomyositis, scleroderma, and SLE.
    - Palmar type are usually seen in SLE.
  - **Vasculitis, palpable purpura,** and **vasculitic ulcers** may occur in SLE and scleroderma.
  - **Raynaud's phenomenon** is associated with scleroderma and SLE.
  - Livedo reticulitis, panniculitis, thrombophlebitis, urticaria, urticarial vasculitis, frontal ("lupus hair") or diffuse nonscarring alopecia, palmar erythema, and bullae are each associated primarily with SLE.

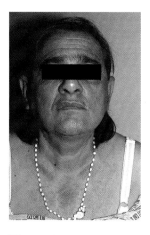

Figure 25.20.
Systemic lupus erythematosus (SLE). "Butterfly rash." Note sparing of the nasolabial creases.

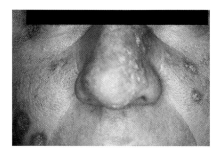

Figure 25.21.
Systemic lupus erythematosus (SLE). Photodistribution at "V" of the neck. Note violaceous color that is suggestive of connective tissue disease.

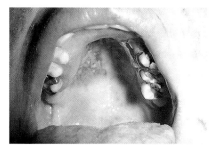

Figure 25.22.
Discoid lesions (chronic cutaneous lupus erythematosus [CCLE]). Erythematous, scaly, disc-shaped plaques.

Figure 25.23.
Systemic lupus erythematosus (SLE). Oral ulcerations on hard palate.

DISTRIBUTION OF LESIONS

- Lesions tend to occur in **sun-exposed areas** such as the face, dorsa of the forearms, hands, and "V" of the neck.
- CCLE (discoid LE) lesions may be on the **head, neck,** or **oral mucosa** or be **widespread**.
- On the **lower extremity**, livedo reticularis (Figure 25.24) and vasculitic ulcers (Figure 25.25) may be seen.
- On the **hands**, violaceous plaques that spare the skin overlying the joints are characteristic of SLE; whereas the skin over the joints is affected in dermatomyositis.
- Also on the **hands,** periungual telangiectasias, palmar erythema (Figure 25.26), palmar telangiectasias, and ulcerated vasculitic lesions on the fingertips (Figure 25.27) may be seen.

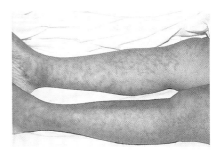

Figure 25.24.
Systemic lupus erythematosus (SLE). Livedo reticularis.

CLINICAL MANIFESTATIONS

- Fatigue, fever, or malaise may be the presenting nonspecific symptoms.
- Eighty-five percent of patients have one or more cutaneous problems.
- Signs or symptoms are related to the specific organ involved (e.g., arthralgia).
- Flare of lupus is common during pregnancy.
- The following hematologic abnormalities may be associated with systemic lupus: idiopathic thrombocytopenic purpura (ITP); hemolytic anemia; leukopenia; clotting abnormalities, which may be related to the anticardiolipin syndrome; rheumatoid arthritis; Sjögren's syndrome; seizures; and multiple chronic spontaneous abortions.

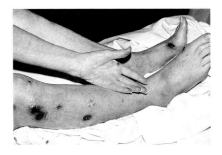

Figure 25.25.
Vasculitic ulcers on the legs.

DIAGNOSIS

- Diagnosis is based on **clinical features**.
- **Biopsy** of a lesion shows atrophy, liquefaction degeneration, edema, lymphocytic infiltrate, and fibrinoid degeneration of blood vessel walls and connective tissue.

Laboratory evaluations

- ANA titers are positive in 95% of patients with SLE.
- Anti-dsDNA (antibody to native double-stranded DNA) is present in 60 to 80% of patients and is more specific for SLE.
- Affected patients have anti-Sm antibody.
- Antiphospholipid antibodies are present in 25% of patients.
- The erythrocyte sedimentation rate is elevated.
- Hypocomplementemia occurs in 70% of patients and is noted especially when there is renal involvement.
- The lupus band test (LBT) involves the direct immunofluorescence of uninvolved, non–sun-exposed skin. When positive, it is suggestive of the presence of renal disease. The LBT has been largely supplanted by the aforementioned serologic tests.

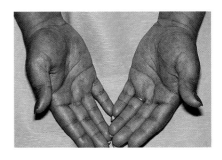

Figure 25.26.
Palmar erythema.

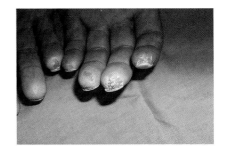

Figure 25.27.
Vasculitic lesions on fingertips.

DIFFERENTIAL DIAGNOSIS

- **Rosacea**
  - Presence of papules and pustules
  - No systemic symptoms
  - Negative ANA titers
- **Seborrheic dermatitis**
  - Responds readily to topical steroids
  - No systemic symptoms
  - Negative ANA titers
- **Other connective tissue diseases**
- **Other photosensitivity conditions**, such as polymorphous light eruption
- **Other causes for renal, hematologic, and CNS diseases**

MANAGEMENT

Management of sun-related symptoms
- Avoidance of sun exposure
- Use of broad-spectrum sunscreens (see Appendix 2)

Management of CCLE, mucosal, and alopecic lesions
- Topical or intralesional steroids
- Antimalarials hydroxychloroquine (Plaquenil) and chloroquine

Management of severely ill patients
- Systemic steroids
- Immunosuppressive drugs, such as azathioprine and cyclophosphamide

---

- According to the American Rheumatologic Association, a person has SLE if four or more of the following criteria are present:
  1. "Butterfly" rash
  2. CCLE (discoid LE) lesions
  3. Photosensitivity
  4. Oral ulcers
  5. Arthritis in two or more joints
  6. Serositis
  7. Renal disorder
  8. Neurologic disorder
  9. Hematologic disorder
  10. Immunologic disorder: anti-DNA, anti-Smith antibody, or a false biologic-positive syphilis serologic result
  11. ANAs
- **Lupus nonspecific lesions** such as telangiectasias, palmar erythema, vasculitis, Raynaud's phenomenon, livedo reticulitis, panniculitis, thrombophlebitis, and urticaria may also be seen in the absence of, or be precursors to, a connective tissue disease.

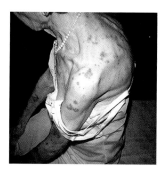

Figure 25.28.
Subacute lupus erythematosus (SCLE). (Courtesy of Herbert A. Hochman, MD)

BASICS

- Subacute lupus erythematosus (SCLE) tends to be **less severe than SLE** and rarely progresses to renal or CNS involvement.
- SCLE occurs most commonly in young and middle-age white women.
- Patients may have some of the American Rheumatologic Association criteria for SLE, but serious disease is uncommon.

DESCRIPTION OF LESIONS (Figure 25.28)

- Lesions are papulosquamous and closely resemble psoriasis or pityriasis rosea.
- Lesions are often annular and heal without scarring.

DISTRIBUTION OF LESIONS

There is a **photodistribution** of lesions on the upper trunk, "V" of the neck, and extensor surfaces of the arms and hands.

DIAGNOSIS

- **Anti-SS-A** (anti-Ro) and **anti-SS-B** (anti-La) **antibodies** are often found. (The absence of these antibodies does not exclude the diagnosis.)
- **Low titers of ANA** may be present.

CLINICAL MANIFESTATIONS

- Fatigue, malaise, and arthralgias
- Dry eyes and dry mouth

DIFFERENTIAL DIAGNOSIS

- Psoriasis
- Pityriasis rosea

MANAGEMENT

- **Avoidance of sun exposure** and the use of broad-spectrum sunscreens (see Appendix 2)
- **Topical steroids**
- **Antimalarials**
- **Dapsone, gold, retinoids, thalidomide,** and **immunosuppressive drugs**

POINTS TO REMEMBER

- Patients with SCLE have a better prognosis than patients with SLE.
- All patients with SCLE should be monitored for systemic disease.

CHRONIC CUTANEOUS LUPUS ERYTHEMATOSUS (DISCOID LE)

BASICS

- Chronic cutaneous lupus erythematosus (CCLE) consists of scarring plaques.
- Only 10% of patients with CCLE are estimated to have SLE.
- If the initial workup of patients who present solely with localized lesions of CCLE shows no evidence of SLE, then those patients are considered to have a low risk (approximately 5%) of development of SLE.
- CCLE lesions develop in approximately 25% of patients with SLE at some time in the course of their disease.

DESCRIPTION OF LESIONS

- Lesions begin as well-defined erythematous plaques that evolve into atrophic disc-shaped plaques, characterized by scale, accentuated hair follicles, follicular plugging, and a combination of hypopigmentation and hyperpigmentation.
- Lesions may become hypertrophic (hypertrophic CCLE).
- CCLE typically involves the scalp, producing a scarring alopecia (Figure 25.29).

DISTRIBUTION OF LESIONS

- CCLE may be **localized** to the face, external ears, and scalp or **widespread** with lesions below the neck (Figure 25.30).
- **CCLE variant** is **lupus panniculitis** (lupus profundus), an inflammation of subcutaneous tissue.

CLINICAL MANIFESTATIONS

- CCLE is generally asymptomatic.
- It may itch or be tender.
- Rarely, squamous cell carcinoma develops in hypertrophic chronic CCLE lesions.

DIAGNOSIS

Clinical appearance is confirmed by a **punch biopsy** of the skin.

DIFFERENTIAL DIAGNOSIS

- Sarcoidosis
- Lichen planus
- Psoriasis
- Tinea corporis

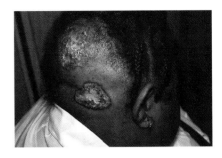

Figure 25.29.
Chronic cutaneous lupus erythematosus (CCLE). Scarring alopecia.

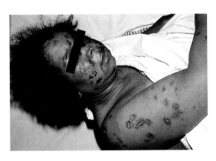

Figure 25.30.
Chronic cutaneous lupus erythematosus (CCLE). Widespread lesions.

MANAGEMENT

- Avoidance of sun exposure
- Use of broad-spectrum sunscreens (see Appendix 2)
- Potent topical steroids
- Intralesional steroid injections in CCLE lesions that are resistant to topical therapy
- Antimalarials hydroxychloroquine (Plaquenil) and chloroquine, dapsone, immunosuppressive agents, oral retinoids, thalidomide, and tetracycline or erythromycin combined with niacinamide

POINT TO REMEMBER

Most patients with CCLE do not have SLE. Even so, many patients having been given the diagnosis of CCLE describe themselves as having "lupus" and are convinced that they have the more serious disease.

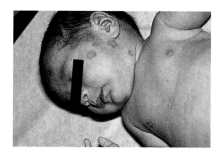

Figure 25.31.
Neonatal lupus erythematosus (NLE).
Annular erythematous plaques look like
"ringworm."

BASICS

- Neonatal lupus erythematosus (NLE) is a **rare autoimmune syndrome** that affects 1 to 2% of infants born of mothers who are anti-Ro (SS-A) antibody positive.
- Mothers may show any of the signs or symptoms of connective tissue disease at the time of birth of the affected infant; however, some features of Sjögren's syndrome or lupus erythematosus (e.g., dry mouth, dry eyes, arthralgias) ultimately develop in the majority of these women. This may occur many years after the birth of the child; however, in most of these women, SLE does not develop.

DESCRIPTION OF LESIONS

- The rash of NLE is a benign, self-limited eruption that appears at birth and tends to disappear by approximately 6 months of age.
- The rash is characterized by annular (ringlike) erythematous plaques or smaller erythematous patches that generally occur at birth or several days after birth (Figure 25.31).

CLINICAL MANIFESTATIONS

- NLE is characterized by either benign skin disease or congenital heart block, or both, in approximately 10% of the cases.

- Involvement of joints, kidneys, and CNS is rare, and the criteria of the American Rheumatologic Association for SLE are not fulfilled.
- **Congenital heart block**, which is complete in 90% of patients, presents a 20% mortality risk and often requires the insertion of a pacemaker. The onset of heart block generally occurs a few weeks before term and is seen at birth.
- Unlike the skin lesions, the cardiac problems associated with NLE are permanent.

MANAGEMENT

Cutaneous manifestations
- Low-potency, nonfluorinated **topical steroids**
- Avoidance of sun exposure

Heart block
- Experimental therapy using **dexamethasone**, which crosses the placental barrier, has been used to treat heart block in utero with minimal success.
- **Pacemaker** implantation is frequently required.

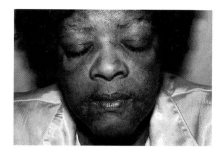

Figure 25.32.
Dermatomyosis. Heliotrope rash around the eyes associated with periorbital edema.

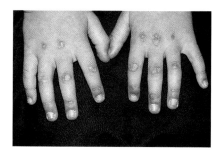

Figure 25.33.
Dermatomyosis. Gottron's papules; violaceous flat-topped papules located on the joints of the fingers.

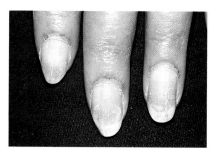

Figure 25.34.
Dermatomyosis. Periungual telangiectasias.

BASICS

- Dermatomyositis is an **inflammatory skin and muscle disease** that is related to polymyositis; in fact, both conditions are considered to be the same disease except for the presence or absence of the rash.
- The female to male ratio is 2:1.
- An autoimmune etiology, which may be initiated by a virus in genetically susceptible people, has been proposed as a possible cause of dermatomyositis. As a result, antibodies that attack the skin and muscle are produced.
- An overlap syndrome with scleroderma or lupus **(mixed connective tissue disease)** is characterized by the presence of anti-ribonucleoprotein (anti-RNP) antibodies.
- Adults with dermatomyositis appear to have an **increased risk of malignancies.** The skin disease often follows the clinical course of exacerbations and remissions of the cancer. Most malignancies are the common cancers (e.g., colon cancer, breast cancer) that are expected in a general aging population.
- Skin without detectable muscle disease is known as **amyopathic dermatomyositis.**

DESCRIPTION OF LESIONS

- The **heliotrope rash** consists of a red or violaceous coloration around the eyes and is associated with periorbital edema (Figure 25.32). (The change in color may be a subtle clinical finding, particularly in dark-skinned patients.)
- **Gottron's papules** consist of erythematous or violaceous flat-topped papules on the dorsa of the hands (Figure 25.33). Lesions are located on the **joints of the fingers**; they begin as papules and later become atrophic and hypopigmented.
- **Poikiloderma** is a characteristic rash of dermatomyositis, consisting of telangiectasia, atrophy, hyperpigmentation and hypopigmentation.
- **Periungual telangiectasias** is shown in Figure 25.34.
- **Calcinosis cutis** is seen in the juvenile form of dermatomyositis.

DISTRIBUTION OF LESIONS

- Poikiloderma occurs on the **extensor aspects** of the body, **upper back, forearms,** and **"V" of the neck.** Atrophic lesions occur particularly on the **knees** and **elbows.**
- Gottron's papules occur on the **dorsum of the hands,** involving the knuckles (SLE spares the knuckles).
- Periungual telangiectasias are noted on the **proximal nail folds.**
- Heliotrope rash occurs in the **periorbital area.**

CLINICAL MANIFESTATIONS

- Progressive, bilateral, symmetrical, proximal muscle weakness develops, as suggested by difficulty brushing or combing hair and standing from a seated position.
- Muscle tenderness or pain is usually not a symptom.
- Photosensitivity is evidenced in areas of poikiloderma.
- Arthralgias occur in 33% of patients.
- There may be possible features of an overlap syndrome.
- Pulmonary fibrosis affects 10% of patients, particularly in the presence of anti-Jo 1 or anti-PL 12 antibodies.
- Vasculitis may be seen.
- Myocardial disease may be an associated finding.
- Dysphagia may occur.

DIAGNOSIS

- **Skin biopsy** is often nonspecific but generally suggestive of a connective tissue disease.
- **Increase of creatine phosphokinase levels** is often a reliable indicator of muscle disease activity.
- **Aldolase levels** may be also increased.
- **Electromyography** may aid in diagnosis.
- **Muscle biopsy** may aid as well.
- **Autoantibodies,** such as anti-DNA, anti-RNP, and anti-Ro, may be found.

DIFFERENTIAL DIAGNOSIS

- SLE
- Mixed connective tissue disease or overlap syndrome
- Other myopathies, when only the muscle is involved

MANAGEMENT

Skin
- Avoidance of sun exposure
- Use of broad-spectrum sunscreens (see Appendix 2)
- Antimalarial drugs
- Low-dose oral methotrexate

Systemic symptoms
- Physical therapy
- Systemic steroids (when used for systemic symptoms, may also improve skin conditions)
- Immunosuppressive therapy, including low-dose oral methotrexate
- Intravenous high-dose γ-globulin

POINT TO REMEMBER

The adult form of dermatomyositis may be associated with internal malignancies; patients older than age 50 years should be evaluated for the evidence of malignancy.

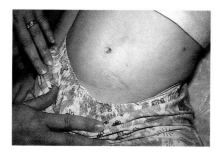

Figure 25.35.
Morphea. Ivory-colored plaque with a "lilac" border.

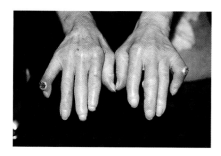

Figure 25.36.
Scleroderma. Tapered shiny, stiff, waxy fingers. Note vasculitic ulcers.

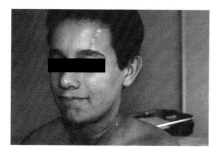

Figure 25.37.
Morphea. En coup de sabre.

BASICS

- Scleroderma is an **autoimmune connective tissue disease** in which excess collagen results from an increase in number and activity of fibroblasts. Induration and thickening of the skin result.
- Microvasculature abnormalities and inflammation also occur and result in the obliteration of vessels in the skin, kidneys, heart, lungs, and gastrointestinal system.
- The etiology of scleroderma is unknown. As in lupus, scleroderma may be seen either in a systemic or localized cutaneous form.
  - **Localized scleroderma**, or **morphea**, is limited to the skin and has rarely been reported to progress to systemic scleroderma. The female to male ratio is 3:1.
  - **Systemic scleroderma** may be divided into:
    - **CREST syndrome**, which accounts for 90% of the cases of systemic sclerosis, is a relatively benign variant with a delayed appearance of visceral involvement.
    - Progressive systemic sclerosis (PSS) is a chronic multisystem disease that affects the skin and internal organs and has a poor prognosis.
    - In systemic sclerosis, there is a female to male ratio of 4:1.

DESCRIPTION OF LESIONS

Morphea
- Localized, indurated, hairless plaque with a characteristic "lilac" border (Figure 25.35)
- Single or multiple
- White, ivory, or hyperpigmented permanent scars from healed lesions

CREST syndrome and PSS
- Acrosclerosis, or ill-defined, indurated fibrotic skin, which occurs peripherally and gradually involves the forearms
- Sclerodactyly, which is thickened, sausage-shaped digits in which the skin becomes tight and bound down. Gradually, the skin becomes shiny, stiff, waxy, and atrophic (Figure 25.36).

DISTRIBUTION OF LESIONS

- In **morphea**, lesions are commonly found on the **trunk**; they may become widespread (**generalized morphea**), linear (**linear morphea**), or have the characteristic frontoparietal distribution (**en coup de sabre**; Figure 25.37).
- In **CREST syndrome**, the cutaneous involvement is usually limited to **acral areas** (hands, feet, face, and forearms).
- In **PSS**, there is often **widespread**, progressive disease.

CLINICAL MANIFESTATIONS

- **Morphea** (localized scleroderma) is generally asymptomatic, usually "burning out" spontaneously and leaving a scar.
- **CREST syndrome** consists of the following:
  - *C*alcinosis cutis, most commonly occurring on the palms, fingertips, and bony prominences
  - *R*aynaud's phenomenon
  - *E*sophageal dysfunction
  - *S*clerodactyly ("claw deformity")
  - *T*elangiectasia (macular lesions) on the face, lips, palms, back of hands, and trunk

- **PSS** manifestations include the following:
  - Raynaud's phenomenon is often an early symptom, consisting of pain and a characteristic sequence of color changes of the distal fingers from white to purple to red in response to cold exposure.
  - There is diffuse involvement and symptoms secondary to the tightening of the skin, with difficulty opening the mouth and loss of manual dexterity; later, there are contractures of the hands, painful fingertip ulcers resulting from vasculitis, and shortening of fingers resulting from distal bone resorption (Figure 25.38).
  - Esophageal dysfunction, dysphagia, bloating, and diarrhea occur.
  - Systemic symptoms include shortness of breath, difficulty in swallowing, and arthralgia.
  - There is a masklike facies.
  - Rapid progression of kidney disease, reduced breathing capacity, cardiac disease, and renal failure are possible.

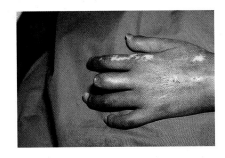

Figure 25.38.
Scleroderma. Note shortened finger resulting from distal bone resorption.

DIAGNOSIS

Morphea
- Diagnosis is generally made on **clinical grounds** and **skin biopsy**.
- Serology is generally negative.

CREST syndrome
- Diagnosis is generally made on **clinical grounds**.
- Positive **anticentromere antibody** is seen in 70% of patients.

PSS
- Diagnosis is generally made on **clinical grounds**.
- **Scl-70** is present in approximately 30% of patients.

DIFFERENTIAL DIAGNOSIS

- Other connective tissue diseases
- Mixed connective tissue disease
- Overlap syndromes

MANAGEMENT

- Treatment is mainly **symptomatic**.
- There is **no effective treatment for morphea**.
- CREST syndrome and PSS are difficult to treat. The following agents have been used with little success:
  - Systemic steroids
  - D-penicillamine
  - Immunosuppressive drugs
  - Photopheresis

POINTS TO REMEMBER

- CREST syndrome has a more favorable prognosis than PSS, although visceral involvement may occur late in the course of the disease.
- Therapy for systemic scleroderma should include full range-of-motion exercises.
- There is some evidence that some European cases of morphea may be the result of *Borrelia burgdorferi* infection. This has not been demonstrated in the United States.

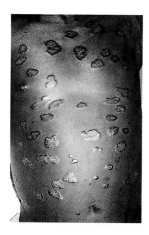

Figure 25.39.
Cutaneous sarcoidosis. Widespread, darkly pigmented dermal plaques.

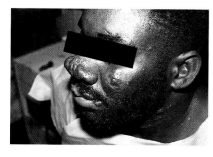

Figure 25.40.
Cutaneous sarcoidosis. Dermal nodules in a periorificial distribution (i.e., around mouth, eyes, and nares). Note sarcoidal lesions arising in scars of the neck.

BASICS

- Sarcoidosis is an example of a systemic disease in which cellular granulomatous infiltrates produce dermal skin lesions.
- Sarcoidosis is a chronic multisystem disease of unknown etiology. Most often it presents with bilateral hilar adenopathy, pulmonary infiltration, eye lesions, and arthralgias; less commonly, there is involvement of the spleen and salivary and lacrimal glands as well as gastrointestinal and cardiac manifestations.
- Sarcoidosis is seen most commonly in young adults, particularly in blacks in the United States and South Africa. It is also more common in Scandinavians.
- Of patients with sarcoidosis, 20 to 35% have cutaneous involvement.

DESCRIPTION OF LESIONS

Specific lesions of cutaneous sarcoid

- Dermal papules, nodules, or plaques that are brown or violaceous in color (Figure 25.39)
- Annular, serpiginous, or atrophic lesions
- Lupus pernio, which consists of reddish-purple plaques around the nose, ears, lips, and face (Figure 25.40)
- Subcutaneous nodules (Darier-Roussy nodules)

Nonspecific cutaneous lesions associated with sarcoid

- EN in acute sarcoidosis (see the section on "Erythema Nodosum" in this chapter)
- Ichthyosis

DISTRIBUTION OF LESIONS

- Lesions may appear **periorificial** (e.g., around the eyelids, nasal ala, tip of nose, earlobes, lips).
- They can also appear in old **scars** anywhere on the body.
- Scalp lesions may produce a scarring alopecia.
- Ichthyosiform and EN lesions may appear on the **pretibial area**.

CLINICAL MANIFESTATIONS

- Skin lesions are generally asymptomatic; however, they are often of great cosmetic concern because they occur commonly on the face.
- EN associated with sarcoidosis generally resolves spontaneously and suggests a better prognosis.

CLINICAL VARIANTS

- **Löfgren's syndrome** (EN and arthritis)
- **Heerford syndrome** (fever, parotitis, uveitis, and facial nerve palsy)

DIAGNOSIS

- "Apple jelly" nodules are seen upon **blanching lesions** with a glass slide (diascopy) (Figure 25.41).
- **Skin biopsy** demonstrates noncaseating granulomas.
- Chest film demonstrates **bilateral hilar adenopathy** and other characteristic changes.

Laboratory evaluations
- Elevated angiotensin-converting enzyme (ACE) levels
- Hypergammaglobulinemia
- Hypercalcemia

DIFFERENTIAL DIAGNOSIS

- Granuloma annulare (see Chapter 5 "Eruptions of Unknown Cause")
- Cutaneous tuberculosis (lupus vulgaris)

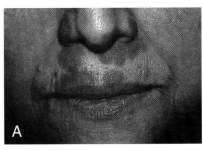

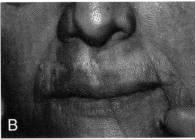

Figure 25.41.
(*A*) Cutaneous sarcoidosis. Reddish-violaceous plaques (*B*) that display an "apple jelly" coloration upon diascopy performed with a glass slide.

MANAGEMENT

- Potent **topical steroids**; occlusion, if necessary
- **Intralesional steroid injections**
- Oral **antimalarial agents** for unresponsive or widespread disease
- **Prednisone**, short-term
- Low-dose **methotrexate**

POINTS TO REMEMBER

- Systemic steroids should not be routinely used to treat cutaneous lesions; rather, potent topical steroids, intralesional steroids, or oral antimalarials should be tried first. If possible, systemic steroids are best reserved for more serious systemic involvement.
- Oral antimalarials can lead to irreversible retinopathy and blindness. **Eye examination** is necessary before and during therapy.

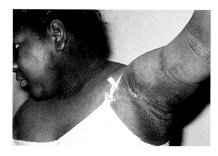

Figure 25.42.
Acanthosis nigricans (AN). Widespread black, leathery plaques.

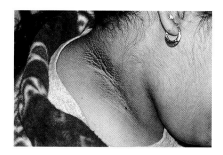

Figure 25.43.
Acanthosis nigricans (AN). Linear, alternating dark and light pigmentation that becomes more apparent when the skin is stretched.

BASICS

- Acanthosis nigricans (AN) is a characteristic **hyperpigmented skin pattern** that occurs primarily in flexural folds. The skin is thought to darken and thicken as a reactive phenomenon to a circulating growth factor or factors.
- AN is best understood when divided into two main groups: **benign** and **malignant**.
- Most cases of AN are of the benign variety, which includes idiopathic AN and AN associated with obesity. AN can be seen in endocrinologic disorders such as insulin-resistant diabetes, Stein-Leventhal syndrome, Cushing's disease, Addison's disease, pituitary tumors, pinealomas, and hyperandrogenic syndromes with insulin resistance. AN is sometimes drug-related, most commonly secondary to glucocorticoid, nicotinic acid, diethylstilbestrol, or growth hormone therapy. AN may also be inherited without any disease associations.
- Malignant AN is associated with an internal malignancy, usually an intraabdominal adenocarcinoma. These patients generally have a poor prognosis. Malignant AN is sometimes seen before the onset of the cancer and can be associated with recurrences and metastases.

DESCRIPTION OF LESIONS

- AN generally presents with a gradual evolution of symmetric tan or brown to black leathery or velvety plaques (Figure 25.42). The plaques are sometimes "warty" (papillomatous) and studded with skin tags.
- Linear alternating dark and light pigmentation becomes more apparent when the skin is stretched (Figure 25.43).

DISTRIBUTION OF LESIONS

- The most common sites of involvement are the **axilla, base of the neck, inframammary folds, inguinal areas,** and the **antecubital fossa**.
- The **dorsum of the hands** (especially on knuckles), **elbows,** and **knees** are also common locations.
- Less commonly, **mucous membranes**, the **vermilion border** of the lips, and the **eyelids** can be involved.

CLINICAL MANIFESTATIONS

Lesions are asymptomatic; they are primarily a cosmetic liability.

DIAGNOSIS

Diagnosis is made on a **clinical basis**.

DIFFERENTIAL DIAGNOSIS

There is little confusion with other disorders.

MANAGEMENT

Treatment is generally not effective. However, several patients with AN were placed on a ketogenic diet, which resulted in a resolution of their lesions.

 POINT TO REMEMBER

Malignant AN generally has a sudden onset but is otherwise clinically similar in appearance to benign AN. An instance of greatest concern is when AN suddenly arises in a nonobese adult with no family history of AN.

LIPID ABNORMALITIES

Lipid abnormalities are manifested in the skin as depositional disorders characterized by skin lesions that are produced by materials or cells deposited in the skin secondary to a systemic disease. Metabolic diseases such as lipid disorders may cause deposition of cholesterol and other lipids in the skin producing **xanthomas**.

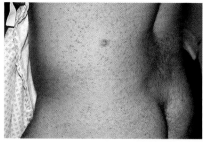

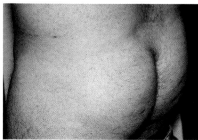

Figure 25.44.
Eruptive xanthomas. (*A*) Patient is a 28-year-old man with a triglyceride level of 31,000 and cholesterol level of 580. (*B*) Same patient after 2 months of a low-fat diet and the cholesterol-lowering drug, gemfibrozil.

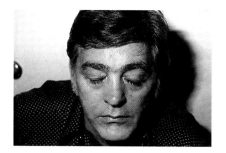

Figure 25.45.
Xanthelasma. Periorbital yellow–orange plaques.

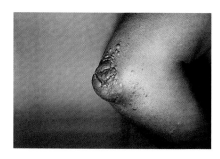

Figure 25.46.
Tuberous xanthomas.

BASICS

- Abnormalities of lipid metabolism, with high circulating levels of various lipoproteins, can result in **deposition of cholesterol and other lipids in the skin, tendons, and other organs**.
- Xanthomas result from the deposition of cholesterol and other lipids found in histiocytes in the skin and tendons. There is also a high correlation between lipoproteinemia and the development of atherosclerosis.
- Lipoprotein abnormalities have been classified into **primary (genetic) lipoproteinemia** and **secondary lipoproteinemia** resulting from underlying diseases.
  - Primary lipoproteinemias are genetic disorders of the lipid metabolism with the following characteristics:
    - Type I familial lipoprotein lipase deficiency: elevated chylomicrons
    - Type II-a familial hypercholesterolemia: elevated low-density lipoproteins (LDLs)
    - Type II-b familial hyperlipidemia: elevated LDLs and very-low-density lipoproteins (VLDLs)
    - Type III familial dysbetalipoproteinemia: elevated (intermediate-density lipoproteins [IDLs])
    - Type IV endogenous familial hypertriglyceridemia: elevated triglycerides
    - Type V familial combined hyperlipidemia: elevated chylomicrons and elevated VLDLs
  - Secondary hyperlipoproteinemias result from disturbances in cholesterol and triglyceride metabolism caused by cholestatic liver disease, diabetes mellitus, pancreatitis, multiple myeloma, and nephrotic syndrome. These disorders may mimic any of the genetic lipoprotein abnormalities and may produce similar xanthomatous deposits in tissues.

DESCRIPTION OF LESIONS

- **Eruptive xanthomas** are smooth, yellow, papular lesions (2 to 5 mm). There is sometimes a red halo around the lesions (Figure 25.44).
- **Planar xanthomas** are flat to slightly palpable yellow lesions.
- **Xanthelasma** (xanthoma palpebrarum) is a form of planar xanthoma (Figure 25.45).
- **Tuberous xanthomas** are small (0.5 cm) to large (3 to 5 cm) firm yellow papules and nodules (Figure 25.46).
- **Tendinous xanthomas** are subcutaneous thickening of tendons and ligaments.

DISTRIBUTION OF LESIONS

- Eruptive xanthomas appear most frequently over the **knees, elbows**, and **buttocks**.
- Planar xanthomas are found in the **palmar creases** but may also be **generalized**.
- Xanthelasma lesions are usually found on the **eyelids** and **medial canthus**.
- Tuberous xanthomas are found on the **elbows, knees**, and **buttocks**.
- Tendinous xanthomas affect the **Achilles tendon, extensor tendons** of the wrists, elbows, and knees.

CLINICAL MANIFESTATIONS

- **Eruptive xanthomas** appear suddenly over the extensor surfaces and pressure points. These lesions are usually seen in association with high levels of triglycerides (2000 to 4000 mg/dl). Uncontrolled DM is a common underlying cause of eruptive xanthomas, and pancreatitis is a possible complication of hypertriglyceridemia.

- **Planar xanthomas** are usually asymptomatic. Palmar xanthomas are seen with type III lipoproteinemia. Diffuse planar xanthomas are found in patients with multiple myeloma.
- **Xanthelasma** lesions grow slowly over years. More than 50% of patients with xanthelasma have normal lipoprotein levels.
- **Tuberous xanthomas** also are slow growing. They are associated with familial hypercholesterolemia but can also occur in patients with high triglyceride levels.
- **Tendinous xanthomas** occur in patients with hypercholesterolemias.

DIAGNOSIS

- Diagnosis is made by **clinical evaluation** of skin and subcutaneous lesions.
- **Skin biopsy** is confirmatory for xanthomas.

Laboratory evaluations
- Fasting blood levels of triglycerides and cholesterol should be determined.
- Lipoprotein electrophoresis demonstrates specific lipoprotein abnormalities.
- Skin biopsy of xanthomas demonstrates collections of lipids in foamy histiocytes in the dermis.
- Blood glucose levels rule out diabetes mellitus.
- Serum amylase levels rule out pancreatitis.
- Serum protein electrophoresis rules out multiple myeloma.

DIFFERENTIAL DIAGNOSIS

- **Eruptive xanthomas** must be differentiated from **cutaneous sarcoid papules** and **cutaneous histiocytosis**.
- **Tuberous xanthomas** can be confused with **rheumatoid nodules** and **subcutaneous granuloma annulare**.

MANAGEMENT

- Patients with lipid disorders and xanthomas must be appropriately evaluated for primary and secondary lipoprotein abnormalities. **Treatment of the underlying cause** may reverse eruptive and tuberous xanthomas over a period of time.
- **Dietary restrictions** and **cholesterol-lowering drugs** may reverse some changes associated with hypercholesterolemia.
- Xanthelasmas of the eyelids can be removed by application of 25 to 50% **trichloracetic acid**, local **electrodesiccation**, or laser surgery.

PART IV

Dermatologic Procedures

CHAPTER 26

BASIC PROCEDURES

Fredric Haberman and Herbert P. Goodheart

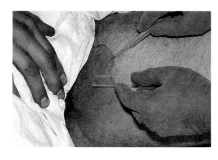

Figure 26.1

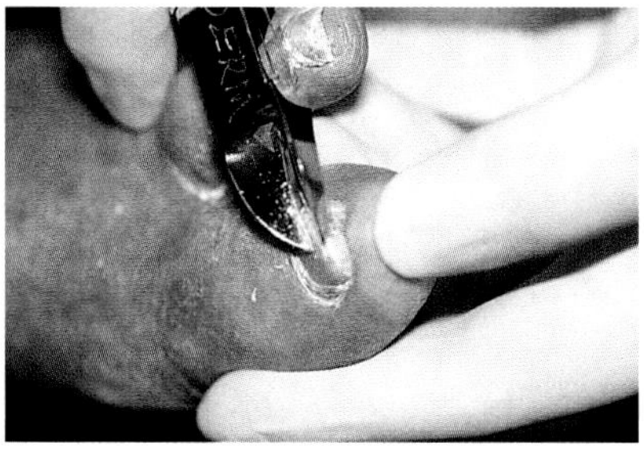

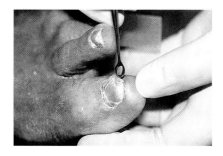

Figure 26.2

HOW TO PERFORM A POTASSIUM HYDROXIDE (KOH) TEST

- The KOH examination has the advantage of providing an **immediate diagnosis** of a superficial fungal infection, rather than waiting weeks for fungal culture results.
- It is a simple, rapid method used to detect fungal elements in the skin, nails, and hair.

COLLECTION

Collection is optimally performed when no surface artifacts (such as topical medications) are present (Table 26.1).

TABLE 26.1. COLLECTION OF SAMPLE FOR KOH EXAMINATION

SKIN	NAILS	HAIR
Gently scrape scale from active border with a #15 scalpel blade or edge of a glass slide (Figure 26.1).	Trim nail (Figure 26.2). Use a #15 scalpel or a 1 to 2 mm curette under the nail surface (Figure 26.3).	Pluck broken hairs with forceps or use a toothbrush to obtain scale and hairs (Figure 26.4).

PREPARATION

- A KOH solution such as Swartz-Lamkins Fungal Stain or KOH with dimethyl sulfoxide (DMSO) is used.
- A **thin layer** of scale, or scale plus hair, is gathered on the slide and covered with a coverslip.
- Using an eyedropper, a single drop of a KOH solution is placed at the edge of the coverslip and allowed to spread under it by capillary action (Figure 26.5).
- It is heated gently with a lighter or match until bubbling begins.
- Excess KOH solution is blotted with paper.

OBSERVATION (Figures 26.6–26.13)

- Examine under low-light intensity (condenser down).
- Begin with low-power scan first to identify scale and possibly hyphae.
- Use high power to confirm presence of hyphae or spores.

CULTURE

- Fungal cultures are placed on Sabouraud's agar or dermatophyte test medium (DTM) and incubated for 1 to 4 weeks (Figures 26.14 and 26.15).
- Recent clinical laboratory improvement act (CLIA) guidelines may require the practitioner to use outside laboratory facilities when conducting fungal cultures.

Figure 26.3

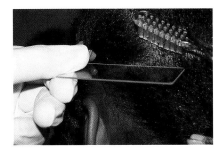

Figure 26.4

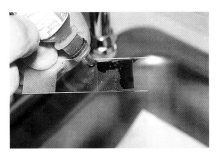

Figure 26.5.
KOH solution placed on slide with eyedropper.

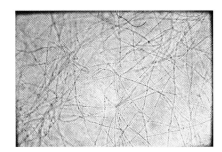

Figure 26.6.
Dermatophyte. Note the filamentous branching hyphae.

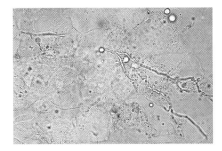

Figure 26.7.
Dermatophyte. Note the wavy-branched hyphae with uniform widths coursing over cell borders.

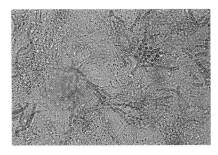

Figure 26.8.
Tinea versicolor. Note the short, stubby hyphae ("spaghetti") and the clusters of spores ("meatballs").

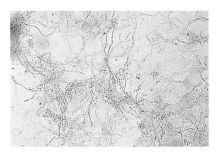

Figure 26.9.
Candida. Spores and pseudohyphae.

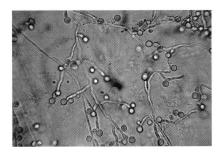

Figure 26.10.
Candida. Pseudohyphae with budding spores.

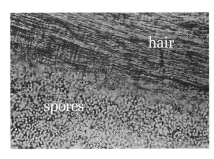

Figure 26.11.
Ectothrix. Note the spores *outside* the hair shaft.

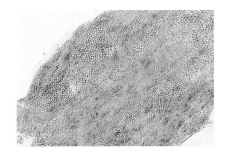

Figure 26.12.
Endothrix. Note the spores *inside* the hair shaft ("a sack of marbles").

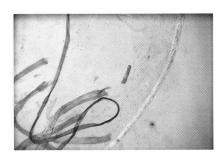

Figure 26.13.
Artifact. Note the clothing fibers on the *left* and the single hair shaft on the *right*.

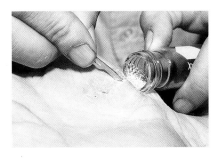

Figure 26.14.
Culture collection onto Sabouraud's agar.

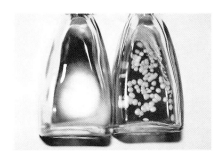

Figure 26.15.
Fungal culture using dermatophyte test medium (DTM). Note positive result on the *left* as indicated by the color change from yellow to red and the monomorphous colony growth. On the *right* there are discrete mucoid growths of a yeast contaminant, despite the false-positive color change to red.

TZANCK PREPARATION

A Tzanck preparation is used to aide in the diagnosis of herpes simplex, herpes zoster, and varicella.

TECHNIQUE

1. A fresh, intact vesicle or bulla, which has been present for less than 24 hours, is preferred.
2. After swabbing the lesion with an alcohol prep, the blister is unroofed by piercing it with a #11 blade or a needle, followed by blotting with a gauze sponge.

3. The underlying moist base of the lesion is then scraped with a #15 scalpel blade, and a thin layer of material is spread onto a glass slide.
4. The specimen is then air dried and stained with a supravital stain such as Giemsa, Wright's, or methylene blue, which is left on for 1 minute.
5. The specimen is then gently flooded with tap water for 15 seconds to remove any remaining stain.
6. Examine initially under a 40x magnification and then a 100x magnification. Oil immersion helps to identify the characteristic multinucleated giant cells (Figure 26.16).

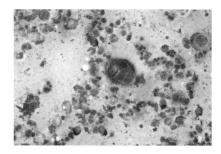

Figure 26.16.
Positive Tzanck preparation demonstrating the multinucleated giant cells. Note the presence of nuclei of normal keratinocytes, which are the size of neutrophils.

BASICS

- There are various skin biopsy techniques available to the practitioner: shave biopsy, scissor or snip biopsy, punch biopsy, and excisional biopsy. The surgical tools and approaches will vary according to size, shape, depth, and site of the biopsy.
- Obtaining the amount of tissue sample that will provide adequate information about the disease is the most important factor to keep in mind when deciding on the proper biopsy technique.
- The biopsy specimen site should not be chosen indiscriminately. The site should be evaluated according to the clinical impression, lesion location, estimated depth of the pathology, planned tissue studies, and the ensuing cosmetic result. The choice of biopsy technique requires some knowledge of where the pathology is likely to be located.

SHAVE BIOPSY

USES

- Used in the diagnosis and therapeutic removal of superficial (epidermal and upper dermal) skin lesions, such as melanocytic nevi, warts, seborrheic and solar keratoses, pyogenic granulomas, skin tags, and other benign tumors
- Used to obtain biopsy specimens to confirm skin disease before a more definitive surgical procedure (e.g., basal or squamous cell carcinoma)
- Useful for flattening and diagnosing nevi, particularly in the facial area

ADVANTAGES

- Fast and economical
- Generally excellent cosmetic results
- Useful for difficult-to-reach sites (e.g., ear canal, orbit of the eye)
- Advantageous in areas of poor healing (e.g., the lower leg in elderly or diabetic patients)

DISADVANTAGES

- Not indicated for lesions that extend into the fat layer
- Not indicated when a full-thickness biopsy is necessary (e.g., in inflammatory dermatoses)
- Should not be performed on a suspected melanoma because of the difficulty in clinically appreciating the maximal thickness or extent of the lesion

TECHNIQUE

- Anesthetize the area adjacent to the lesion with an injection into the superficial dermis with either 0.5% or 1% plain lidocaine using a 27- or 30-gauge needle. If necessary, epinephrine in a 1:100,000 or 1:200,000 dilution can be used.
- Local anesthesia with lidocaine creates a wheal and elevates the lesion above the surrounding skin (Figure 26.17).
- Traction applied with the thumb and index finger of the free hand on either side of the lesion stabilizes it (Figure 26.18).
- A #15 scalpel blade is placed flat on the skin. The blade is drawn through the lesion in a sawing motion with smooth strokes parallel to the skin's surface.
- Traction is released when the lesion becomes sufficiently free (Figure 26.19).
- Small forceps with teeth are used to hold and elevate the lesion to complete the "shave" and then deliver it to a bottle of formalin.
- Jagged edges can be "feathered" with electrocautery or further shaving.
- Hemostasis may be rapidly achieved with the use of Monsel's Solution (ferric subsulfate) applied with a cotton pledget (Q-Tip). Hemostasis is best achieved if the field is wiped dry of blood.

SCISSOR (SNIP) AND EXCISION BIOPSY

USES

A variety of lesions can be removed from the skin in a short time period. Certain elevated or pedunculated lesions, such as warts, nevi, seborrheic keratoses, and skin tags are ideally suited for removal with scissors. Many can be precisely removed level to the skin.

ADVANTAGES

- The technique is fast and economical.
- Many lesions can be removed in one visit.
- It can frequently be performed without anesthesia.

DISADVANTAGES

There are no disadvantages, except for the possibility of obtaining an inadequate amount of tissue if a specimen is to be sent for histopathology.

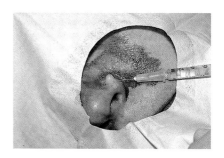

Figure 26.17.
Local anesthesia creating a wheal that elevates the lesion above the surrounding skin.

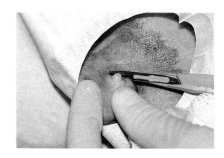

Figure 26.18.
The lesion is stabilized with the free hand.

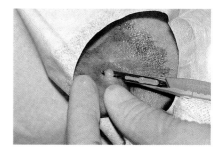

Figure 26.19.
The blade flat on the skin is drawn through the lesion.

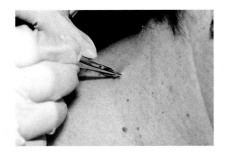

Figure 26.20.
Snip excision of a skin tag.

TECHNIQUE

- Thin, small lesions may be snipped off without any anesthesia; larger lesions require local anesthesia.
- The lesion is gently held by small forceps without teeth and pulled to cause slight tenting of the epidermis and upper dermis (Figure 26.20). A curved iris scissor with fine points may be used to snip off the lesion.
- The base of the lesion may be lightly electrodesiccated or a styptic (e.g., Monsel's Solution) may be applied to cause hemostasis. Stinging or burning may result if the lesion has not been anesthestized. Local pressure is also effective in preventing blood flow.
- A slight elevation or irregularity of the margin is easily trimmed away with scissors.

PUNCH BIOPSY

A punch biopsy is performed by using a cylindric cutting instrument ("punch") in a 3- to 4-mm size to remove all or part of a lesion.

ADVANTAGES

- The specimen obtained is uniform.
- It is an effective method to evaluate inflammatory skin diseases.
- It is an efficient biopsy method for full-thickness skin.
- There is rapid healing of the operative site.
- Skin closure establishes a barrier to infection almost immediately following the procedure.

DISADVANTAGES

- The sample may not adequately show the entire lesion; a second technique (i.e., an elliptical biopsy) may be necessary for adequate demonstration of tumor architecture.
- This method is not suitable for lesions primarily located in the subcutaneous tissue.

TECHNIQUE

- Cleanse lesion and surrounding skin with 70% isopropyl alcohol.
- Anesthetize the area with an injection into the deep dermis with either 0.5% or 1% plain lidocaine using a 27- or 30-gauge needle. If necessary epinephrine in a 1:100,000 or 1:200,000 dilution can be used (Figure 26.21).
- Stretch the skin at a 90° angle to the natural wrinkle lines.
- Gently push the punch downward into the dermis; while advancing it slowly, twirl it back and forth until it gives. Caution should be used over thin tissue or vital structures (Figure 26.22).
- It is important to push the punch deep enough to obtain underlying fat tissue for an adequate sample.
- Withdraw the punch along with the tissue sample. If the sample does not come out with the punch, it may be cut at the base while depressing the surrounding skin.
- Remove the tissue specimen using the forceps with teeth, and then cut the specimen if necessary with iris scissors. Be careful not to squeeze the specimen and distort the tissue sample (Figure 26.23).
- Place firm pressure on the circular skin wound to curtail bleeding.
- A single suture for closure is all that is usually necessary (Figure 26.24).

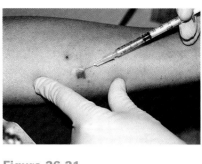

Figure 26.21.
Punch biopsy. Local anesthesia.

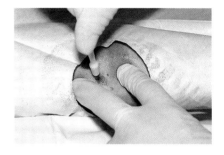

Figure 26.22.
Punch biopsy. Traction of surrounding skin while the punch is rotated.

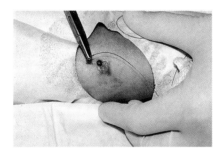

Figure 26.24.
Punch biopsy. Closure.

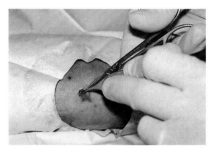

Figure 26.23.
Punch biopsy. Sample is cut with iris scissors.

BASICS

- Electrodesiccation and curettage (ED&C) is used to remove or destroy many types of benign superficial skin lesions, such as warts, seborrheic keratoses, solar keratoses, pyogenic granulomas, and skin tags.
- Electrodesiccation employs monopolar high-frequency electric currents to destroy the lesions; curettage is a scraping or scooping technique performed with a dermal curet, which has a round or oval sharp ring. In experienced hands, ED&C is often used as a method to treat skin cancers, such as small basal cell and squamous cell carcinomas.
- **Electrodesiccation without curettage** (as an alternative to shave procedures previously described) is often used to eliminate warts, skin tags, and spider angiomas and to flatten lesions (e.g., melanocytic nevi).
- Conversely, **curettage without electrodesiccation** may also be used to remove many of these epidermal lesions.

ADVANTAGES

- Fast and economical
- Useful for difficult-to-reach sites (e.g., ear canal, orbit of the eye)
- Useful in areas of poor healing (e.g., the lower leg in elderly or diabetic patients)
- Secondary infection uncommon

DISADVANTAGES

- ED&C is a "blind" procedure; margins of lesions can only be guessed.
- Cosmetic results are unpredictable; hypopigmentation and scarring may result.
- Healing by second intention takes 2 to 3 weeks, which is longer than healing after an excisional procedure.
- Curettage used for a biopsy specimen is discouraged.

CURETTAGE

TECHNIQUE

- Anesthetize the area adjacent and subjacent to the lesion with an injection into the superficial dermis of either 0.5% or 1% plain lidocaine using a 27-or 30-guage needle. If necessary, epinephrine in a 1:100,000 or 1:200,000 dilution can be used.
- The local anesthetic creates a wheal and elevates the lesion above the surrounding skin.
- Apply traction with the thumb and index finger of the free hand on either side of the lesion to stabilize it and keep it taut.
- A sharp curette is held like a pencil and, with the thumb, drawn through the tissue with strokes pushed away from the surgeon until an adequate amount of tissue is removed (usually when the dermis is reached; Figure 26.25).
- After wiping the field dry of blood, hemostasis is obtained by using Monsel's Solution.

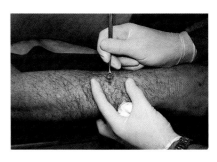

Figure 26.25.
Curettage.

ELECTRODESICCATION

Electrodesiccation may be used before or after curettage, or used alone. It causes superficial destruction with a charring of the skin.

TECHNIQUE

- This procedure is performed after local anesthesia. Very small lesions (e.g., skin tags) may be electrodesiccated without anesthesia provided that a very low current is used.
- To prevent unnecessary tissue damage, electrodesiccation should be utilized with the lowest possible settings appropriate for an intended lesion.
- If a biopsy of the lesion is required, a shave biopsy should precede any electrodesiccation.

BASICS

- Excisions are used to obtain tissue samples for biopsy specimens and for removing many benign and cancerous lesions.
- Excisional biopsies may be performed on discrete lesions, such as cysts, basal or squamous cell carcinomas, malignant melanoma, and other solitary tumors and nevi. An **incisional biopsy** is the incomplete or partial removal of a lesion that may be too big or poorly located to perform a complete excision (e.g., a suspected melanoma that is too large to remove).

ADVANTAGES

- Excision provides more extensive tissue samples than a punch biopsy.
- Margins of submitted tissue can be examined for possible involvement (e.g., basal cell carcinoma, squamous cell carcinoma, melanoma).
- It often affords a definitive cure for many benign and malignant lesions.

DISADVANTAGES

- The procedure is time-consuming and less economical than shaves and snips.
- It usually requires a return visit for suture removal.

TECHNIQUE FOR AN ELLIPTICAL EXCISION

- The best cosmetic results are achieved by placing the lines of incision in or parallel to the relaxed skin tension lines. This is demonstrated by observing wrinkle lines and the effect of pinching the skin.
- Once a direction for the long axis of the ellipse is decided, the ellipse should be drawn around the lesion before use of a local anesthetic. This minimizes tissue distortion, which may cause difficulty in subsequent planning of the ellipse. A gentian violet dye or surgical skin marker can be used to mark the skin. The excision should have a length: width ratio of at least 3:1, and the apices should be at an angle of 30°.
- The area is anesthetized by local infiltration with lidocaine and epinephrine 1:100,000.
- A #15 scalpel blade can be used to make the incision. The scalpel is held in the dominant hand, and the index finger and thumb of the other hand are placed on either side of the incision. This pushes the skin under tension downward and away from the scalpel (Figure 26.26).
- The incision should be started using the point of the scalpel and held in a vertical position at the apex of the ellipse. The belly of the scalpel then should be used along the side of the ellipse as the incision is elongated.
- The scalpel should cut through the full thickness of the skin, including the upper subcutaneous fat, in order to obtain an optimal tissue sample for histologic examination.
- The tissue is dissected, free of the underlying fat, after incisions have been made on both sides of the ellipse. Forceps with teeth can be used to hold the apex of the skin that is being removed. The ellipse is dissected further by using curved, blunt-tipped scissors (e.g., Steven's tenotomy or gradle scissors), making certain that the plane of the dissection is at the same level throughout.
- Sutures can be used for direct edge-to-edge wound closure. It may be necessary to undermine the surrounding skin to obtain the best skin closure and to minimize suture tension. Subcutaneous sutures may be placed after undermining, which allows the edges of the wound to be approximated in order to close the wound.
- Meticulous hemostasis must be achieved after undermining.

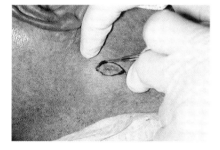

Figure 26.26.
Excision.

UNDERMINING

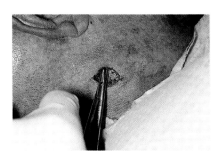

Figure 26.27.
Undermining.

TECHNIQUE

- Undermining is performed using blunt-tipped scissors while the skin edge is elevated by forceps with teeth or a skin hook.
- Scissors are advanced to the desired degree and opened to stretch the underlying skin (Figure 26.27).
- If necessary, this procedure is repeated several times to achieve the desired skin mobility for wound closure.
- Any remaining tissue septa should be removed using the open blades of the scissors.
- Undermining is most effective when performed at the level of superficial fat tissue. This reduces the possibility of injury to nerves and blood vessels in the facial and neck areas.
- Wound repair is facilitated if an adequate ellipse has been formed, the edges are perpendicular to the skin, and skin lines are followed. Wounds should be closed in layers.
- The closure of dead space is necessary when large, subcutaneous vacuities have been created, as occurs following removal of subcutaneous cysts.
- Dermal, buried sutures are important on areas of the body that overlie large muscle groups, such as the upper trunk.

SUTURE MATERIAL

- Choice of suture material depends on the size and degree of tension on the wound and the area of placement.
- For facial or limb areas, Vicryl or Dexon sutures are suitable for proper wound closure; 5-0 or 6-0 synthetic (Prolene or Ethilon) are recommended for the face.
- On the upper trunk, greater skin support is required for proper wound closure. Therefore, Maxon or PDS sutures are recommended; 3-0 or 4-0 are preferred.

WOUND CLOSURE

- The method of **"halving"** is the most effective technique for wound closure. "Halving" allows for equal distribution of wound tension. Simple, interrupted skin sutures are most commonly used in this procedure.
  - The first suture is placed in the center of the ellipse.
  - The second and third sutures are placed in the centers of the remaining wound lengths.
  - This procedure is repeated until the wound is completely closed.
- Pressure dressings and skin closure bandages provide additional support for immediate wound care. Dry, sterile gauze covered with paper tape can help maintain cosmetic results.
- Suture removal depends on wound tension, area of location, and depth of placement. Generally, facial sutures may be removed in 5 days.
  - Sutures in the trunk and extremities are removed in 1 to 2 weeks.

- Infections following simple skin surgery are unusual, and administration of systemic antibiotics is generally unnecessary.
- Small amounts of necrosis normally occur in wound healing.
  - Meticulous hemostasis during surgery is essential.
  - Hemostasis can be achieved with a pressure dressing, which is applied for 24 hours. This will help to eliminate dead space.
  - Hemostasis induced by electrosurgery, suture ligature, or cautery always produces tissue necrosis.
  - Wound healing is delayed when there is extensive necrosis.
- When wounds are closed with a considerable amount of tension or the patient has been taking steroids, sutures should be nonabsorbable and buried (nylon or Prolene) or have prolonged tensile strength (PDS, Dexon, Vicryl). Under the former conditions, skin sutures may be left in place for longer time periods.
- External splinting using tape provides additional support until the tensile strength of the wound increases after suture removal.
- Exercise that stretches the skin should be avoided to minimize spreading of the scar.

- An occlusive dressing (perforated plastic film or sheet with an absorbable pad) or pressure dressing should be applied when necessary.
- After 24 hours, the patient can remove the dressing and compress the wound with tap water or 1:3% hydrogen peroxide. The hydrogen peroxide mechanically softens the wound and removes any debris.
- A topical antibiotic, such as bacitracin, is applied to the surface of the wound before applying a clean, occlusive dressing.
- The patient repeats this procedure daily at home until the wound is covered with fresh epidermis.
- Patients are advised to return for a follow-up if there is any pain, swelling, tenderness, purulent drainage, discharge, or bleeding of the wound.
- Postoperative pain is usually negligible, and patients are advised to call the surgeon should any pain occur.

BASICS

- Cryosurgery entails the destruction of tissue by freezing in a controlled manner, producing a sharply circumscribed necrosis. Tissue destruction results from inter- and extracellular ice formation, denaturing liquid protein complexes, and cell dehydration. A repeat freeze–thaw cycle results in more cellular damage than a single cycle.
- Liquid nitrogen (LN_2) at $-195.8°C$ is the standard agent used. It is applied with a cotton swab, cryospray gun, or a cryoprobe and is stored in a special vacuum container.
- Cryosurgery should only be undertaken when a confident, clinical diagnosis is made. It is most commonly used on warts and solar keratoses.

ADVANTAGES

- Cryosurgery is an inexpensive, rapid, and simple technique that does not require complicated apparatus.
- Anesthesia is usually not necessary.
- Postoperative pain is minimal.
- Bleeding is not a problem during or after treatment.
- Sutures are not necessary, and scarring is generally minimal or absent.
- Cryosurgery is helpful for some skin conditions in patients who are HIV positive. These include patients with molluscum contagiosum, condylomata acuminatum, Kaposi's sarcoma, and warts.

DISADVANTAGES

- Cryosurgery is not well tolerated by very young children.
- Multiple treatments may be necessary.
- It is not as useful on lesions below the knee because of a possible recuperation period of several months, especially in elderly patients.
- Scarring will occur, particularly if lesion is overzealously frozen or if the patient tends to heal with hypertrophic scars or keloids.
- Postinflammatory pigmentary alterations may occur; more often hypopigmentation will result because of the destruction of melanocytes.

TECHNIQUE

- Local anesthetic is generally not required.
- For smaller lesions, cryosurgery is performed by treating the center of the lesion and allowing the freeze to spread laterally.
- The length of time for the application varies, depending on the thickness of the lesion. Standardization of freeze times is difficult to categorize for the treatment of benign and premalignant lesions. The goal is to produce, with either the swab or spray technique, a solid ice ball that extends visibly 2 mm onto normal skin.

Cotton-tip applicator technique

- Place LN$_2$ in a Styrofoam cup.
- Dip a cotton/wool swab into the cup.
- Touch the lesion with the saturated cotton-tipped applicator, applying a minimal amount of pressure, and create a 2- to 3-mm zone of freeze around the lesion for a total of 4 to 5 seconds (Figure 26.28).
- The skin will turn white. Care must be taken to avoid dripping onto surrounding, normal skin.

Cyrospray technique

- A hand-held cryogun, which operates under a working pressure of approximately 6 psi, is the standard instrument. Nozzle attachments with apertures of varying diameter for spray application are available (the "A" nozzle applies the greatest amount of spray; the "D" applies the least amount and is used for delicate work; Figure 26.29).

POSTOPERATIVE COURSE AND WOUND CARE

- Mild-to-moderate swelling may develop at the lesion site.
- A blister or blood blister may form within 24 hours and resolve in 2 to 7 days (Figure 26.30).
- The lesion site can be cleansed with soap and water several times during the day during the exudative stage. The site does not have to be covered.
- The lesion site starts to dry at the end of the exudative stage and will then slough.
- A crust, which loosens spontaneously, commonly occurs.

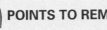

POINTS TO REMEMBER

- Stubborn warts are sometimes defeated by frequent (usually once monthly) treatments with LN$_2$ (Figure 26.31).
- It is best to under-freeze lesions; they can be retreated at a later date.
- The patient should be told that it may take 4 to 5 weeks for the wart to disappear.

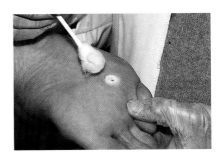

Figure 26.28.
Application with a cotton pledget.

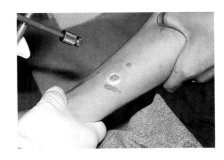

Figure 26.29.
Cryotherapy of warts with a cryospray gun.

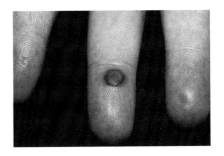

Figure 26.30.
A hemorrhagic blister 24 hours after treatment of a wart.

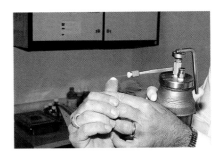

Figure 26.31.
Application with a cryogun apparatus (freezing the lesion at a right angle may lessen the pain).

CHAPTER 27

HIGHLY SPECIALIZED PROCEDURES

Fredric Haberman and Herbert P. Goodheart

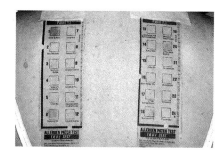

Figure 27.1.
T.R.U.E test patches, which are removed after 48 hours.

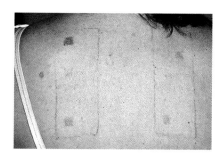

Figure 27.2.
Final reading at 96 hours showing reactions to various allergens.

BASICS

Patch testing is a method used to help diagnose allergic contact dermatitis. It is usually not performed until a thorough history has exhausted possible allergens or if a rash persists, despite treatment and avoidance of a suspected allergen.

TECHNIQUE

The allergens most commonly responsible for allergic contact dermatitis are standardized and available commercially (e.g., T.R.U.E. Test).

- The allergens, which are fixed in dehydrated gel layers, are taped against the skin of the back for 48 hours and then removed (Figures 27.1 and 27.2).
- The area is examined for evidence of contact dermatitis. A final reading at 96 hours is suggested because delayed hypersensitivity reactions may take longer than 48 hours to appear.
- The presence of erythema, papules, and vesicles (i.e., an acute eczematous reaction) is considered to be strongly positive of allergic contact dermatitis. A bullous reaction is considered as extremely positive of allergic contact dermatitis.
- Interpretation of patch test results and correlation with clinical findings requires experience and is generally performed by dermatologists.
- A much larger battery of less common allergens are available commercially or may be prepared individually.

BASICS

Phototherapy is the use of ultraviolet light (UV) to treat various skin diseases. Patients receive a controlled dose of UV while standing in a booth lined with high-output bulbs (Figure 27.3).

INDICATIONS

- **UVB** (ultraviolet B) is most often used to treat psoriasis; however, it is also useful for certain patients with eczema, parapsoriasis, mycosis fungoides, pityriasis rosea, pruritic eruptions of HIV infection, and intractable pruritus resulting from renal failure.
- **PUVA** is an acronym for **p**soralen and **u**ltraviolet light, type **A**. It involves the combined use of an oral or topical psoralen and UVA light. It is most often used for psoriasis, but it is also sometimes helpful in treating parapsoriasis, mycosis fungoides, eczema, and vitiligo.
- **RePUVA** treatment uses an oral retinoid such as acitretin and PUVA in combination. It is used to help clear psoriasis with less cumulative UVA exposure than if PUVA is used alone.

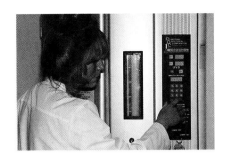

Figure 27.3
Ultraviolet therapy light box.

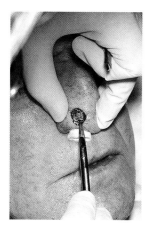

Figure 27.4.
First stage of excision of lesion. (Slide courtesy of Michael J. Mulvaney, MD)

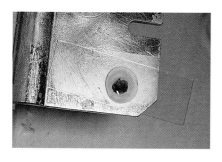

Figure 27.5.
Excised tissue color-coded, then evaluated by frozen section. (Slide courtesy of Michael J. Mulvaney, MD)

BASICS

- Mohs' micrographic surgery is a microscopically controlled method of removing skin cancers that allows for controlled excision and maximum preservation of normal tissue.
- Mohs' surgery is time-consuming, expensive, and may require extensive reconstruction of surgical wounds; however, it provides the most reliable method in determining adequate margins, has a high cure rate of between 98 to 99% for basal cell carcinomas, and preserves the maximum amount of normal tissue around the cancer.

INDICATIONS

Mohs' surgery is most suited for:
- Recurrent basal and squamous cell carcinomas, particularly those seen on the face
- Excessively large or invasive carcinomas
- Carcinomas with poorly delineated clinical borders
- Carcinomas within an orifice (e.g., ear canals or nostrils)
- Carcinomas in locations where preservation of normal tissue is extremely important (e.g., tip of the nose, eyelids, ala nasi, ears, lips, glans penis)
- Carcinomas in locations known to have a high rate of recurrence (e.g., ala nasi, nasal labial fold, medial canthus, pinna, postauricular sulcus)
- Morpheaform or sclerotic (desmoplastic) basal cell carcinomas
- Lesions of the finger or penis

TECHNIQUE

- Tissue is excised in a circular pie-shaped fashion (Figure 27.4), then it is systematically mapped and examined by means of frozen sections.
- While the patient waits in the examination room, tissue is submitted to a histotechnician for the surgeon to review (Figure 27.5).
- Excisions are repeated in the areas proven to be cancerous until a complete cancer-free plane is reached (Figure 27.6).
- This procedure may occur in one or more stages until a tumor-free section is reached.
- Surgical wounds may be left to heal by secondary intention or are corrected by plastic reconstructive procedures (Figure 27.7).

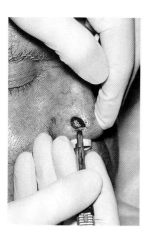

Figure 27.6.
Second stage of excision of lesion because first had positive margins. (Slide courtesy of Michael J. Mulvaney, MD)

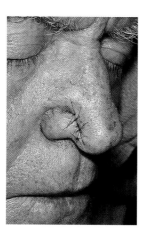

Figure 27.7.
Primary closure after second stage was free of malignancy. (Slide courtesy of Michael J. Mulvaney, MD)

FACIAL PEELS

BASICS

Chemical peels produce a controlled, partial-thickness chemical burn of the epidermis and upper dermis. Regeneration of the peeled skin results in fresh, organized epidermis and a new 2- to 3-mm band of dense and compact collagen in the dermis.

INDICATIONS

- Removal of fine wrinkles
- To treat hyperpigmentation (e.g., melasma)
- Improvement of acne
- Destruction of solar keratoses and lentigines

CLASSIFICATION

Chemical peels are classified as deep, medium, or superficial, depending on the depth of penetration of the specific agent used.

DEEP PEELS

This type of peel extends to the deep dermis using phenol (carbolic acid), which causes rapid denaturation of the surface keratin and other proteins in the epidermis and upper dermis to a depth of 2 to 3 mm. Phenol provides dramatic, longer-lasting results in fine wrinkles and hyperpigmentation; however, there is potential for rapid absorption, which could cause cardiac dysrhythmias.

MEDIUM-DEPTH PEELS

These are performed with trichloroacetic acid (TCA) alone, or in conjunction with Jessner's solution (a combination of salicylic acid, lactic acid, and resorcinol). Medium-depth peels are used for lightening hyperpigmentation and afford some improvement in wrinkles and solar keratoses. Medium and deeper peels are best performed on light-skinned people to avoid the risk of postinflammatory hyperpigmentation.

SUPERFICIAL PEELS

Glycolic acid, TCA, or Jessner's solution are used to improve pigmentary abnormalities, acne, fine wrinkling, lentigines, melasma, and solar keratoses in the outer papillary dermis.

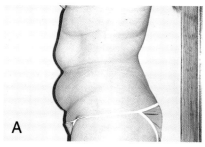

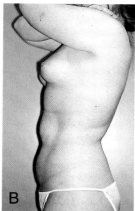

Figure 27.8.
(*A*) Before liposuction; (*B*)
5 months later.

BASICS

Liposuction involves the removal of subcutaneous fat from the skin by means of a microcannula that is attached to a high-powered suction device. Traditional methods of fat removal required large excisions and resulted in large scars; liposuction results in minimal scarring.

USES

- Body contouring
- Gynecomastia (male breasts)
- Removing unwanted fat deposits in the abdomen (Figure 27.8)
- Various areas of the body, including the "spare tire," hips, lateral and inner thighs, chin, and submental areas, neck, anterior axillary fat folds, proximal posterior arms, knees, calves, and ankles
- Removal of more localized fat deposits, such as lipomas

BASICS

- Fat transplantation is used as a soft tissue correction for cosmetic and reconstructive problems.
- Fat transplantation can be performed as an adjunct to liposuction surgery.

USES

- Facial wrinkles
- Facial aging changes, such as nasolabial folds, furrows, central cheek depressions, glabellar furrows, and diffuse age-related lipoatrophy
- Facial scar corrections, such as those associated with acne, en coup de sabre hemiatrophy (see Figure 25.37), and cosmetic defects resulting from traumatic injury
- Nonfacial corrections, such as the rejuvenation of the hands, body contour defects, liposuction-induced depressions, and traumatic scars

TECHNIQUE

- Syringe extraction and injection (microlipoinjection) of autologous fat involves the harvesting and subcutaneous implantation in the desired location.
- If additional fat is needed for a future procedure, the extra fat from the first harvesting may be stored for 6 months in a freezer.

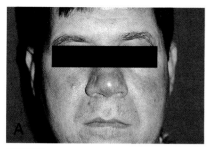
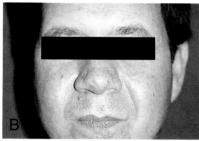

Figure 27.9.
(A) Preoperative erythema of nose and cheeks; (B) 2 months postoperative pulsed-dye laser treatment.

BASICS

- Laser therapy uses the principles of selective photothermolysis. It is based on the principle that chromophores (or targets) in the skin, such as hemoglobin and melanin, can be selectively destroyed by lasers that emit light at particular wavelengths and pulsed durations. The localized absorption of laser light energy, with the subsequent production of heat in the target, causes selective damage without destruction of the normal surrounding and overlying skin.
- The carbon-dioxide (CO_2) laser is the most widely used form of laser therapy. It serves as a cutting and vaporizing tool. For many applications, the laser remains an alternative tool that produces treatment results similar to less expensive standard therapeutic procedures.

INDICATIONS

Laser therapy is most suited for:
- Vascular lesions such as hemangiomas, port-wine stains, and facial telangiectasias (Figure 27.9)
- Removal of unwanted pigmented lesions (e.g., lentigines)
- Warts, extensive condyloma acuminata, stretch marks, and hypertrophic scars
- Rhinophyma, actinic keratoses, and actinic cheilitis
- Tattoo removal
- Facial resurfacing
- Hair removal

LASER RESURFACING

- Recently, the development of pulsed CO_2 lasers allows for ablation or vaporization of thin layers of skin, layer-by-layer, producing a much narrower zone of cutaneous, dermal damage than the continuous-wave systems, which were previously used.
- Selective absorption in water-containing tissue, such as the epidermis, can be achieved; in a duration shorter than 1 msec, the pulsed CO_2 systems have the advantage of limited penetration, confining thermal damage. As a result, sufficient energy is delivered to ablate, rather than to burn tissue.

- Indications for cutaneous laser resurfacing include wrinkles in the perioral, periorbital, and zygomatic areas and for actinic keratoses and other epidermal lesions. It is also used for wrinkles of the forehead, nasolabial folds, and diffuse facial lentigines.
- Although facelifts and blepharoplasties remain the treatments of choice for sagging skin, the latest CO_2 laser technology has added to the approach for facial rejuvenation of wrinkles.

LASER TREATMENT OF PIGMENTED LESIONS

Because cutaneous pigment absorbs light and a wide spectrum of wavelengths (ranging from approximately 400 to 1000 nm), many different lasers can be used to treat pigmented lesions. The laser target is the melanosome, the cellular organelle that contains melanin. The pigmented lesions, which are generally responsive to laser, include lentigines, freckles, some café au lait macules, and various pigmented nevi.

LASER TREATMENT OF TATTOOS

Several tattoo-specific lasers are available for treatment. Because of multiple ink colors, various compositions of dyes used, and the different types of tattoos that can be obtained, response to laser treatment is not uniform. The selection of laser for treating tattoos should be determined by the type of tattoo and ink colors present. Different lasers can treat different color pigments.

LASER-ASSISTED HAIR REMOVAL

This method involves the delivery of laser light directly to the hair follicle target. Its purported advantage lies in the enhanced selectivity and, thus, effectiveness in permanently eradicating hair or slowing hair regrowth. It is associated with minimal patient discomfort. Long-term efficacy of this procedure has not been proven.

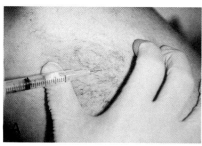

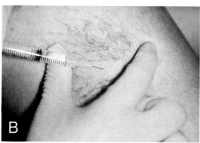

Figure 27.10.
(*A*) Hypertonic saline injection into lumen of telangiectatic vessel; (*B*) blanching reaction.

BASICS

- "Spider veins," or telangiectatic leg veins, are telangiectatic vessels that range from 0.1 to 1.0 mm in diameter; they are red to cyanotic in color. Destruction is primarily for cosmetic concerns; however, a rare complaint of a dull throbbing or burning sensation may be reported.
- Sclerotherapy is defined as the introduction of a foreign substance into the lumen of a vessel, causing thrombosis and subsequent fibrosis. The mechanism of action for sclerosing agents occurs from endothelial damage, which results in exposure of subendothelial collagen fibers, thrombus formation, and fibrosis.

TECHNIQUE

- Usually a 30-gauge needle is used to introduce the agent within the vessel wall (Figure 27.10).
- Detergent-sclerosing agents, such as **sodium morrhuate, sodium tetradecyl sulfate (STS),** and **Polidocanol (POL),** cause endothelial damage through interference with the cell surface lipids.
- **Hypertonic saline** causes dehydration of endothelial cells through osmosis, resulting in endothelial destruction.

HAIR TRANSPLANTATION

BASICS

- Hair transplantation is most often performed to improve the appearance of androgenetic alopecia; less commonly, hair is transplanted to replace areas of the scalp that have scarred from chemical or thermal burns or from inflammatory dermatoses, such as cutaneous lupus erythematosus.
- Hair transplantation is based upon the principle of donor dominance, wherein multiple punch autografts are transferred from one location to another in the same person. Usually, the donor grafts are taken from the occipital area and sides of the scalp where hairs rarely fall out. Grafts are then are transplanted to the alopecic scalp, where they tend to grow in a normal manner.
- A **scalp reduction** procedure (i.e., excision of bald skin) can markedly reduce the extent of alopecia that it is necessary to correct by using hair transplantation.

TECHNIQUE

Minigrafts and micrografts have been a major advancement in the technique of hair replacement surgery. In contrast to the standard grafts of 4.0 or 4.5 mm, a micrograft consists of 1 or 2 hairs, and a minigraft contains between 3 and 8 hairs. These are placed in a recipient area to enhance the appearance of the frontal hairline. To refine the frontal hairline, 1.5- and 2.0-mm minigrafts can also be used. Minigrafts can also be used for the entire replacement procedure to produce a thinned but natural appearance (Figure 27.11).

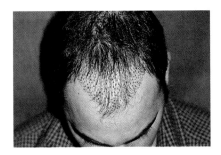

Figure 27.11.
Multiple minigrafts.

BASICS

Dermabrasion is the process in which skin is resurfaced by planning or sanding with a rapidly rotating abrasive tool, such as a diamond fraise, wire brush, or serrated wheel.

INDICATIONS

Dermabrasion is used for the removal of:
- Postacne scars (non–ice-pick variety)
- Surgical and traumatic scars
- Tattoos
- Wrinkles
- Actinic keratoses
- Adenoma sebaceum (angiofibromas of tuberous sclerosis)
- Rhinophyma

TECHNIQUE

- Local lidocaine anesthesia is used via nerve blocks.
- A diamond fraise or wire brush is spun at a high speed in order to slowly remove the entire epidermis and upper dermis.
- Residual portions of the skin, sweat ducts, and hair follicles proliferate and re-epithelize the smooth planed surface of the skin.
- The duration of time until complete re-epithelialization after dermabrasion is between 7 and 10 days, with the use of dressings, such as Biobrane and Vigilon.
- Postinflammatory pigmentary alterations may occur after healing.

COLLAGEN AND BOTOX

COLLAGEN

BASICS

- Collagen is a soft tissue implant that is used for the treatment of wrinkles, furrows, augmentation of the lips, and soft acne scars with sloping borders (i.e., not ice-pick scars). It has also been used to treat painful corns and calluses.
- Bovine collagen implants are the most commonly used filling agent. Solubilized bovine collagen consists of 95% type I collagen and 5% type III collagen.
- It is currently available as three separate products and packaged in prefilled syringes that already contain lidocaine as the local anesthetic. The agents are Zyderm I, Zyderm II, and Zyplast (a glutaraldehyde cross-linked collagen form that shrinks less and lasts longer).

TECHNIQUE

- After appropriate skin testing, collagen is injected into the dermis with a 30-gauge needle.
- Periodic maintenance injections are necessary because collagen becomes degraded by the body.

BOTOX

BASICS

Botulism toxin has been used for facial hemispasm, strabismus, and blepharospasm. It is now being used to treat frown lines that have been "worn into the skin" as a result of a lifetime of contractions of the muscles of facial expression.

TECHNIQUE

- The botulism toxin is diluted with saline.
- Very small quantities are injected into the intended muscle, or muscles, of facial expression in 2 or 3 sessions to produce a temporary loss of muscle tone.
- The procedure has few side effects and **is reversible**.
- Cosmetic denervation with botulism toxin occurs within 5 to 7 days, resulting in a reduction of the lines of facial expression.
- The effects wear off in 3 to 5 months, at which time another injection is required.
- The toxin is expensive.

DIAGNOSIS BY SITE, WITH AGE, SEX, SKIN TYPE, GENETIC, HEALTH, AND ENVIRONMENTAL CONSIDERATIONS

- We live in an era in which it is difficult to categorize people with respect to race, culture, age, and even sex at times. There is also a broad range of variation in social, cultural, and health characteristics within racial or ethnic populations themselves. The future will certainly make these distinctions more complex. Groupings of this kind also carry the potential handicap of political correctness. Notwithstanding these difficulties, it would be an important omission not to include these categorical designations, despite the risk of overgeneralization.
  - Many skin conditions tend to favor particular parts of the body (e.g., psoriasis favors the elbows and knees, while recurrent herpes simplex returns predictably to the vermilion border of the lip).
  - Certain dermatoses are seen more commonly in patients of a particular age (e.g., dry skin, drug rashes, and skin cancer in the elderly; viral exanthems in the very young; seborrheic dermatitis in infants and postadolescents.)
  - There are diseases that have a predilection for one sex (e.g., systemic lupus erythematosus in women, tinea cruris in men). The reported higher frequency of acne and androgenetic alopecia in women may be more of a reflection of a higher cosmetic demand for treatment of these conditions in affluent countries, rather than a higher incidence.
  - Skin pigmentation will often determine an individual's sun-sensitivity and tendency to have skin cancer (the lighter the skin, the more prone to sunburn and skin cancer). There are also a number of ethno-racial heritable differences: rosacea is found more commonly in fair-skinned northern Europeans, eczema in Asians, folliculitis of the scalp in adult Blacks, tinea capitis in African American children, and pemphigus vulgaris is seen disproportionately in Jewish people.
  - Immunocompromised patients are prone to develop viral infections (e.g., molluscum contagiosum or herpes zoster in HIV-infected patients, warts in patients with organ transplants or undergoing immunotherapy). Immunocompromised patients are also prone to certain skin cancers associated with viruses (e.g., epidemic Kaposi's sarcoma).
  - The role of environmental factors such as pollution, ultraviolet radiation, toxins, food, occupation, and life-style must be considered; for example, inner-city African Americans and Hispanics who live in poor neighborhoods tend to have more atopic dermatitis, while whites, poor and rich alike, tend to manifest head lice and scabies.

- These tendencies often afford valuable diagnostic clues. The following tables provide the most probable diagnosis considering the following variables: body region, age, sex, and skin type; they are confined to only those conditions discussed in this book. The list is by no means comprehensive, but hopefully will serve as a starting point in helping to make a diagnosis.

SCALP

AGE GROUP	DISEASE	OCCURS MOST PREDOMINANTLY*
INFANT	Seborrheic dermatitis ("cradle cap")	
	Atopic dermatitis	Positive atopic history
	Tinea capitis	African Americans; urban environment
	Congenital melanocytic nevi	Whites
TODDLER/TEEN	Tinea capitis	African Americans
	Traction alopecia	African Americans; women
	Alopecia areata	
	Pediculosis capitis (head lice)	Whites in United States; common in Africa; incidence is higher in women
	Acquired melanocytic nevi	Whites; onset in puberty
ADULT	Dandruff	Whites; uncommon in dark-skinned people
	Seborrheic dermatitis	Whites; uncommon in dark-skinned people
	Lichen simplex chronicus	Blacks; other dark-skinned people; positive atopic history
	Psoriasis	Whites
	Androgenetic alopecia	Whites
	Traction/chemical alopecia	African Americans; women
	Chronic cutaneous lupus erythematosus (discoid LE)	African Americans; women
	Folliculitis	Blacks; men and women
	Cysts	
OLDER ADULT	Seborrheic keratosis	Whites
	Actinic keratosis	White/fair-skinned balding men
	Basal cell carcinoma	White/fair-skinned men
	Squamous cell carcinoma	White/fair-skinned balding men

* Blank spaces indicate insufficient data.

AGE GROUP	DISEASE	OCCURS MOST PREDOMINANTLY*
INFANT	Atopic dermatitis	Positive atopic history
	Seborrheic dermatitis	
	Acne neonatorum	Males
TODDLER	Warts	
	Impetigo	
TEEN	Acne vulgaris	Both sexes
	Cystic acne	Males
	Acquired melanocytic nevi	Whites; onset in puberty
ADULT	Adult acne	Women; may continue beyond age 40
	Rosacea	Northern Europeans; white/fair-skinned people
	Perioral dermatitis	White/fair-skinned people; women
	Telangiectasias	White/fair-skinned people
	Postinflammatory pigmentary alteration	Dark-skinned people, east Asians
	Sunburn, photoreaction, etc	White/fair-skinned people
	Chronic cutaneous lupus erythematosus (discoid LE)	African Americans; women
	Seborrheic dermatitis	Whites; men
	Herpes simplex	
	Warts	
	Melasma	Women; Hispanics, African Americans, East Indians
	Systemic lupus erythematosus	Women; African Americans, Afro-Caribbeans, Native Americans; data insufficient in Asians and East Indians
	Dermatosis papulosa nigrans	African Americans, Afro-Caribbeans, African blacks
	Vitiligo	Equal prevalence, but more obvious in dark-skinned people
	Sarcoidosis of skin	African Americans
	Eczematous dermatitis	
	Contact dermatitis	
	Tinea faciale	
	Acquired nevi	Whites
	Basal cell carcinoma	White/fair-skinned people
	Sebaceous hyperplasia	White/fair-skinned people
OLDER ADULT	Basal cell carcinoma	White/fair-skinned people
	Solar keratosis	White/fair-skinned people
	Seborrheic keratosis	Whites
	Squamous cell carcinoma	White/fair-skinned people
	Solar lentigo	White/fair-skinned people, east Asians
	Lentigo maligna, lentigo, maligna melanoma	White/fair-skinned people
	Herpes zoster	

* Blank spaces indicate insufficient data.

EYES (PERIORBITAL AREA)

AGE GROUP	DISEASE	OCCURS MOST PREDOMINANTLY*
INFANT/TODDLER/TEEN	Molluscum contagiosum (especially eyelids)	
	Atopic dermatitis	Positive atopic history
ADULT	Eczema (excluding contact dermatitis)	Positive atopic history
	Contact dermatitis	Whites
	Seborrheic dermatitis	Whites; men
	Xanthelasma	
	Acrochordons (skin tags)	Obese individuals; pregnant women
	Angioedema	
	Sarcoidosis	African Americans
	Dermatomyositis	
OLDER ADULT	Basal cell carcinoma	White/fair-skinned people

* Blank spaces indicate insufficient data.

EARS

AGE GROUP	DISEASE	OCCURS MOST PREDOMINANTLY*
INFANT	Atopic dermatitis	Positive atopic history
TODDLER/TEEN	Atopic dermatitis	Positive atopic history
ADULT/OLDER ADULT	Psoriasis	Whites
	Seborrheic dermatitis	Whites; men
	Solar keratosis	White/fair-skinned men
	Basal cell carcinoma	White/fair-skinned men
	Keloid of earlobe	African Americans; women
	Squamous cell carcinoma	White/fair-skinned men
	Chronic cutaneous lupus erythematosus (discoid LE)	African Americans; women

* Blank spaces indicate insufficient data.

NOSE

AGE GROUP	DISEASE	OCCURS MOST PREDOMINANTLY*
TEEN	Acne	
	Compound nevi	Whites
ADULT/OLDER ADULT	Rosacea	White/fair-skinned people
	Telangiectasias	White/fair-skinned people
	Solar keratosis	White/fair-skinned people
	Basal cell carcinoma	White/fair-skinned people
	Angiofibroma (fibrous papule of the nose)	

* Blank spaces indicate insufficient data.

MOUTH (ORAL CAVITY), LIPS, TONGUE

AGE GROUP	DISEASE	OCCURS MOST PREDOMINANTLY*
INFANT	Candidiasis ("thrush")	
	Mucous cyst	
	Primary herpes simplex	
TODDLER/TEEN	Recurrent herpes simplex (vermilion border of lips)	
	Aphthous ulcers (aphthous stomatitis)	
	Warts	
ADULT	Recurrent herpes simplex (vermilion border of lips)	
	Aphthous ulcers (aphthous stomatitis)	
	Mucous cyst	
	Erythema multiforme	
	Angular cheilitis (perlèche)	
	Pyogenic granuloma	Pregnant women; children
	Fordyce spots (upper lip)	
	Geographic tongue	
	Hairy leukoplakia	HIV-infected people
	Leukoplakia	Men
	Black hairy tongue	
	Mucous patches (secondary syphilis)	African Americans, Hispanics
OLDER ADULT	Squamous cell carcinoma	Men; tobacco use; sun exposure; white/fair-skinned men
	Venous lake	

* Blank spaces indicate insufficient data.

NECK

AGE GROUP	DISEASE	OCCURS MOST PREDOMINANTLY*
TODDLER/TEEN	Atopic dermatitis	Positive atopic history
ADULT	Lichen simplex chronicus (posterior neck and occipital scalp)	Positive atopic history
	Prurigo nodularis (posterior neck and occipital scalp)	Positive atopic history
	Contact dermatitis	
	Photoreaction ("V" of neck)	Fair-skinned people
	Folliculitis	
	Pseudofolliculitis barbae	Black men, beard area
	Acne keloidalis (posterior neck and occipital scalp)	Black men
	Acanthosis nigricans	Blacks; obese individuals
	Cysts	

* Blank spaces indicate insufficient data.

AGE GROUP	DISEASE	OCCURS MOST PREDOMINANTLY*
INFANT	Atopic dermatitis	Positive atopic history
	Seborrheic dermatitis	
	Exanthems	
	Impetigo	
	Varicella (chickenpox)	
	Scabies	Whites
	Molluscum contagiosum	
	Insect bites (papular urticaria)	
TODDLER/TEEN	Varicella (chickenpox)	
	Pityriasis rosea	
	Tinea corporis	
	Nevi	Whites
	Tinea versicolor	Young adults; common in tropical latitudes
	Vitiligo	More apparent in dark-skinned people
	Acne (cystic)	Whites; men
ADULT	Pityriasis rosea	
	Drug reaction	Elderly; HIV-infected people
	Fixed drug reaction	Higher prevalence in India, Africa, and Scandinavia
	Psoriasis (guttate)	Whites; East Africans
	Tinea versicolor	Young adults; common in tropical latitudes
	Atopic dermatitis, nonspecific eczematous dermatitis	
	Secondary syphilis	African Americans, Hispanics
	Tinea corporis	
	Parapsoriasis, mycosis fungoides	
	Nevi	Whites
	Dysplastic nevi	White/fair-skinned people; often a positive family history
	Malignant melanoma	White/fair-skinned people
	Keloids	Blacks
	Acne scars	Whites; men
	Morphea	Women
	Urticaria	
	Dermatographism	
	Eruptive xanthomas (especially on the buttocks)	Diabetics and individuals with high cholesterol and triglyceride levels
	Folliculitis/furunculosis (especially on the buttocks)	
	Epidemic Kaposi's sarcoma	HIV-infected people
	Disseminated herpes zoster	HIV-infected people
	Striae distensae	Immunocompromised people; malignancy
		Pregnant women
OLDER ADULT		
	Herpes zoster	
	Drug reactions	
	Seborrheic keratosis	Whites
	Cherry angioma	Whites
	Solar keratosis	White/fair-skinned people
	Basal cell carcinoma (often superficial or pigmented)	Whites
	Xerosis (asteatotic eczema)	

* Blank spaces indicate insufficient data.

AXILLAE (tinea corporis is rare here)

AGE GROUP	DISEASE	OCCURS MOST PREDOMINANTLY*
INFANT	Atopic dermatitis	Positive atopic history
	Scabies	Whites
ADULT	Intertrigo, irritant dermatitis	
	Folliculitis, furunculosis, hidradenitis suppurativa	
	Irritant/contact dermatitis	
	Inverse psoriasis	Whites
	Striae distensae	
	Acanthosis nigricans	Blacks; obese individuals
	Candidiasis	Diabetics
	Acrochordons (skin tags)	Pregnant women; obese individuals

* Blank spaces indicate insufficient data.

INGUINAL AREA

AGE GROUP	DISEASE	OCCURS MOST PREDOMINANTLY*
INFANT	Diaper rash (secondary candidiasis)	
	Seborrheic dermatitis	
	Atopic dermatitis	Positive atopic history
	Warts (condyloma acuminata)	
TEEN	Tinea cruris	Males
	Atopic dermatitis	Positive atopic history
ADULT	Tinea cruris	Men
	Intertrigo	
	Inverse psoriasis	Whites
	Atopic dermatitis	Positive atopic history
	Acrochordons (skin tags)	Obese individuals; pregnant women
	Folliculitis, furunculosis, hidradenitis suppurativa	
	Candidiasis	Diabetics; unusual in healthy adults

* Blank spaces indicate insufficient data.

ARMS

AGE GROUP	DISEASE	OCCURS MOST PREDOMINANTLY*
INFANT/TODDLER	Atopic dermatitis	Positive atopic history
	Follicular eczema	Blacks; positive atopic history
	Insect bite reaction (papular urticaria)	
	Keratosis pilaris (deltoid area)	
	Sunburn, photoreaction	White/fair-skinned people
ADULT	Atopic dermatitis	
	Chronic eczematous dermatitis, prurigo nodularis	
	Insect bite reaction	
	Sunburn, photoreaction	White/fair-skinned people
	Psoriasis	Whites
	Tinea corporis	
	Scabies (flexor wrists)	Whites
OLDER ADULT	Seborrheic keratosis (flat type)	Whites
	Lentigo, solar	White/fair-skinned people
	Solar keratosis	White/fair-skinned people
	Basal cell carcinoma	White/fair-skinned people
	Squamous cell carcinoma	White/fair-skinned people
	Malignant melanoma	White/fair-skinned people
	Purpura (dorsum)	
	Xerosis, asteatotic eczema	

* Blank spaces indicate insufficient data.

HANDS (PALMS)

AGE GROUP	DISEASE	OCCURS MOST PREDOMINANTLY*
INFANT	Scabies	Whites
	Atopic dermatitis	Positive atopic history
TODDLER/TEEN	Scabies (between digits)	Whites
	Hand, foot, and mouth disease	
	Warts	
	Pyogenic granuloma	
ADULT/OLDER ADULT	Dyshidrotic eczema (often on sides of fingers)	Frequently positive atopic history
	Tinea manum, or id reaction	
	Psoriasis (hyperkeratotic or pustular)	
	Scabies (web spaces between digits)	Whites
	Secondary syphilis	Hispanics, Blacks
	Warts	
	Erythema multiforme	

* Blank spaces indicate insufficient data.

HANDS (DORSA)

AGE GROUP	DISEASE	OCCURS MOST PREDOMINANTLY*
INFANT	Atopic dermatitis	Positive atopic history
TODDLER/TEEN	Warts	
	Granuloma annulare	
	Pyogenic granuloma	
ADULT	Contact dermatitis	
	Atopic dermatitis	Positive atopic history
	Chronic eczematous dermatitis	
	Warts	
	Psoriasis	Whites, East Africans
	Vitiligo	More obvious in dark-skinned people
	Candidiasis (web spaces between digits)	Diabetics
	Granuloma annulare	Women
	Scabies (web spaces between digits)	Whites
	Systemic lupus erythematosus (between joints)	Women
	Dermatomyositis (on joints)	Women
	Scleroderma	Women
OLDER ADULT	Seborrheic keratosis (flat type)	Whites
	Lentigo, solar	Whites
	Basal cell carcinoma (less common here)	Whites
	Squamous cell carcinoma	Whites
	Malignant melanoma	Whites

* Blank spaces indicate insufficient data.

NAILS AND SURROUNDING TISSUE

AGE GROUP	DISEASE	OCCURS MOST PREDOMINANTLY*
INFANT	Congenital nail disorders	
TODDLER/TEEN	Trauma (e.g., nail biting, habit tic)	
	Warts	
	Herpes simplex (whitlow)	
	Pyogenic granuloma	
	Periungual fibroma	Tuberous sclerosis
ADULT	Onycholysis	Female
	Psoriasis	Whites
	Onychomycosis	Often a family history
	Aging nails, split and brittle nails	
	Green nails	Women
	Paronychia (acute and chronic)	Women
	Digital mucous cyst	
	Trauma (subungual hematoma, habit tic deformity)	
	Acral lentiginous melanoma	Although melanoma is rare in this location, it is the principal type of malignant melanoma in Blacks and Japanese.

* Blank spaces indicate insufficient data.

PENIS

AGE GROUP	DISEASE	OCCURS MOST PREDOMINANTLY*
INFANT/YOUNG TEEN	Atopic dermatitis	Positive atopic history
ADULT	Condyloma acuminata	Sexually active young adults
	Trauma, irritant dermatitis	
	Seborrheic dermatitis,	
	Nonspecific balanitis	
	Lichen planus	
	Scabies	
	Herpes simplex	Sexually active young adults
	Molluscum contagiosum	Sexually active young adults and HIV patients
	Pearly penile papules	Normal finding
	Psoriasis	Whites
	Primary syphilis (chancre)	African Americans, Hispanics
	Chancroid	Men; high prevalence in sub-Saharan Africa and seen in patients with HIV and other sexually transmitted diseases

* Blank spaces indicate insufficient data.

SCROTUM (tinea is rare in this location)

AGE GROUP	DISEASE	OCCURS MOST PREDOMINANTLY*
INFANT/TODDLER	Diaper rash	
	Atopic dermatitis	Positive atopic history
	Cutaneous candidiasis	
ADULT	Scabies	Whites
	Lichen simplex chronicus	
	Atopic dermatitis	
	Irritant dermatitis	
	Angiokeratoma (Fordyce spots)	
	Epidermoid cysts	

* Blank spaces indicate insufficient data.

VULVA (tinea is rare here)

AGE GROUP	DISEASE	OCCURS MOST PREDOMINANTLY*
INFANT/TODDLER	Diaper rash	
	Atopic dermatitis	Positive atopic history
	Cutaneous candidiasis	
ADULT	Lichen simplex chronicus, irritant dermatitis	
	Angiokeratoma (Fordyce spots)	
	Condyloma acuminata	
	Epidermoid cysts	
	Primary syphilis (chancre)	African Americans, Hispanics
	Other sexually transmitted diseases	
	Cutaneous candidiasis	Diabetics; secondary to vaginal candidiasis

* Blank spaces indicate insufficient data.

MONS PUBIS

AGE GROUP	DISEASE	OCCURS MOST PREDOMINANTLY*
ALL AGES	Pediculosis ("crabs")	Sexually active young adults
	Folliculitis/furunculosis	
	Atopic dermatitis	Positive atopic history
	Seborrheic dermatitis	

* Blank spaces indicate insufficient data.

PERIANAL AND INTERGLUTEAL REGIONS

AGE GROUP	DISEASE	OCCURS MOST PREDOMINANTLY*
INFANT/TODDLER	Atopic dermatitis	Positive atopic history
	Warts (condyloma acuminata)	
	Seborrheic dermatitis	
	Diaper rash	
	Vitiligo	Equal prevalence in white- and dark-skinned people, but more obvious in dark-skinned people
ADULT	Atopic dermatitis,	
	Lichen simplex chronicus	
	Neurodermatitis	
	Pruritus ani	
	Seborrheic dermatitis	
	Inverse psoriasis	Whites
	Herpes simplex	Sexually active young adults; HIV-infected people
	Condyloma lata (secondary syphilis)	African Americans, Hispanics
	Condyloma acuminata	Sexually active young adults; HIV-infected people
	Vitiligo	Equal prevalence, but more obvious in dark-skinned people

* Blank spaces indicate insufficient data.

UPPER LEGS

AGE GROUP	DISEASE	OCCURS MOST PREDOMINANTLY*
INFANT/TODDLER	Atopic dermatitis (popliteal fossa in toddlers)	Positive atopic history
	Insect bites	
	Henoch-Schönlein purpura	
TEENS	Flat warts	Women
	Folliculitis	
ADULT	Dermatofibroma	Women
	Psoriasis	Whites, East Africans
	Nummular eczema	
	Malignant melanoma	White/fair-skinned people
	Prurigo nodularis	Positive atopic history

* Blank spaces indicate insufficient data.

LOWER LEGS

AGE GROUP	DISEASE	OCCURS MOST PREDOMINANTLY*
INFANT/TODDLER/TEEN	Atopic dermatitis (popliteal fossa in toddlers)	Positive atopic history
	Insect bites	
	Henoch-Schönlein purpura	
	Benign pigmented purpura	
	Flat warts	Teenage girls who shave their legs
	Folliculitis	
	Ichthyosis	
ADULT/OLDER ADULT	Dermatofibroma	Women
	Psoriasis	Whites, East Africans
	Nummular eczema	
	Malignant melanoma	White/fair-skinned people
	Prurigo nodularis	Positive atopic history
	Lichen simplex chronicus	Positive atopic history
	Stasis dermatitis and ulcers xerosis	Venous insufficiency
	Asteatotic eczema	
	Benign pigmented purpura	
	Purpura, palpable purpura (vasculitis)	Idiopathic or resulting from drugs or disease
	Erythema nodosum	Women; sarcoid, drugs, etc.
	Pretibial myxedema	Women; thyroid disease
	Necrobiosis lipoidica	Women; majority are diabetics
	Pyoderma gangrenosum	Inflammatory bowel disease, gammopathy

* Blank spaces indicate insufficient data.

FEET (DORSA)

AGE GROUP	DISEASE	OCCURS MOST PREDOMINANTLY*
INFANT	Atopic dermatitis	Positive atopic history
TODDLER	Granuloma annulare	
ADULT	Contact dermatitis	
	Lichen simplex chronicus	Positive atopic history
	Tinea pedis ("moccasin" distribution)	
	Epidemic Kaposi's sarcoma	HIV-infected individuals
OLDER ADULT	Stucco keratosis	
	Classic Kaposi's sarcoma	White Jewish men, Mediterranean men

* Blank spaces indicate insufficient data.

FEET (PLANTAR SURFACE)

AGE GROUP	DISEASE	OCCURS MOST PREDOMINANTLY*
INFANT	Atopic dermatitis	Positive atopic history
	Scabies	Whites
TODDLER	Plantar warts	
	Hand, foot, and mouth disease	
ADULT/OLDER ADULT	Tinea pedis (between fourth and fifth toes)	Men; uncommon before puberty
	Chronic tinea pedis (on soles and sides of feet ["moccasin"] type)	
	Dermatitis	Positive atopic history
	Plantar warts	
	Corns, callouses	
	Psoriasis (hyperkeratotic or pustular)	Whites, East Africans
	Erythema multiforme	
	Secondary syphilis	African Americans, Hispanics

* Blank spaces indicate insufficient data.

DISEASES THAT MAY HAVE A GENERALIZED DISTRIBUTION

AGE GROUP	DISEASE	OCCURS MOST PREDOMINANTLY*
INFANT	Seborrheic dermatitis (Leiner's disease)	
	Atopic dermatitis	Positive atopic history
	Exanthems	
TODDLER/TEEN	Atopic dermatitis	Positive atopic history
	Exanthems	
	Alopecia areata (universalis)	
ADULT	Atopic dermatitis	Positive atopic history
	Drug eruption	Older adults; HIV-infected people
	Exfoliative dermatitis (erythroderma)	Men
	Psoriasis	Whites
	Mycosis fungoides (Sézary syndrome)	
	Erythema multiforme	
	Toxic epidermal necrolysis	

* Blank spaces indicate insufficient data.

PATIENT HANDOUTS

Appendix 2 provides patient handouts in English and Spanish. The Spanish translation of the English patient handout is located on the back of the English version. English headings are boxed in green, and Spanish headings are boxed in red.

Apéndice 2 provee informes para el paciente en inglés y en español. La traducción en español se encuentra al reverso del inglés. Los capítulos españoles se dibujan en cajas rojas y los capítulos ingleses se dibujan en cajas verdes.

The patient handouts may be photocopied directly from the book and given to individual patients as necessary.

INFORMATION AND INSTRUCTIONS FOR ACNE PATIENTS

- Acne is the most common skin problem of teenagers, but it is not limited to that age group. It can begin before adolescence in both sexes or in adulthood, especially in women.
- Acne tends to run in families and is caused by the reaction of the skin's oil glands to sex hormones. Patients with acne usually have normal levels of these hormones, but their oil glands are more sensitive to the hormones and sometimes produce increased amounts of oil. Certain bacteria beneath the skin, acting on the oil, form irritating substances. When the openings to the oil glands become clogged, these irritating substances lead to the formation of blackheads, whiteheads, pimples, or cysts.
- Acne is not caused by foods; however, some individuals may occasionally find that certain foods, such as chocolate or greasy food, may make their acne worse. In these instances, these foods should be avoided.
- Acne is not caused by dirt, and a patient with acne usually does not have to wash his or her face more that once or twice a day.
- Acne can be aggravated by a number of things. Emotional stress may worsen acne, and women often have flares before their menstrual cycle. Hair pomades and greasy cosmetics tend to clog pores and may worsen acne. Picking and squeezing of pimples is harmful and can lead to scars. The treatment prescribed specifically for you will consist of one or more of the following therapies (Table A2.1).

- Acné es un problema de la piel más común en adolescentes, pero no es limitado a ese grupo de edad. Puede comenzar antes de la adolecencia en ambos sexos o en la edad adultos, especialmente en mujeres.
- Acné tiende a correr en familias y es causado por la reacción de las glándulas de aceite en la piel y a hormonas de sexo. Los pacientes con acné tienen generalmente los niveles normales de estas hormonas, pero glándulas de aceite son más sensibles para ellos, y producen a veces las cantidades aumentadas de aceite. Ciertas bacterias bajo la piel, siguiendo del aceite, forman substancias molestas. Cuándo las aperturas de las glándulas de aceite llegan a ser atascadas, estas substancias molestas dirigen a la formación de poros negros, de poros blancos, de barros, o de quistes.
- Acné no es causado por alimentos; sin embargo, algunos individuos pueden encontrar ocasionalmente que ciertos alimentos, tal como chocolate o alimento grasiento, pueden hacer su acné peor. En estos casos, estos alimentos se deben evitar.
- Acné no es causado por tierra, y por un paciente con acné generalmente no tiene que lavar su cara más que un par de veces un día.
- Acné puede ser agravado por varias cosas. El tensión nerviosa puede empeorar el acné, y las mujeres a menudo tienen estallos antes de su ciclo menstrual. Pomadas de cabello y cosméticos grasientos tienden a atascar reflexiona y puede empeorar el acné. Apretar los barros es inocuo y pueden dirigir a cicatrices. El tratamiento prescrito específicamente para usted se compondrá de uno o más de las terapias siguientes (Tabla A2.1).

TABLE A2.1 TREATMENT OF ACNE

TREATMENT	HOW THEY WORK	HOW TO USE THEM	POSSIBLE SIDE EFFECTS
RETINOIDS	Differin Gel, Differin Lotion, and Retin-A preparations dry and peel the outer layer of skin to loosen blackheads and whiteheads. They also help to clear the red pimples and white pustules. Improvement of acne may take up to 2 to 3 months, and the condition may actually **appear to worsen** in the first few weeks. This does not mean that the preparation is not working, and it should not be discontinued. The apparent worsening is the result of deeper lesions coming to the surface; they will eventually clear.	Use a pea-size amount of the preparations once nightly at bedtime. Apply to the entire face from the hairline to the jaw line, avoiding the areas around the corners of the eyes and mouth. People with fair, sensitive, or dry skin, especially in winter months, can begin using it every other night, and gradually increase the frequency after 2 to 3 weeks.	•Burning •Stinging •Irritation These side effects may occur in the first 2 to 3 weeks. A mild soap such as Dove may be used for a routine facial washing, but avoid too much washing. A moisturizer may be used as necessary. Excessive sun exposure should be avoided. If you plan to be out in the sun, especially if you are fair skinned, an appropriate sunscreen should be applied beforehand. It is generally advised not to apply topical retinoids during pregnancy, even though there have been no proven problems with their use. **STOP** using the preparation and contact your health care provider if excessive redness, burning, or irritation develop.
BENZOYL PEROXIDE	Benzoyl peroxide agents such as Oxy-5, Clearsil, Desquam-X, and Fostex cause the skin to dry and peel. Benzoyl peroxide destroys the bacteria that help cause acne.	Apply once or twice daily to the entire face, or as directed.	•Redness •Scaling •Itching These side effects may occur in the first few weeks and gradually lessen. Benzoyl Peroxide may bleach clothing. **STOP** using the preparation and contact your health care provider if excessive redness, burning, or irritation develops.
TOPICAL ANTIBIOTICS	Cleocin T and Cleocin Gel and the erythromycins, such as A/T/S, Eryderm, Erygel, Emgel, etc., are topical antibiotic preparations. They act primarily by reducing the inflammatory lesions (red pimples and pus pimples) of acne.	Apply each morning and evening to the affected areas and to other areas where your acne usually occurs. Gently wash with a mild soap and pat dry before application. Makeup may be used over these preparations. After control occurs (time varies for each patient), use may be decreased or discontinued. This decision should be discussed with your health care provider.	•Redness •Peeling •Burning •Drying These side effects can occur, especially in patients with sensitive skin, and may be controlled by reducing the frequency of application.

Continued on page 427

TABLA A2. 1 RATAMIENTO DE ACNÉ

EL TRATAMIENTO	CÓMO ELLOS TRABAJAN	PARA CÓMO USARLOS	POSIBLES EFECTOS DE LADO
RETINOIDS	Differin Gel, las preparaciones de Loción y Retina de Differin secan y pelan la capa exterior de piel para aflojar poros negros y poros blancos. Ellos ayudan también limpiar los barros rojos y pustules blancos. La mejora de acné puede tomar a 2 a 3 meses, y en las primeras pocas semanas, la condición puede **aparecer verdaderamente** al peor. Esto no significa que la preparación no trabaja, y no se debe discontinuar. El empecrarse aparente está debido a la venida más profunda de lesións a la superficie, ellos limpiarán eventualmente.	Use una cantidad del tamaño de guisante de las preparaciones una vez por la noche en la hora de acostarse. Aplique a la cara entera del nacimiento de pelo, a la línea de la mandíbula, evitando las áreas alrededor de los rincones de los ojos y la boca. La gente .con la piel feria, sensible o seca, especialmente en meses de invierno, lo puede comenzar a usar cada dos noches, y aumentar gradualmente la frecuencia después de 2 a 3 semanas	•Ardiente •Picar •Irritación Estos efectos de lado pueden ocurrir en el primer 2 a 3 semanas. Un jabón templado tal como "Dove" se puede usar para un lavar facial rutinario, pero evitar también mucho lavar. Un hidradante se puede usar como sea necesario. La exposición excesiva del sol se debe evitar. Si usted esta planeando para estar fuera en el sol, y es pecialmente si usted es pelado justamente, un protector de sol apropiado se debe aplicar antes de estar afuera. Se avisa generalmente que no aplicar topical retinoids durante el embarazo, aunque no habido los problemas con el uso. No use la preparación y avisa su proveedor del cuidado de la salud si la piel de arder, rojado excesivo, o la irritación desarrollan.
PEROXIDO DE BENZOYL	Los agentes del peróxido del Benzoyl tal como Oxy-5, Clearsil, Desquam X, y Fostex para la causa de la piel secar y pelar. El peróxido de Benzoyl destruye las bacterias que ayudan la causa de acné.	Aplique una o dos veces diario a la cara entera, o cuando dirigido	•Enrojecer •Escalar •Estos efectos de lado pueden occurir en las primeras semanas y gradualmente dismiuir. Cuidado porque el medicamento puede blanquear su ropas. Para de usando la preparación y avisa su proveedor del cuidado de la salud si ardiente o irritación desarrollan.
TOPICAL ANTIBIOTICS	Cleocin T y Cleocin Gel así como también el erythromycins, tal como UN/T/S, Eryderm, Erygel, Emgel, etc., son las preparaciones de antibiótico de topical. Ellos actúan principalmente reduciendo las lesiónes de inflammación (barros rojos y ɔus) de acné.	Aplique cada mañana y el anochecer a las áreas afectadas, así como también a otras áreas donde su acné ocurre generalmente. Suavemente lava con un jabón y la palmadita templados seca antes de la aplicación. La constitución se puede usar sobre estas preparaciones. Después que el control ocurre (tiempo varía para cada individuo), el uso se puede disminuir o puede ser discontinuado. Esta decisión se debe discutir con su proveedor del cuidado de la salud.	•Enrojecer •Pelar •Ardiente •Estos efectos de lado pueden ocurrir, especialmente en pacientes con sensible de la piel, y se puérde controlar con reduciendo la frecuencia de aplicaciónes.

Continued on page 428

TABLE A2.1 TREATMENT OF ACNE *Continued*

TREATMENT	HOW THEY WORK	HOW TO USE THEM	POSSIBLE SIDE EFFECTS
BENZAMYCIN GEL	Benzamycin Gel combines benzoyl peroxide with the topical antibiotic erythromycin. This combination appears to work better than using each of them separately.	Apply once or twice per day, as tolerated. Refrigerate to maintain potency.	As with benzoyl peroxide and topical antibiotics, mild to moderate irritation may occur.
ORAL ANTIBIOTICS	Antibiotics, such as tetracycline or erythromycin, are used to kill the bacteria that form irritating products from the oil made in oil glands.	Tetracycline should be taken with water on an empty stomach and at least 1 hour before or 2 hours after a meal. Tetracycline should not be taken by pregnant women. If you are pregnant or planning pregnancy, please inform your health care provider. Minocycline and doxycycline are types of tetracycline, but they do not have to be taken on an empty stomach.	Birth control pills may be affected by tetracycline and erythromycin. If you are taking or planning to take oral contraceptives, tell your health care provider. In sun-sensitive individuals, tetracycline can cause a faster and more severe sunburn in some instances. Erythromycin, which can cause gastrointestinal upset, may be taken with meals.

TABLA A2. 1 RATAMIENTO DE ACNÉ *Continua*

EL TRATAMIENTO	CÓMO ELLOS TRABAJAN	PARA CÓMO USARLOS	POSIBLES EFECTOS DE LADO
BENZAMYCIN GEL	Benzamycin Gel combina el peróxido de benzoyl con el erythromycin de antibiótico de topical. Esta combinación aparece trabajar mejor que usar cada uno de ellos separadamente.	Aplique un par de veces por día, cuando tolerado. Refrigere el medicamento para mantener la potencia.	Con el peróxido de benzoyl y antibióticos de topical, templado a moderar irritación puede ocurrir.
ANTIBIOTICS ORAL	Antibióticos, tal como tetracycline o erythromycin, se usan para matar las bacterias que forman los productos molestos del aceite hecho en glándulas de aceite.	Tetracycline se debe tomar con agua en un estómago vacío, y por lo menos 1 hora antes, o 2 horas después, una comida. Tetracycline no debe ser tomado por mujeres embarazadas. Si usted está embarazada or planeando el embarazo, informa por favor su proveedor del cuidado de la salud. Minocycline y doxycycline son ambos tipos de tetracycline, no tienen que ser tomado en un estómago vacío.	Las píldoras del control de la natalidad pueden ser afectadas también por tetracycline y erythromycin. Si usted toma o está planeando tomar anticonceptivos orales, avisa su proveedor del cuidado de la salud. En los individuos que son sensibles al sol, tetracycline puede causar una quemadura de sol más rápida y más severa en algunos casos. Erythromycin, que puede causar el contratiempo de gastrointestinal, se puede tomar con comidas.

ATHLETE'S FOOT (*TINEA PEDIS*)

Athlete's foot is a very common skin infection caused by a fungus. It is seen mostly in men and teenage boys. The fungus that causes athlete's foot is not very contagious, but it tends to grow in a warm, moist, sweaty environment as is found in shoes and sneakers. There are several types of athlete's foot:

ACUTE TOE WEB INFECTION

This is the most common type of athlete's foot. There is peeling and sometimes cracking of the skin usually between the last two toes, which can spread to neighboring toes if it is not treated. Itching, burning, and sometimes pain may occur with this type. The infection may also be associated with a bad odor.

Treatment
- Over-the-counter topical fungal medications such as Lotrimin and Micatin creams applied twice daily are very effective. If necessary, a prescription topical or oral antifungal agent may be prescribed to you by your health care provider.
- Wetness, oozing, or cracking of the skin between the toes may be soothed and dried by using Burow's solution (Domeboro or Bluboro) applied as wet compresses for 20 minutes twice daily. The Burow's solution can be obtained without a prescription. It is made by dissolving 1 packet or tablet in an 8-ounce glass of cool or lukewarm water.
- Topical antifungal agents are then applied after soaks.

Prevention
The aim of prevention is to decrease wetness and friction by frequent change of socks and use of absorbant powders such as Zeasorb A-F or talcum powder and drying the area with a hair dryer after bathing

THE "MOCCASIN," OR DRY TYPE

This is a scaly, sometimes reddish condition that appears on the soles of the feet. It is usually not very itchy, but sometimes the skin thickens and cracks and becomes painful. The infection can also involve the toenails. You should be aware that these symptoms can be the result of causes other than tinea, such as psoriasis or eczema.

Treatment
Treatment, if necessary, may require oral antifungal agents in addition to topical agents. The moccasin and toenail type of athlete's foot is the most difficult type to cure. Recurrence is common after therapy and can lead to long-term infection.

El pie del atleta es una infección muy común de piel causada por un hongo. Se ve en su mayor parte en hombres y adolescentes. El hongo que causa pie de atleta no es muy contagioso, pero tiende a crecer en un ambiente húmedo y suderoso como se encuentra en zapatos y zapatos de lona. Hay varios tipos de infección del pie de atleta:

LA INFECCION AGUDA DE MEMBRANA DEL DEDO

Esto es el tipo más común de pie de atleta. Allí pela y agrieta a veces de la piel generalmente entre los últimos dos dedos, que puede esparcir a los otro dedos, si no se trata. Un picar, ardor, y a veces dolor puede ocurrir con este tipo. La infección se puede asociar también con un olor malo.

El tratamiento
- Sobre el mostrador los medicamentos de hongo topical tal como Lotrimin y Micatin de cremas aplicados dos veces son diariamente muy efectivos. Si necesario, un topical por recieta o tabletas oral de antihongo pueden ser dados a usted por su proveedor de cuidado de salud.
- Empapado o agrietar de la piel entre los dedos se pueden aliviar y pueden ser secados usando la solución de Burow (Domeboro o Bluboro) compresas mojadas aplicadas por 20 minutos dos veces diariamente. La solución de Burow se puede obtener sin una recieta. Es hecho disolviendo 1 paquete o tableta de 8 onzas de agua refresca o agua tibia.
- Entonces aplica los agentes de antihongo topical después que se remojes los pies.

La prevención
La puntería de la prevención deberá disminuir el empapado y fricción por el cambio frecuente de calcetines (medias) y uso de polvos de absorbant tal como Zeasorb A-F o polvo de talcum y secante el área con un secador de pelo después de bañar

EL "MOCCASIN," O SECA EL TIPO

Esto es una condición a veces rojiza, costras que aparece en las suelas de los pies. Generalmente no es muy picante, pero a veces la piel espesa y agrieta y llega a ser doloroso. La infección puede implicar también en las uñas de los pies. Usted debe estar enterado que estos síntomas pueden estar debido a causas de otra manera tal como psoriasis, tinea o eczema.

El tratamiento
El tratamiento, si necesario, puede requerir a agentes orales de antihongo además de agentes de topical. El tipo de moccasin y las uñas de los pies del pie de atleta es el tipo más difícil de curar. La reaparición es común después que la terapia y puede dirigir a una infección por tiempo largo.

PREVENTION OF OUTBREAKS OF ATOPIC DERMATITIS (ECZEMA)

- Wear nonirritating clothing (cotton) next to the skin, rather than wool, which may trigger itching.
- Reduce overbathing, which tends to dry the skin; lukewarm water should be used.
- Use mild, moisturizing soaps, or nonsoap cleansers, such as Cetaphil Lotion.
- Try to avoid using soap on red or itchy skin (many people are mistakenly led to believe that "good soaps" may actually help inflamed skin).
- A topical cortisone preparation, such as _____, should be applied once or twice daily, or as needed.
- A milder topical cortisone preparation, such as _____, is recommended for use on the face and in skin folds such as the diaper area, groin, and underarms. It is applied once or twice dialy, or as needed.
- Topical cortisone preparations **should be applied only to inflamed, itchy skin**.
- Areas that no longer itch and were darkened or lightened by the rash tend to return to their original color over a period of time. These areas should not be treated with cortisone preparations.
- Use of topical cortisone preparations should be stopped when the skin is healed and **not used to prevent new outbreaks**.
- Avoid excessive dryness or overheating; a bedroom humidifier or air conditioner may help to avoid dramatic changes in climate that may trigger outbreaks.
- Moisturizers, particularly in the dry winter months may be applied immediately after bathing in order to "seal" water in the skin.
- Sometimes, moisturizers may actually be irritating or interfere with healing, especially if they are applied to inflamed skin.
- Elimination of house dust mites may bring some relief.
- Although some foods may provoke attacks, avoiding or eliminating them will not bring a lasting improvement or cure.
- Skin tests and allergy shots may actually bring on attacks of atopic dermatitis.

- Lleve la ropa (algodón) que no sea irritante a la piel, mejor que la llana, que puede provocar picazón.
- Reduzca demasiado bañarse, porque tiende a secar la piel; agua tibia se debe usar.
- Uses los jabones templados y que contienen hidradantes, o un jabon suplente, tal como Loción de Cetaphil.
- La prueba para evitar usando el jabón en la piel roja o picante (muchas personas son dirigidas erróneamente creer que esos "jabones buenos" pueden ayudar verdaderamente piel inflamada).
- Una preparación de cortisone de topical, tal como _____, debe ser aplicado un par de veces diario, o cuando necesitado.
- Una preparación más templada de cortisone de topical, tal como _____ es recomendado para el uso en la cara y en los dobleces en la piel tal como el área de pañal, la ingle, y axilas. Se aplica un par de veces diario, o cuando sea necesitado.
- Las preparaciones del cortisone de topical deben ser aplicadas **sólo a la piel inflamada** y picante.
- Las áreas que no tienen a picar y se oscurecieron o fueron aligerado por el sarpullido, tienden a volver a su color original sobre un período de tiempo. Estas áreas no se deben tratar con preparaciones de cortisone.
- El uso de la preparaciones del cortisone de topical se debe parar cuando la piel se cura y **no es usado para prevenir los epidemias nuevos**.
- Para evitar la sequedad o recalentaro excesivo; un humedecedor de dormitorio o con aire acondicionador pueden ayudar a evitar los cambios dramáticos en el clima que puede provocar las epidemias.
- Uses hidradantes, particularmente en los meses secos de invierno se puede aplicar inmediatamente después de bañar "mantener" agua en la piel.
- A veces, hidradantes pueden hacer la piel verdaderamente irritando o interviene con la curación, especialmente si son aplicados a la piel inflamada.
- La eliminación de acarido de polvo de la casa puede traer algún alivio.
- Aunque algunos alimentos puedan provocar los ataques, evitar o eliminarlos no traerán una mejora remedio o el curación.
- Las pruebas de la piel y inyección de allergia pueden causar verdaderamente los ataques de dermatitis de atopica.

BUROW'S SOLUTION

WHAT IS IT USED FOR?

Burow's solution is a preparation that helps to dry up and control weeping, oozing, and infected skin conditions.

WHERE DO I GET IT?

Purchase a box of Burow's solution (Domeboro, Bluboro). It is available in most chain pharmacies and does not require a prescription. It may come as a powder in packets, tablet form, or as a concentrated solution that must be diluted.

HOW DO I USE IT?

Dissolve 1 packet or tablet in an 8-ounce glass of cool or lukewarm water. Either soak the affected areas in the solution or make a wet compress using a cloth moistened by the solution and leave it in place for 30 minutes to 1 hour. Do this three to four (3–4) times each day. Continue to use until all lesions are dry.

¿PARA QUE ES USADO?

La solución de Burow es una preparación que ayuda a secarse y controlar la secreción y las condiciones infectadas de la piel.

¿DONDE YO LO PUEDO OBTENER?

Compre una caja de la solución de Burow (Domeboro, Bluboro). Está disponible en la mayoría de las farmacias y no requiere una recieta. Puede venir como en un polvo en paquetes, forma de tableta, o cuando una solución concentrada que se debe diluir.

¿COMO LO USO YO?

Disuélvase 1 paquete o tableta en 8 onzas de agua refresca o agua tibia. Empape las áreas afectadas en la solución o hace una compresa mojada usando una tela humedecida con la solución y te lo dejas puesto para 30 minutos a 1 hora. Haga esto tres a cuatro (3–4) veces cada dia. Continúe usar hasta que todo las lesións sea secado.

DRY SKIN

- Moisturizers do not add water to the skin, but do help retain, "lock in," or trap water that is absorbed while bathing. Therefore, applying a moisturizer when the skin is still damp will help seal in the absorbed water.
- There are many over-the-counter preparations available such as Aquaphor, Eucerin, Alpha Keri, Cutemol, Lubriderm, Moisturel, Vaseline Petroleum Jelly, Vaseline Dermatology Formula, cocoa butter, and, believe it or not, Crisco shortening, which may serve as an effective, inexpensive moisturizer.
- Some of these products come in ointment and cream bases, some are lotions, and others contain alpha-hydroxy acids. The decision about which product to use involves personal choice, ease of application, cost, and effectiveness.
- Lac-Hydrin 12% Lotion or Cream, which is available by prescription only, is very effective for scaly skin.
- Low- to medium-potency topical steroids are valuable for treating itchiness and redness, when necessary. In severe cases, or if fissuring (a crack in the skin) is present, stronger topical steroids may be prescribed.
- Take less frequent and shorter showers and baths using lukewarm water.
- Use mild soaps such as Dove, Basis, or a soap substitute such as Cetaphil Lotion.
- Excessive use of any soap is to be avoided, especially on affected areas.
- Band-Aids can be helpful to promote healing of fissures.
- Wear lined gloves while washing dishes.
- Protect yourself from outdoor cold exposure by wearing gloves, hats, and so forth.
- The value of room humidifiers is probably overestimated.
- Drinking large amounts of fluid is also of questionable value.
- Vitamins also have not been shown to be of any benefit; in fact, overingestion of vitamin A can produce a dry skinlike condition.

- Hidradantes no aumenta la agua en la piel, pero ayuda retiene, trampa la agua de que se absorbe mientras bañándose. Por lo tanto, aplicar un hidradante cuando la piel está todavía húmeda ayudará para mantener la agua absorbida.
- Hay muchos sobre el mostrador preparaciones disponibles tal como Aquaphor, Eucerin, Alpha Keri, Cutemol, Lubriderm, Moisturel, Vaseline Petroleum Jelly, Vaseline Dermatology Formula, mantequilla de cacao, y,creo o no, el acortamiento de Crisco, que puede servir como un hidradante efectivo y económico.
- Algunos de estos productos entran las bases de pomada y crema, algunos son lociones, y los otros contienen los ácidos de hydroxy alfa. La decisión acerca de cuál el producto para usar implica personal selecto, la comodidad de la aplicación, del costo, y de la eficacia.
- Hydrin de Lac 12% de Loción o la Crema, que está disponible por la prescripcíon sólo, es muy efectivo para la piel escamosa.
- Bajo- al steroids del topical de la potencia del medio son valioso en tratar picazón y rojizo, cuándo necesario. En casos severos, o si grietas (una grieta en la piel) es steroids más fuerte presente de topical se puede prescribir.
- Tome menos tempo de chaparrones y baños y reducir el uso de agua tibia.
- Use los jabones templados tal como Dove, Basis, o un jabón suplente tal como Loción de Cetaphil.
- El uso excesivo de cualquier jabón deberá ser evitado, especialmente en áreas afectadas.
- Vendajes puede ser promover a la curación de grietas.
- El uso de guantes forrado mientras lavando platos.
- Protéjase de la exposición fría del aire afuera por llevar guantes, los sombreros, etcétera.
- El valor de humedecedores de habitación es probablemente sobreestimado.
- Beber las cantidades grandes del líquido es también muy importante.
- Las vitaminas también no se han mostrado para ser de ningún beneficio; de hecho, sobre ingestión de vitamina un puede producir una piel seca–como la condición.

HAND ECZEMA

Most people who have hand rashes have inherited this tendency. Often they, or family members, have dry, sensitive, scaly, red skin or blistery hands, or possibly asthma, hay fever, sinus or other allergies. Other people may develop a hand rash from overexposure to irritating substances (e.g., hairdressers, cement workers), while others develop a contact dermatitis or allergic reaction from allergenic substances (e.g., latex gloves in health care personnel). An evaluation may involve careful history taking and possible patch testing with chemicals or substances that might be the source of the rash.

TREATMENT

- Usually a potent topical steroid cream or ointment, such as _____, is prescribed to be applied once or twice daily. This should **not be applied to your face**.
- Stubborn cases may require covering the medicated preparation with plastic wrap (e.g., Saran Wrap), which is held in place with tape or by wearing vinyl gloves. This helps the medicine penetrate the skin and is left on overnight or for several hours.
- If your rash only involves one or two fingers, only these fingers need be treated in this manner. This occlusion, or wrapping, should only be done under the direction of your health care provider.
- Severe cases are sometimes treated with antibiotics and oral cortisone.

PREVENTION

- Use lukewarm water, mild cleansers, or soap substitutes.
- Avoid latex gloves; have protective vinyl gloves at work and at home.
- Avoid irritants.
- Make liberal use of moisturizers (especially in the cold, dry months).
- Wear gloves in cold weather.
- Band-Aids are helpful in healing fissured (cracked) fingers.

La mayoría de la gente que tienen los sarpullidos de mano han heredado esta tendencia. A menudo ellos, o miembros de familia, tienen seca, piel, o manos con ampollas, sensible escamosa y roja o posiblemente asma, la fiebre de sinus y otro allergies. Otra gente puede desarrollar un sarpullido de mano de la exposición excesiva a substancias molestas (por ejemplo, peluqueros, trabajadores de cemento), mientras los otros desarrollan una dermatitis del contacto o la reacción alérgica de substancias de allergénica (por ejemplo, guantes de plástico en ella personal del cuidado de la salud). Una evaluación puede implicar tomar una cuidadosa historia y probar el posible remedio con sustancias químicas o substancias que quizás sean la fuente de su sarpullido.

EL TRATAMIENTO

- Generalmente una crema poderosa de steroid de topical o pomada, tal como _____, es prescrito para ser aplicado un par de veces diariamente. Esto no se debe de ser aplicado a su cara.
- Los casos tercos pueden requerir cubrir la preparación del medicado con plástico envuelve (e. g. Saran Wrap), que se tiene en el lugar con cinta o por llevar guantes de vinilo. Esto ayuda la medicina penetrar la piel y se deja durante la noche o por varias horas como lo pueda tolerar.
- Si su sarpullido sólo implica uno o dos dedos, sólo estos dedos serán tratada en esta manera. Este occlusión, o envolviendo, sólo debe ser hecho abajo la dirección de su provider del cuidado de la salud.
- Los casos severos se tratan a veces con antibióticos y cortisone oral.

LA PREVENCION

- Use agua tibia, tintoreria templadaso, o los substitutos del jabón.
- Evite guantes làtex; tenga guantes de vinilo en el trabajo y en casa.
- Evite irritantes.
- Haga el uso liberal de hidradantes (especialmente en el tiempo frío y los meses de las temperaturas seca).
- Lleve guantes durante el tiempo frío.
- Auxiliado vendas son útiles en la curación de dedos con grietas (agrietados).

GENITAL WARTS (CONDYLOMA ACUMINATUM)

- Genital warts, or condyloma acuminatum, are a very common sexually transmitted disease. The warts are usually smooth or cauliflowerlike growths caused by a virus, the human papilloma virus (HPV), and they occur in the regions of the penis, vagina, vulva, cervix, and anus. These warts are caused by specific types of HPV (there are more than 70 known to date) and probably are not caused by the same virus that causes the type common wart, which can be found on any part of the body, especially on the hands and feet. It is thought that most genital warts are spread by sexual contact; however, recent evidence suggests that nongenital spread of the virus can also occur.
- These warts have a fairly long incubation period and may appear several weeks or even years after sexual contact. Therefore, it is difficult to determine the origin of the infection in patients who have had multiple sexual partners.
- The diagnosis of genital warts is often simple; however, when they are very small and difficult to see, they may be confused with normal structures of the skin. Often, careful examination using good lighting and magnification is necessary to see them. In women, evidence of the viral infection may be detected during a routine pelvic examination or Pap smear. Magnification using a special fiberoptic lens, called a culdoscope, may be used by gynecologists to more easily detect them in the vagina and on the cervix.

TREATMENT

- Treatment is often difficult because there is no specific agent, antibiotic, antiviral, or otherwise, that destroys the virus.
- Methods that are currently used include the following.
  - **Podophyllum** is a liquid medication applied by health care providers.
  - **Imiquimod** and **Condylox** are medications that may be self-applied.
  - **Electrodesiccation** utilizes a direct electric current to destroy the warts after local anesthesia is used.
  - **Cryodestruction** (freezing) is accomplished with liquid nitrogen.
  - **Bichloro-** and **trichloroacetic acids** may be applied.
  - **Laser therapy** is another method to destroy the warts.
  - **Interferon** is available as an injectable method of treatment. It is expensive, has more side effects and may not offer any great advantage over the other treatments.
- The biggest problem is the tendency for the warts to recur, whichever method is used. It is impossible to predict who will have recurrences. Sometimes, the warts will disappear without treatment, depending upon the affected individual's immune system.
- HPV (the wart virus) has been associated with precancerous changes in the uterine cervix; these precancerous changes as a result of HPV are also known as dysplasia.

- Verrugas genitales, o acuminatum de condyloma, es una enfermedad sexualmente transmitida muy común. Las verrugas es generalmente liso o los crecimientos como de coliflor causados por un virus, el virus (HPV) humano de papilloma, y ellos ocurren en las regiones del pene, de vagina, de vulva, del útero, y de ano. Estas verrugas es causado por específicos tipos de HPV (hay sobre 70 conocido a la fecha) y probablemente **no es causados por el mismo virus que causa el tipo común verruga**, que se puede encontrar en caulquier parte del cuerpo, especialmente en las manos y pies. Se piensa que la mayoría de las verrugas genitales es propagada por el contacto sexual; sin embargo, la evidencia reciente sugiere esa extensión de no genitales del virus puede ocurrir también.
- Estas verrugas tiene un período bastante largo de la incubación y puede aparecer varias semanas o aún años después del contacto sexual. Por lo tanto, es difícil de determinar el origen de la infección en los individuos que han tenido múltiples asocios sexuales.
- El diagnóstico de las verrugas de genitales es a menudo sencillo; sin embargo, cuando ellos son muy pequeños y difíciles de ver, ellos pueden ser confundidos con estructuras normales de la piel. A menudo, usar cuidadoso de examen con la iluminación y la ampliación buenas son necesarias para verlos. En mujeres, la evidencia de la infección de viral se puede discernir durante un examen rutinario de pelvic o un papanicolaou. Usar de ampliación un lente especial de fiberóptico, llamado un "culdoscope", puede ser usado por ginecólogos para más discernirlos fácilmente en el vagina y en el útero.

EL TRATAMIENTO

- El tratamiento es a menudo difícil porque no hay medicamentos específicos, como tal antibiótico, antiviral, ni de otro modo, que destruye el virus.
- Los métodos que se usan actualmente incluyen:
  - **Podophyllum** es un medicamento líquido aplicado por proveedor de cuidado de salud.
  - **Imiquimod** y **Condylox** son medicamentos que puede ser aplicado por uno mismo.
  - **Electrodesiccation** utiliza una corriente eléctrica directa para destruir el verrugas después que anesthesia local sea uso.
  - **Cryodestruction** (helado) se hecho con líquido de nitrógeno.
  - **Bichloro-** y **los ácidos de trichloroacetic** se pueden aplicar.
  - **La terapia del laser** es otro método de destruir las verrugas.
  - **Interferon** está disponible como un método de tratamiento de inyección. Es costoso, tiene más lado realiza y no puede ofrecer ninguna ventaja magnífica sobre los otros tratamientos.
- El problema más grande es la tendencia para las verrugas de volver a ocurrir, cualquier método sea usado. Es imposible predecir quién tendrá reapariciones. A veces, las verrugas desaparecerán sin el tratamiento, dependiendo sobre el afectó sistema inmune de individuo.
- HPV (el virus de verrugas) se ha asociado con cambios de precanceroso en el útero de uterine, que se sabe también como "dysplasia".

HERPES ZOSTER ("SHINGLES")

Herpes zoster (shingles) is caused by the same virus that causes varicella (chickenpox). The varicella-zoster virus first occurs as chickenpox, which is usually seen in childhood; later it returns as herpes zoster caused by a reactivation of the same virus. Reactivation into shingles may be associated with illness or occurs with no obvious cause. The pain of herpes zoster is thought to be the result of the nerve damage caused by the virus spreading to the skin.

Special Instructions _____

_____

Las palabras en *cursivo* son términos en inglés.

Herpes (*shingles*) zoster es causado por el mismo virus que causa varicella (*chicken-pox*). El virus de zoster de varicella ocurre primero como *chickenpox*, que se ve generalmente en la niñez; luego vuelve como herpes zoster causado por una reactivación del mismo virus. La reactivación (*Shingles*) se puede asociar con la enfermedad, u ocurrir sin la ningúna causa. El dolor con herpes zoster se piensa que es debido al daño de nervio causado por el virus que esparce a la piel.

Las Instrucciones especiales _____

_____

INSECT REPELLENTS

- The most effective insect repellent is the compound diethyltoluamide **(DEET)**. It is effective against mosquitoes, ticks, mites, black flies, and chiggers (Table A2.2).
- Serious reactions to DEET are rare, and even allergic reactions and irritation are not common. Use caution when applying DEET to atopic dermatitis (eczema) because irritation and absorption are more likely to occur.
- DEET should be used sparingly and should be reapplied only when needed. In children, reapplications should be avoided, if possible.
- **DEET should be kept out of the hands of small children; ingestion may cause seizures and even death.** Application to the hands or face in children may result in unwanted ingestion of DEET.
- For backyard activities, products containing 10 to 30% DEET are recommended for adults, and products with less than 10% are best for children.

PERMETHRIN

- Permethrin is actually an insecticide rather than an insect repellent. It is effective against ticks, fleas, and blackflies.
  - Elimite, a 5% cream, contains permethrin and is used to treat scabies.
  - Nix, a 1% lotion, is used to treat lice.
- When used as a repellent, permethrin is applied to clothing and not directly to the skin.
- The **combination of DEET** on exposed skin **and permethrin** on clothing provides an excellent method of protection.

AVON SKIN SO SOFT

- Avon Skin So Soft, which is actually a bath oil, affords some short-term protection against mosquitoes.
- It appears to work by nature of its stickiness, which traps the wings of mosquitoes.

CITRONELLA

- Citronella is a natural oil that offers limited protection against mosquitoes.
- It is available in lotions, sprays, candles, and incense sticks.

INSECT REPELLENTS COMBINED WITH SUNSCREENS

- Recently, insect repellents and sunscreens are often combined.
- It is not clear if this combination decreases the efficacy of either or both products.
- For effective sun protection, it is now recommended that supplementary sunscreens be applied if necessary.

- El repelentes del insecto más efectivo es el compuesto de diethyltoluamide (**DEET**). Es efectivo contra mosquitos, contra las garrapatas, contra acaridos, y contra moscas negras (Tabla A2.2).
- Las reacciones peligrosas de DEET son raras, e incluso las reacciones y la irritación alérgicas no son comunes. Use el cuidado cuando aplicando DEET al dermatitis (eccema) del atopic porque irritación y absorción son más probables de ocurrir.
- El DEET se debe usar frugalmente y debe ser aplicado sólo cuando sea necesario. En niños, aplicacións se debe evitar, si es posible.
- **El DEET no ser debe entrar en las manos de niños pequeños; ingestión puede causar los ataquees e incluso la muerte.** La aplicación a las manos o la cara en niños puede tener como resultado ingestion no deseado de DEET.
- Para actividades de traspatio, los productos que contienen 10% a 30% de DEET son recomiendo para adultos, y para los productos con menos de 10% son mejores para niños.

PERMETHRIN

- El Permethrin es verdaderamente un insecticida que un repelentes de insecto. Es efectivo contra garrapatas, contra las pulgas, y contra las moscas negras.
- El Elimite es un medicamento de un 5% de crema, contiene permethrin y se usa para tratar las dillas.
- El Nix, es otro medicamento es un 1% de loción, se usa para tratar piojos.
- Cuando se usa como un repelentes, permethrin es aplicado a la ropa y no directamente a la piel.
- La **combinación de DEET** en la piel y **permethrin** en la ropa proporciona un método excelente de la protección.

EL PRODUCTO DE AVON "SKIN SO SOFT"

- "Skin so soft," que es verdaderamente un aceite de baño, proporciona alguna protección corto contra los mosquitos.
- Aparece trabajar por la naturaleza porque es pegajoso y atrapa las alas de los mosquitos.

CITRONELA

- La Citronela es un aceite natural que ofrece la protección limitada contra los mosquitos.
- Está disponible en lociones, en rocíos, en velas, y en los palos de incienso.

EL REPELENTES DE INSECTOS COMBINADO CON EL PROTECTOR DE SOL

- Recientemente, repelentes de insecto y protector de sol a menudo se puede combinar.
- No es confirmado si esta combinación disminuye la eficacia de ambos productos.
- Para la protección efectiva del sol, ahora se recomienda que el protector de sol suplementario sea aplicado si necesario.

TABLE A2.2. COMMERCIALLY AVAILABLE INSECT REPELLENTS CONTAINING DEET

PREPARATIONS WITH UP TO 10% DEET ARE BEST FOR USE IN CHILDREN MORE THAN 2 YEARS OF AGE	10 %–30% PREPARATIONS ARE GOOD FOR BACKYARD USE	40%–50% PREPARATIONS ARE FOR LONGER EXPOSURES, SUCH AS HIKING OR CAMPING	55%–100% PREPARATIONS HAVE A HIGHER RISK OF ADVERSE REACTIONS
•Cutter •Skedaddle •Skintastic	•Cutter Backyard •OFF!	•Muskol Spray •Ticks OFF!	•Repel •OFF! Sportsman •Muskol Liquid •Permethrin (best agent for use against ticks; use on clothing, tents, and equipment)

DEET = diethyltoluamide.

TABLA A2.2. CONTENER COMERCIALMENTE DISPONIBLE DE INSECTO REPELENTES DEET

LAS PREPARACIONES CON HASTS 10% DE DEET SON MEJOR PARA EL USO EN NIÑOS MEJORES QUE 2 AÑOS DE EDAD	10 %–30% LAS PREPARACIONES SON BUENAS PARA EL USO DEL TRASPATIO	40%–50% LAS PREPARACIONES SON PARA EXPOSICIONES MÁS LARGAS, TAL COMO EXCURSIONISMO O ACAMPAR	55%–100% LAS PREPARACIONES TIENEN UN RIESGO MÁS ALTO DE REACCIONES ADVERSAS
•Cortador •Skedaddle •Skintastic	•Cutter Backyard •OFF!	•Muskol Spray •Ticks OFF!	•Repele •LEJOS! El deportista •Líquido de Muskol •Permethrin (mejor agente para el uso contra garrapatas; el uso en la ropa, en las tiendas dé campaña , y en el equipo)

TICKS AND LYME DISEASE

- You'll be able to spot ticks more easily if you wear light-colored clothing.
- Tuck your pants into your socks or boots.
- Wear closed shoes.
- Spray insect repellent that contains 25 to 30% diethyltoluamide (DEET) onto clothing, especially pants from knees to cuff, and on exposed skin.
- Walk in the center of trails to avoid tall grass and brush.
- Inspect your children for any new "freckles."
- Use tick and flea repellent on your dogs and cats.
- Dogs can get Lyme disease, showing symptoms of joint stiffness
- If you find a tick attached, remove it carefully.
  - Using a steady force, remove the attached tick with tweezers, gently grasping the tick by the head, not the body, as close as possible to the skin.
  - Avoid force that may crush it, then carefully pull it straight out.

- Usted será capaz de notar las manchas de garrapata más fácilmente si usted lleva el coloró claro de ropa.
- Métase sus pantalones en los calcetines (medias) o las botas.
- Uses zapatos cerrados.
- Rocíe repellent de insecto que contenga 25% a 30% de DEET (diethyltoluamide) en toda su ropa, especialmente en pantalones cortos, y rocie la piel expuesta tambien.
- Trate de caminar en el centro de rastros y paseos para evitar las hierbas alta y los arbustos.
- Inspeccione a sus niños en busca de marcas que se parescan a pecas nuevas.
- Use repellent de garrapatas y pulgas en sus perros y gatos.
- Los perros pueden obtener la enfermedad de Lyme, los síntomas son articulación rígidas.
- Si usted encuentra una garrapata conectada al cuerpo, quítela con cuidado.
  - Con fuerza constante, quite la garrapata conectada al cuerpo con pinzas, suavemente agarre la garrapata por la cabeza, no el cuerpo, tan cerca de la piel que sea posible.
  - Evite mucha fuerza la cual puede aplastarla, cuidadamente retirela derecho.

PITYRIASIS ROSEA

- Pityriasis rosea is a harmless rash of unknown cause that has a predictable course. It tends to occur in the spring and fall and is seen mostly in young adults and older children, but may be seen at any age. It is not contagious, and it is very rare for it to occur in the same patient more than once.
- Typically, pityriasis rosea begins with the larger **"herald,"** or **"mother," patch**, which resembles, and is most often mistaken for, "ringworm" (a fungal infection of the skin). In several days to 2 weeks, the herald patch is followed by many smaller scaly patches on the chest, back, sides of the neck, and the upper parts of the arms and legs. Often a "Christmas tree" pattern is noted on the chest and back. The rash, which may itch, usually disappears within 6 to 8 weeks.

- Rosea de pityriasis es un sarpullido inofensivo de la causa desconocida que tiene un curso previsible. Tiende a ocurrir en la primavera y el otoño y sea visto en un mayor parte en adultos jóvenes y niños, pero puede ser visto en cualquier edad. No es contagioso, y es muy raro para ocurrir en el mismo individuo más de una vez.
- Típicamente, rosea de pityriasis comienza con el "**heraldo**" más grande, o **"madre," mancha**, que se parece, y es muy a menudo erróneo con la infección, "ringworm" (una infección de hongo de la piel). En varios días a 2 semanas, la mancha de heraldo es seguido por muchas manchas escamosos más pequeños en el pecho, la espalda, los lados del cuello, y de las partes superiores de los brazos y las piernas. A menudo se parece a un modelo de "árbol de Navidad" se nota en el pecho y la espalda. El sarpullido, que puede picar, generalmente desaparecer dentro de 6 a 8 semanas.

DIRECTIONS FOR TAKING PREDNISONE

Modified from Sandra S. Mamis, RPA-C

- You should take prednisone with meals or right after meals to avoid an upset stomach.
- Possible side-effects include a short-term weight gain because of fluid retention, a possible change in your mood, and disturbance of your sleep.
- Prednisone can increase blood sugar levels in people with diabetes.

DIRECTIONS

Name of Drug: Prednisone
Strength: 5 mg
Schedule: The number on the schedule refers to the number of tablets to be taken at the designated time

Patient Name:________________________

Day **A.M. (Morning)** **P.M. (Evening)**

Monday ____
Tuesday____
Wednesday____
Thursday____
Friday____
Saturday____
Sunday____

Monday____
Tuesday____
Wednesday____
Thursday____
Friday____
Saturday____
Sunday____

Monday____
Tuesday____
Wednesday____
Thursday____
Friday____
Saturday____
Sunday____

Provider Name:__________________ Date:__________________

Modificado por Sandra S. Mamis, RPA C

- Usted debe tomar prednisone con comidas o derecho después de la comida para evitar un mal estómago.
- Los efectos posibles del lado incluyen aumento de peso debido a la retención de líquido, un cambio posible en su humor, y en algún interrupción en su sueño.
- Prednisone puede aumentar los niveles de azúcar en su sangre para la gente con diabetes.

LAS DIRECCIONES

El nombre de la Droga: Prednisone
la Fuerza de Prednisone: 5 de mg
Horario: El número en el horario se refiere al número de tabletas para ser tomado en el tiempo designado.

El Nombre del paciente:_____

| día | A.M. (Mañana) | P.M. (Noche) |

El domingo:_____
El lunes:_____
El martes:_____
El miércoles:_____
El jueves:_____
El viernes:_____
El sábado:_____

El domingo:_____
El lunes:_____
El martes:_____
El miércoles:_____
El jueves:_____
El viernes:_____
El sábado:_____

El domingo:_____
El lunes:_____
El martes:_____
El miércoles:_____
El jueves:_____
El viernes:_____
El sábado:_____

Médico:_____   La fecha:_____

SCALE REMOVAL FOR PSORIASIS

SCALP PSORIASIS

If your health care provider has diagnosed scalp psoriasis, it is often necessary to remove thickened scale so as to allow the medications to get to where the action is (i.e., your scalp). Scale may be removed as often as necessary, usually 2 to 3 times per week at the beginning and later whenever the scale builds up again.

Procedure to follow:

1. Wash your hair with your favorite shampoo.
2. Then, while your scalp is still damp, apply salicylic acid in a petrolatum base (sometimes given by prescription), Keralyt, and Hydrisalic Gel, both of which may be obtained without a prescription. These preparations are applied to scaly areas only.
3. Cover your head with a shower cap and leave it on overnight, or leave it on while you are awake for several hours (whichever is more convenient for you).
4. Shampoo the area again.
5. Other recommended medication(s), such as _____, may now be applied.

PSORIASIS IN HAIRLESS AREAS

1. Soak the area(s) to be treated for 5 minutes.
2. Rub in a thin film of salicylic acid in petrolatum such as Keralyt or Hydrisalic Gel.
3. Cover the area with a plastic wrap (e.g., with Saran Wrap, Handi-Wrap, a Baggie).
4. Remove the plastic wrap the next morning, and wash the area with soap and water.
5. If irritation occurs, stop the treatment temporarily and then resume every other night after the irritation clears.
6. Use as necessary when the scale builds up again.
7. Other recommended medication(s), such as _____, may be applied after the scale is cleared away.

PSORIASIS DEL CUERO

Si su proveedor del cuidado de la salud ha diagnosticado psoriasis de cuero, es a menudo necesario quitar la escala espesada para permitir que los medicamientos para llegar a donde la acción es (en otras palabras, su cuero). La escala se puede quitar tantas veces como necesaria, generalmente 2 a la vez de 3 por la semana al principio y mas tarde, cuando la escala construye otra vez.

   Aquí está cómo:
1. Lave el cabello con su champú favorito.
2. Entonces, mientras su cuero todavía húmedo, aplica el ácido de salicylic en una base de petrolatum (generalmente dado por recieta). Keralyt y Hydrisalic Gel se pueden obtener sin una recieta. Estas aplicaciones se aplican a las áreas escamosas solamente.
3. Cubra la cabeza con una tapa de chaparrón y lo dejas puesto durante la noche, o puede dejar puesto durante usted está despierto por varias horas (el que es más conveniente para usted).
4. El champú el área otra vez.
5. Otro medicamiento (s) recomendado, tal como _____,
   ahora puede ser aplicado.

PSORIASIS EN AREAS SIN PELO

1. Empape el área (s) para ser tratada para 5 minutos.
2. Frote una aplicación delgada del ácido de salicylic en el petrolatum o Hydrisalic Gel.
3. Cubra el área con un plástico (por ejemplo, Saran Wrap, Handi-Wrap o un Baggie).
4. Quite el plástico la próxima mañana y lava el área con el jabón y el agua.
5. Si irritación ocurre, para el tratamiento temporariamente y entonces reasume cada dos noches después que la irritación sea mejorado.
6. Use como sea necesario cuando la escala construye otra vez.
7. Otro medicamiento (s) recomendado, tal como _____
   se puede aplicar después que la escala se mejorado.

PREVENTION OF RHUS DERMATITIS (POISON IVY, OAK, SUMAC)

- Learn to recognize the plants—"leaves of three, let it be."
- If your work or hobbies involve frequent exposure to poisonous plants, try a **barrier cream** such as IvyGuard or Stokogard **before exposure**.
- If you have been exposed to the plant or its oil, wash with soap and cold water as soon as possible.
- Carefully remove all exposed clothing and wash it.
- **The rash is not contagious**; you cannot spread the rash to others or spread it on yourself by touching the blisters or fluid.
- Over-the-counter topical steroids such as Cortaid are not strong enough to relieve severe itching and inflammation.
- Vaccines and other immunizations given orally or by "shots" may be very risky and often fail to work.

- Aprenda a reconocer las plantas—"las hojas de tres, permiten ser."
- Si su trabajo o los pasatiempos implican la exposición frecuente a plantas tóxicas, trata **una crema que contienga agente para barrera** tal como Guardia de Hiedra o Stokogard **antes de la exposición**.
- Si usted ha sido expuesto a la planta o su aceite, lava el àrea con el jabón y con agua fría tan pronto que sea posible.
- Quite detenidamente toda la ropa y lava lo.
- **El sarpullido no es contagioso**; usted no puede esparcir del sarpullido, ni otros lo puede esparció en usted mismo tocando las ampollas o el líquido de la ampollas.
- Sobre el contra steroids de topical tal como Cortaid no están fuerte suficiente en aliviar picazón e inflamación severos.
- Las vacunas o otras inmunizaciones dados oralmente o por inyección puede ser muy arriesgado y a veces falla de trabajar.

HOW TO USE SALICYLIC ACID (DUOFILM) TO TREAT WARTS

1. Soak the area to be treated for 5 minutes before applying salicylic acid. Duofilm and Occlusal are salicylic acid products that may be obtained without a prescription. You'll save time by doing the soaking while you're taking your usual bath or shower.
2. Dry the area to be treated.
3. Use a toothpick to make sure the Duofilm is applied to the wart only.
4. When dry, cover the area with a waterproof tape such as Johnson & Johnson Waterproof Tape. If you are using Occlusal, the tape is not necessary because Occlusal acts as a waterproof barrier.
5. Do this every day unless there is uncomfortable irritation or pain and then stop for 1 day or more before continuing.
6. The length of time for treatment is different for everybody, and the only way to know if your wart is gone is to stop applying the medication (usually after 6 to 8 weeks) and see if the wart returns.
7. If the wart returns, you can use the medication again for a longer time period or see your health care provider.

1. Remojar el área para ser tratada para 5 minutos antes de aplicar el ácido de salicylic. Duofilm y Occlusal son los productos que contiene ácidos de salicylic que se pueden obtener sin una receta. Usted salvará tiempo haciendo el remojar mientras usted toma su baño o el chaparrón usuales.
2. Seque el área para ser tratada.
3. Use un palillo de dientes para cerciorarse que el Duofilm sea aplicado a la verruga nada más.
4. Cuándo el área está secado y la medicina aplicado, cubre el área con una cinta impermeable tal como Johnson & Johnson Waterproof Tape. Si usted usa Occlusal, la cinta no es necesaria desde que Occlusal actúa como una barrera impermeable.
5. Haga esto todos los días a menos que hay irritación o dolor incómodos. Si tienes estos síntomas entonces parada por 1 día o más antes de continuar.
6. El duración de tiempo para el tratamiento es diferente para todos, y la única manera de saber si su verruga sea ido, usted deber parar aplicar el medicamento (generalmente después de 6 a 8 semanas) y ver si las verrugas regresado.
7. Si las verrugas regresan, usted puede usar el medicamento otra vez por un período más largo de tiempo o ver su proveedor del cuidado de la salud.

SUN PROTECTION TIPS

Modified from Recommendations of the Skin Cancer Foundation

- Avoid sun exposure during the hours between 10 A.M. and 4 P.M., when the sun is strongest.
- Wear protective headgear such as a hat with a wide brim or a baseball cap; wear long-sleeved shirts and long pants.
- Apply a sunscreen at least 30 minutes before sun exposure.
- Apply sunscreens even on cloudy, hazy days.
- Be aware of reflected light from sand or snow.
- Use a sunscreen with a sun protection factor (SPF) of 15 or greater to prevent burning (Table A2.3).
  - If you have very fair skin that never tans but always burns, have a history of skin cancer, or are at a high risk for skin cancer, apply a SPF 30 or greater sunscreen, even in the winter months.
  - If you tan easily, you may use a lower SPF number.
- Apply sunscreens liberally and frequently at least every 2 hours, as long as you stay in the sun and reapply after swimming or perspiring.
- Lips are also sun sensitive, so use special lip coating sunscreens that have a waxy base.
- Choose a waterproof sunscreen.
- Choose a broad-spectrum sunscreen that blocks UVB (ultraviolet light midrange spectrum—the burning rays) and UVA (ultraviolet light long wavelength—the more penetrating rays that promote wrinkling and aging).
- So-called "nonchemical," opaque, physical sunscreens, such as titanium dioxide and zinc oxide, provide good coverage, are waterproof, and cause fewer allergic reactions than other sunscreens.
- Preparations that dye the skin (self-tanning products) do not offer any sun protection, unless combined with a sunscreen.
- Moisturizers that contain built-in sunscreens usually have a lower SPF.
- Avoid tanning parlors.
- Keep infants out of the sun.
- Teach children sun protection at a young age.
- Wear UV-blocking sunglasses.
- Certain drugs can make you more likely to burn, such as tetracycline, thiazide diuretics, and certain oral antidiabetic medications.
- Remember, there is no such thing as a healthy tan!

Modificado por las Recomendaciones de la Fundación del Cancer de la Piel

- Evite la exposición del sol durante las horas entre 10 de la mañana y 4 de la tarde, cuando el sol es más fuerte.
- Lleve gorros tal como un sombrero con un borde ancho o una tapa del béisbol; lleve camisas de mangas largas y pantalones largos.
- Aplique un protector de sol por lo menos 30 minutos antes de la exposición del sol.
- Aplique un protector de sol aún los días nublados y nebulosos.
- Ser consciente de la luz reflejada de la arena o la nieve.
- Use un protector de sol con un SPF (el factor de la protección del sol) de 15 o más grande para prevenir quemaduras (Tabla A2.3).
- Si usted tiene piel muy blanca que nunca curte pero siempre quemaduras, tiene una historia del cancer de piel, o está en un riesgo alto para el cancer de piel, aplica un SPF 30 o un protector de sol más grande, aún en los meses de invierno.
- Si usted curte fácilmente, usted puede usar un número más bajo de SPF.
- Aplique protector de sol liberalmente y frecuentemente por lo menos cada 2 horas, tan largo como usted permanece en el sol y haré lo después de nadar o transpirar.
- Los labios son también sol sensible, así que usan protector del sol para los labios que tiene una base cerosa.
- Escoja un protector de sol impermeable.
- Escoja un protector de sol con el espectro ancho que bloquea ambos UVB (los rayos del ardor) y UVA (los rayos más penetrantes que promueven arrugar y envejecimiento).
- Llamado "no sustancia química," opaco y físico el protector de sol, tal como bióxido de titanium y óxido de zinc, proporcionan el alcance bueno, es impermeable, y causa menos reacciones alérgicas que otro protector de sol tiene.
- Las preparaciones que tiñen la piel (los productos que auto curtiendo) no ofrece cualquier protección del sol, a menos que sea combinado con un protector de sol.
- Hidradantes que contiene incorporado en un protector de sol tiene generalmente un SPF más bajo.
- Evite los salones que curten.
- Mantenga los niños fuera del sol.
- Enseñe a los niños a como usar la protección del sol en una edad joven.
- Lleve las gafas de sol bloqueando de UV.
- Ciertas drogas lo pueden hacer más probable de quemarse, tal como tetracycline, diuretics de thiazide, y ciertos medicamentos oral de antidiabeticos.
- ¿Recuerde, no hay tal cosa como un bronceado saludable!

TABLE A2.3. SUNSCREEN RECOMMENDATIONS (SPF 15 OR GREATER)

WATERPROOF SUNSCREENS	FOR OILY SKIN	MOISTURIZER/SUNSCREEN COMBINATIONS	SPORT SUNSCREENS *	FOR SENSITIVE SKIN †	FOR LIP PROTECTION
•Ombrelle 15 (Offers UVB and UVA protection.) •Presun 15, 29, or 46 •Shade 30 or 45 •Almay 15, 25, or 30 •Bain de Soleil All Day 15 or 30 •Bullfrog gel For Kids 36 •Sundown 15, 25, or 30 •Coppertone 15, 25, 30, or 45 •Neutrogena Sunblock 15 or 30 •Solbar 50 •BioSun 15, 30, or 45	•Clinique 15 Oil Free •Presun Active 15 or 30 (alcohol gel–based) •Neutrogena 15 •Presun Facial 15 or 29 •Shade 15 or 25 Oil Free	•Neutrogena Moisture (SPF 15) •Oil of Olay Daily UV Protectant (SPF 15) •Eucerin Daily Facial Lotion (SPF 25) •Almay Moisture Balance Lotion (SPF 15) •Basis Protective Facial Moisturizer (SPF 15)	•Coppertone Sport 15 or 30 •Neutrogena "No-Stick" Sunscreen (SPF 30)	•Almay Super-Sensitive SPF 30 Lotion •Clinique Special Defense Sun Block (SPF 25) •Estee Lauder Advanced Suncare Sunblock (SPF 15 or 25) •Neutrogena Sensitive Skin Sunblock (SPF 17)	•Coppertone Lipkote 15 •Presun 15 Lip Protector •Chapstick Sunblock

SPF = sun protection factor; UVA = ultraviolet light long wavelength; UVB = ultraviolet light midrange spectrum.

* Lotion will not run into eyes with sweating.

† "Nonchemical" sunscreens generally contain titanium dioxide or zinc oxide.

TABLA A2.3. RECOMENDACIONES DEL USO DE UN PROTECTOR DE SOL (SPF 15 O MÁS GRANDE)

SUNSCREENS IMPERMEABLE	PARA LA PIEL GRASIENTA	MOISTURIZER/LAS COMBINACIONES DE SUNSCREEN	SUNSCREENS DEPORTIVO *	PARA LA PIEL SENSIBLE †	PARA LA PROTECCIÓN DE LABIO
•Ombrelle 15 (Las ofertas la protección de UVA y UVB.) •Presun 15, 29, o 46 •Shade 30 o 45 •Almay 15, 25, o 30 •Bain de Soleil All Day 15 o 30 •Bullfrog gel For Kids 36 •Sundown 15, 25, o 30 •Coppertone 15, 25, 30, o 45 •Neutrogena Sunblock 15 o 30 •Solbar 50 •BioSun 15, 30, o 45	•Clinique 15 Oil Free •Presun Active 15 o 30 (alcohol gel–based) •Neutrogena 15 •Presun Facial 15 o 29 •Shade 15 o 25 Oil Free	•Neutrogena Moisture (SPF 15) •Oil of Olay Daily UV Protectant (SPF 15) •Eucerin Daily Facial Lotion (SPF 25) •Almay Moisture Balance Lotion (SPF 15) •Basis Protective Facial Moisturizer (SPF 15)	•Coppertone Sport 15 o 30 •Neutrogena "No-Stick" Sunscreen (SPF 30)	•Almay Super-Sensitive SPF 30 Lotion •Clinique Special Defense Sun Block (SPF 25) •Estee Lauder Advanced Suncare Sunblock (SPF 15 o 25) •Neutrogena Sensitive Skin Sunblock (SPF 17)	•Coppertone Lipkote 15 •Presun 15 Lip Protector •Chapstick Sunblock

* Loción no chocará adentro los ojos con sudar.
† Un Protector del sol "sin químicos" contiene generalmente el bióxido de titanium u óxido de zinc.

TINEA VERSICOLOR

Tinea versicolor is a harmless, noncontagious fungal infection of the skin. The fungus that causes it normally lives on almost everybody in small numbers, but it may grow and cause a discolored rash in some young adults. The color of the rash may vary from white to pink to tan or brown. The rash may last for years, worsening and improving over time. It often becomes more noticeable in the summer months because of heat, sun exposure, and tanning of the skin.

TREATMENT

- Sometimes, you can clear the rash on your own by using medications such as Selsun Blue or Micatin or Lotrimin cream or spray. These preparations are available over-the-counter without prescription and are less expensive when purchased as generic miconazole or clotrimazole.
- The scale of this rash will disappear after a few treatments, but it may take months for your skin color to return to normal. This slow return of color is part of the normal healing process and does not mean that the treatment has failed; however, repeat treatment is often necessary.
- **Treatment is performed as follows:**
  - For mild, limited tinea versicolor, use a topical over-the-counter agent that contains selenium sulfide, such as Selsun Blue. It should be left on for 15 minutes and rinsed off. In addition, apply an antifungal agent such as Micatin (Micatin Spray allows for easy application to the back) once or twice daily. This may be repeated for 3 or 4 weeks. It is also a good idea to repeat this routine before the next warm season or a tropical vacation. If this treatment fails, a prescription medication such as Nizoral Cream or Shampoo or Lamisil Solution in a pump spray may be given to you by your health care provider.
  - For stubborn or widespread disease, a short-term course of antifungal pills may be prescribed for 5 to 10 days.
  - Preventive therapy with selenium sulfide lotion or shampoo or a zinc pyrithione bar (e.g., ZNP Bar) or shampoo (e.g., Head & Shoulders) may be used twice monthly.

Versicolor de Tinea es un infección inofensivo, el infección de hongo de la piel no es contagioso. El hongo que causa versicolor de tinea normalmente vive en casi todos pero en cantidades pequeños. En algunos adultos jóvenes el hongo puede crecer y poder causar un sarpullido descoloraro. El color del sarpullido puede variar de blanco a rosado o curtir o marrón. El sarpullido puede durar por años, empeorar y mejorar con el tiempo. A veces llega a ser más notable en los meses del verano debidos al calentor, la exposición del sol, y curtir de la piel.

EL TRATAMIENTO

- A veces, usted puede curar el sarpullido con usando medicamientos tal como Selsun Blue o Micatin o la crema o el rocío de Lotrimin (más barato genéricamente como miconazole o clotrimazole). Estas preparaciones están disponibles para comprar sin receta.
- La escala de este sarpullido puede desaparecer después con pocos tratamientos, pero puede llevar meses para su color de piel para volver a normal. Este regreso lento del color es parte del proceso curativo normal y no significa que el tratamiento ha fallado; sin embargo, repite el tratamiento quando sea necesario.
- **El tratamiento se realiza como lo seguir:**
  - Para el templado y limitado versicolor de tinea, use un topical sobre la mostrador los agente que contiene sulfide de selenium, tal como Selsun Blue, se debe dejar para 15 minutos y enjuague. Además, aplica una agente de antihongo tal como Micatin (el Rocío de Micatin tiene un aplicación fácil para las espalda) un par de veces diariamente. Esto se puede repetir para 3 o 4 semanas. Es también una idea buena de repetir este rutinario antes del próximo cambio de la temporada o una vacación tropical. Si este tratamiento falla, un medicamento por receta tal como Crema de Nizoral o Champú o la Solución de Lamisil en un rocío o bomba puede ser dado a usted por su proveedor de cuidado de salud.
  - Para la enfermedad peor o esparcida, un curso de plazo corto de píldoras de antihongo se puede prescribir para 5 a 10 días.
  - La terapia impeditiva con loción de sulfide de selenium o champú, o con la barra de pyrithione de zinc (por ejemplo, la Barra de ZNP) o el champú (por ejemplo, Head & Shoulders) puede ser usado dos veces mensualmente.

Page references followed by "t" denote tables

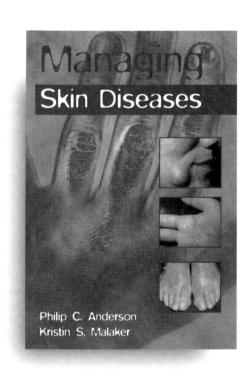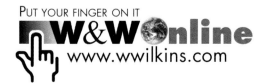